# MEDICAL ETHICS TODAY:

# ITS PRACTICE AND PHILOSOPHY

# MEDICAL ETHICS TODAY:

# ITS PRACTICE AND PHILOSOPHY

from the **BMA's Ethics, Science and Information Division**

| | |
|---|---|
| *Head of Division* | Dr Fleur Fisher |
| *Project Managers* | Dr Natalie-Jane Macdonald (to 31 August 1992) Miss Rosemary Weston |
| *Written and researched by* | Ms Ann Sommerville |
| *Editorial Secretariat* | Ms Henrietta Wallace |
| *Project Secretary* | Mrs Lynne Burton |
| *Technical Editor* | Ms Anne Lloyd |

Published by the BMJ Publishing Group
Tavistock Square, London WC1H 9JR

First printed 1993

**British Library Cataloguing Publication Data**
**A catalogue record for this book is available from the British Library**

ISBN 0–7279–0817–0

Typeset and Printed by
Latimer Trend & Company, Plymouth

# Acknowledgements

*Membership of the Working Party*

Dr J Stuart Horner: Director of Public Health, Preston; Chairman, BMA
Medical Ethics Committee

Dr David Cook: Theologian, Director of Whitefield Institute, Oxford

Mr Karl Fortes-Mayer: Surgeon, Birmingham (until February 1992)

Dr R John Givans: General practitioner, Harrogate

Mr Geoff Hinchley: Registrar, Accident and Emergency, Derby

Dr Caroline M Marriott: Consultant psychiatrist, Antrim

Dr Anne E P Rodway: General practitioner, Sevenoaks; Vice-Chairman,
BMA Medical Ethics Committee

Ms Lydia Sinclair: Solicitor, Legal advisor, MENCAP, London

Dr Michael Wilks: General practitioner, Forensic medical examiner,
London (from July 1992)


*The Medical Ethics Committee*

Throughout all its stages, the book has been supervised by the BMA's
Medical Ethics Committee whose membership includes those listed above
and the following:

Professor Christine M Chapman: Emeritus professor of nursing education,
University of Wales

Dr Peter H Dangerfield: Academic staff, Faculty of Medicine, University
of Liverpool

Professor John Harris: Philosopher, Centre for Social Ethics and Policy,
University of Manchester

Dr Tony Hicklin: Consultant rheumatologist, Crawley

Bishop Crispian Hollis: Theologian, Bishop of Portsmouth

Professor Ian Kennedy: Academic lawyer, King's College, London

Dr George M Mitchell: Clinical pharmacologist, Cardiff

Rabbi Julia Neuberger: Chair, Camden & Islington Community Health
Services NHS Trust, London

Rev Dr John Polkinghorne: Theologian, University of Cambridge

Dr J David Watts: General practitioner, Ayrshire

## *Individuals*

We wish to thank the following for the assistance they gave in the preparation of this report: Dr Priscilla Alderson, Dr James Appleyard, Professor Michael Baum, Mr Ian Bynoe, Mr Maurice Frankel, Dr Brian Hurwitz, Dr Peter Kielty, Ms Barbara Mitchels, Mr Derek Morgan, Mrs Jean Robinson, Dr Stephen Robinson, Dame Cicely Saunders, Professor Gordon Stirrat, Professor Nicholas Wald, Dr Frank Wells, Dr Tom West.

## *Organisations*

The following organisations kindly responded to invitations from the British Medical Association to give written or oral comments: Alzheimers Association, The Association of the British Pharmaceutical Industry, The Association of Police Surgeons, Christian Action Research and Education (CARE), Council of Professions Supplementary to Medicine, Freedom of Information Campaign, Human Fertilisation and Embryology Authority, Macmillan Unit - Christchurch Hospital, Marie Curie Cancer Centre - Glamorgan, Northern Ireland Prison Medical Service, Royal College of Nursing, St Christopher's Hospice, Terrence Higgins Trust.

# Contents

# Introduction

*The aims of the book and how to use it: history of BMA involvement in ethical debate, including the differing roles of the BMA and the General Medical Council: how the advice has been derived.*

## The aims of the book

This book is intended to be a practical guide which reflects contemporary ethical thinking. It is written primarily for doctors but we hope that other people will find it useful. Its approach is patient-centred. Emphasis is given to promoting a balanced partnership between doctors and patients, which means that effective communication (which includes listening to the patient as well as giving him or her information) must be seen as a key component of practical medical ethics. Increasingly, doctors play a role within a team of professionals and so attention is also given to inter-professional dialogue.

The fundamental principles observed by the medical profession remain constant but their application to newly evolving situations requires debate. Each of these chapters centres on ethical questions which doctors raise with the BMA and attempts to show briefly how moral theories can be applied to these common dilemmas. In many cases, doctors' enquiries are more mundane than the ethical issues which philosophers, lawyers and bio-ethicists debate. Since doctors tend to need a quick and workable solution for an immediate case, we focus on a practical response to these common questions but this process inevitably brings in reference to philosophy and law. Abortion, embryo research and euthanasia, for example, raise weighty moral issues which must be explored to some degree although the actual procedures are regulated by law in such a way that most questions about what is practically permissible can be answered briefly. Even superficially simple queries, such as how much information to give a patient, or whether children can choose treatment for themselves, cannot be answered fully without mentioning how legal cases and bio-ethical discussions are influencing medical practice and vice versa.

Furthermore, the prosaic questions cannot be completely separated from the major ethical dilemmas. The way in which those questions are answered, and the dilemmas resolved, must be informed by the same strands of reasoning. The responses to both the day-to-day questions, and the major ethical ones, usually reflects among other things, a judgement about the fundamental nature of the doctor-patient relationship.

Above all, the aim has been to produce a working tool for doctors rather than a philosophical treatise - but without neglecting reference to the broad lines of philosophical thinking. Some would claim that clinical decisions are not amenable to being slotted into patterns of abstract reasoning because they require experience and commonsense and, most of all, they hinge on the particular circumstances of the case. It is certainly true that our approach is eclectic and does not attempt to fit every issue into one or two schools of thought. We are persuaded, however, that even the commonsense approach rests upon some form of reasoned analysis which should be articulated and open to scrutiny. By analysing their own reasoning, doctors and patients will be helped to formulate decisions about newly arising situations, whose ethical implications are as yet unforeseen. The ownership of human tissue and how it can be used provides an example of just such an area of continuing discussion.

## How to use the book

Busy doctors seek prompt and unambiguous advice. Hopefully, the summaries at the end of each chapter will assist in providing this but they should not be considered in isolation from the discussion in the text. Many ethical issues are too sophisticated to be summarised satisfactorily in a few lines: the reader needs to be aware of the underlying parameters of the debate, laid out in the preceding chapter. In many situations, the context of the question and the motives of those involved will influence the response and we have tried to illustrate this by examples or by relevant legal cases.

Previous editions of the BMA handbook featured separate sections on ethical dilemmas upon which no consensus view has been reached. The number of such "continuing dilemmas" has not decreased. In this book, instead of segregating these particularly hard questions from the more humdrum issues, we have attempted to integrate them into one debate and, by reference to accepted ethical principles, point a practical way forward.

For ease of reference, the main areas of discussion are briefly indicated at the beginning of each chapter and a summary of conclusions is given at the end of each chapter. The philosophical basis of the guidance is discussed in chapter 13. It should be noted that each year the BMA produces guidance sheets on a variety of ethical or medico-legal issues. Recent guidance notes on subjects such as advance directives and decision-making for the mentally disordered are summarised where relevant in the text and are available in full from the BMA. A list of guidance notes produced after the publication of this book is also available from the Ethics Department. Published sources are indicated where relevant and summarised in a bibliography. There is a comprehensive index at the end of the book.

In many situations, doctors' legal obligations will overlap with their ethical duties. Where this is the case, brief reference is made to the law. The full legal implications, including explanation of relevant case law and legislation are explored in the companion volume to this book, "Rights and Responsibilities of Doctors", (revised 1992).

## The BMA tradition of publishing ethical advice

Since its inception in the last century, the BMA has aimed to promote standards of good professional practice and contribute to the discussion of ethical issues. One of the objectives outlined in the prospectus advertising the establishment of the Provincial Medical and Surgical Association in 1832 was "the maintenance of the honour and respectability of medicine by defining those elements which ought ever to characterise a liberal profession". The Association changed its title to the British Medical Association in 1856.

The Association appointed its first committee "to bring the subject of medical ethics before the profession" in 1849 and although it was requested to draw up a short code of medical ethics within a year, it found itself unable to do so. Further committees were established to complete the task in 1853 and 1858 but they were no more successful. When the Central Ethical Committee was finally set up in 1902, it wisely rejected a request to draw up an ethical code.

In 1927 the BMA Council again advised against the preparation of an ethical code although the BMA members at the Annual Representative Meeting that year urged it to do so. It was not until 1949 that the Association produced a booklet, "Ethics and Members of the Medical Profession". It was a small, 16-page pamphlet fitting comfortably into a breast pocket and was concerned mainly with relationships between doctors and with members of other professions.

The first BMA handbook of medical ethics was published in 1980 and was immediately revised the following year. A further revision took place in 1984. In 1988, a different approach was taken, resulting in a document that was more comprehensive in many ways but which was criticised by some for failing to provide simple and readily accessible "answers". "Philosophy and Practice of Medical Ethics" forsook the style of its predecessors, which was to give ethical guidance through a list of generally agreed precepts. Instead, it briefly mentioned the influences which give rise to the general moral and ethical order and set out principles as a basis for studying practical problems. Its aim was to help doctors formulate an appropriate ethical response to the individual circumstances of each case rather than to give ready-made answers. The present document is therefore the fifth in this series. It tries to combine the accessibility of advice which doctors appreciated in the early handbooks with a recognition of the diverse currents of thought on many ethical issues. As is discussed in chapter 13, the application of such reasoning to the individual circumstances of each case is something we see as very important.

## Liaison between the BMA and GMC

The BMA is a voluntary, professional association without statutory powers. From its foundation the BMA campaigned for the establishment of a General Medical Council to register and regulate qualified doctors and this came about when the GMC was founded, according to the Medical Act of 1858. In its early years the GMC showed little eagerness to determine and adjudicate upon suitable standards of conduct among registered medical practitioners. In 1886 the GMC was given much wider powers, although it did not issue its first warning about "infamous conduct" until 1893. Like the BMA, the GMC has only begun to publish comprehensive written advice on professional matters relatively recently and has a responsibility to do so under the Medical Act 1978. Unlike the BMA, the GMC, as the statutory regulatory body, has a major sanction to support the implementation of its guidance. The GMC can erase from the medical register the name of any practitioner whom its Professional Conduct Committee finds guilty of serious professional misconduct. The BMA works closely with the GMC in the task of interpreting how broad principles can be applied to the day-to-day problems which occur in medical practice.

Thus, unlike some other countries, where specific aspects of medical ethics have been incorporated into law, the profession in the United Kingdom has functioned largely on the basis of self-regulation in accordance with the guidance published by the GMC. This has perhaps permitted a more flexible system which is capable of responding to change. A continuing aim of the BMA has been not only to keep abreast of such change, but also to anticipate the new ethical dilemmas brought about by technological advance and changing circumstances.

## How this advice has been derived

Despite the emphasis on change, this book continues a tradition. It has been drafted over a two-year period by a Working Party of the BMA's Medical Ethics Committee. The Working Party was established in late 1990 with the ambitious task of conducting a review of the Association's published ethical advice and producing "practical advice with extrapolation of the philosophical principles in order to guide doctors in any aspects of their practice where ethical considerations arise". All of the issues discussed in the book have been scrutinised by the BMA Council and committees within the BMA which represent the interests of particular groups of doctors.

Revision does not necessarily involve radical change and on major issues such as advance directives, contraception for minors, euthanasia and the treatment of malformed infants, this book re-affirms the advice previously issued by the Association. In re-affirming BMA advice, the book tries to show the reasoning which supports such views. The principles which underlie the advice are explained in a more detailed way in the final chapter.

It is evident that society's views on many areas of life are changing, and implicit in the Working Party's mandate was the need for discussion of some topics whose ethical implications had not previously been addressed by the Association in a comprehensive manner. Included in such topics are the ethical issues arising in reproductive technology, the sterilisation of people with learning disabilities, questions involving the autonomy of children and young people, and insights gained from the hospice movement about attitudes towards the dying. Efforts have also been made to address continuing dilemmas in a practical way and to take account of instances where the patient's desires conflict with the doctor's personal moral views.

Clearly, doctors are not a homogeneous group. Attempting to reflect their views and the expectations society has of doctors is a daunting task. This book, like those which preceded it, aims to clarify the continually evolving application of fundamental ethical concepts. Rather than simply reflecting the status quo it ambitiously attempts to look ahead. It does not seek to address, but cannot fail to reflect, wider decisions about morality, which are a matter for society. In an effort to avoid professional insularity, the Working Party in the course of twenty meetings, has taken advice from a wide range of individuals and from representatives of both medical and non-medical organisations. A list of those who have aided the discussion, either orally or in writing, is given at the front of the book. It must be noted that the views reflected in the handbook are not necessarily synonymous with the opinions of those whose advice, knowledge and wisdom we sought, but it is hoped that the benefit gained from the exploration of different viewpoints will be evident and will fuel further debate.

# 1 Consent and Refusal

*Introductory remarks including the importance of shared decision-making within the partnership model; consent and refusal by patient or doctor. Seeking consent, including the purpose and nature of consent; consent forms as an indicator of discussion; the amount of information to be provided in order to facilitate patient consent. When the patient cannot give consent, including incapacitated patients and minors. Pressures on consent, including patients in a position of dependency or restricted choice. Refusal of treatment, including refusal by advance directive, and advice for doctors when patients refuse. Exceptional circumstances, including organ transplantation and circumstances when the treatment is not proposed in the interests of the patient; where treatment has implications for other people. Summary.*

## 1:1 Introduction

### 1:1.1 *The doctor-patient relationship*

The relationship between doctor and patient is based on the concept of partnership and collaborative effort. Ideally, decisions are made through frank discussion, in which the doctor's clinical expertise and the patient's individual needs and preferences are shared, to select the best treatment option. The patient's consent to be examined and to receive treatment is the trigger which allows the interchange to take place. Some people question the emphasis which is currently placed on patient consent, suggesting it implies that the patient is somehow doing the doctor a favour by signifying his or her agreement to be treated. They feel it would be more appropriate to talk about "a request for treatment". Regardless of how it is expressed, the basic premise is that treatment is undertaken as a result of patients being actively involved in deciding what is to be done to them.

### 1:1.2 *Types of relationship*

Two main types of professional relationship exist between doctors and patients.

i)    The most common form of relationship is the therapeutic partnership, discussed above, where a doctor's professional advice is sought about a medical problem. The existence of a continuing relationship means that patient consent to examination and treatment will usually be implicit rather than expressed. Doctors are expected to use their

1

skills to the best of their ability not only to treat the condition which is the subject of the consultation but also to advise how best patients should conduct themselves in order to maintain their health. The doctor is responsible to the patient. In this form of relationship, the doctor should act only in the best interests of the patient, unless these dangerously conflict with a wider duty to society and put other people's health at risk.

In the therapeutic context, patients can choose their doctor. Equally, doctors are free to accept or refuse a patient, subject to the constraints of their professional obligations, such as: i) in an emergency when a doctor is ethically bound to provide urgent treatment and to ensure that arrangements are made for any further treatment, ii) in an isolated community, where the doctor is the only source of medical advice. The situation of doctors who do not wish to accept particularly difficult patients is discussed in 1:1.4.2 below.

ii)    In the second form of relationship the doctor acts as an impartial medical examiner and reports to a third party, for example, when conducting a pre-employment medical or insurance examination. The patient usually has no choice about which doctor is approached by the organisation commissioning the report. The nature of the doctor's role must be clearly explained to the patient. It should also be explained that the tests which are carried out are not for the purposes of health care, and that the information gathered will be used for purposes other than treatment.

Such reports may either be undertaken by the patient's own GP or by a doctor who has no previous professional relationship with the patient. Patients have a statutory right to see reports about them by their GP for insurance or employment purposes. This is discussed further in chapter 9 (sections 9:2 and 9:3). Where the examining doctor is unknown to the patient, the latter may wish to limit the information shared with the doctor. The doctor can only report on the basis of information presented by the patient. The party commissioning the report may request examining doctors to keep their findings secret from the patient. The BMA advises that doctors who do not have a clinical relationship with a patient, nevertheless, ethically owe some duty of care to that patient. Examining doctors who discover some clinical fact significant to the management of the patient's health care which they believe is not known to the patient's own GP, have a duty either to bring it to the attention of the GP or the patient, or to request that the chief medical officer of the insurance company, who receives the report, takes steps to make sure the patient is informed.

### 1:1.3 *The therapeutic relationship*

As a prerequisite to choosing treatment, patients have the right to receive information from doctors and to discuss the benefits and risks of appropriate treatment options. Doctors give medical guidance as to the optimal course of action but must also recognise that patients' responses will not be formed solely on the basis of clinical data but by their circumstances, needs, rational conclusions and irrational emotions. Individuals have varied information requirements, which may focus on different issues from those that doctors think important. Thus, a doctor who seeks guidance about the amount or type of information which should be made available must first listen to the patient and consider, among other things, what it is that the patient wants to know.

Patient consent must be voluntary, free from pressure and arise from a competence to decide. Competence is not a "blanket" concept. Some patients may be able to take some treatment decisions but not others. Incompetent individuals may also have preferences within the scope of the available options and these should be accommodated. Those close to the patient can play an important role in helping the patient decide but no person can consent on behalf of another adult. It is a common misconception that consent by the relatives of an incapacitated patient carries some particular legal weight. The views of those close to the patient are important insofar as it is presumed that these people have the patient's welfare closely at heart and may be able to reflect the patient's known preferences in circumstances when the patient cannot express these.

In many aspects of medicine, the legal and ethical requirements are separate and ethical guidance need make no reference to the law. Consent, however, is an issue which binds the two since failure to seek patient consent is not only a moral failing but also leaves the doctor liable in the crime or tort of battery or in the tort of negligence.[1]

It would be wrong to assume that consent is only relevant when initiating an examination or treatment. Consent is a process and not an event and it is important that there be continuing discussion to reflect the evolving nature of treatment. The BMA has traditionally advised that doctors should be very wary of proceeding with a treatment when there is any doubt regarding the consent of a competent patient. In cases where life or health is seriously at risk, however, the courts have made clear that if there is the slightest doubt about the validity of a patient's refusal of treatment, any apparent refusal should be disregarded. This may give rise to confusion as to the doctor's responsibilities. In this chapter, therefore, we discuss the doctor's ethical duties in response to patient refusal, as well as in the context of consent.

Clearly, the opportunity to consent to treatment is counterbalanced by a right to refuse it. As a result of recent legal cases,[2] increasing attention is now being given to the issue of refusal, which in most cases is quite different from a simple failure to consent or a failure to give valid consent based on adequate information. Society, it is argued, has an interest in ensuring that life and health is preserved. It is assumed that doctors propose treatments with patients' interests in mind. The individual who refuses treatment challenges society's expectations and may expect to be called upon to demonstrate a greater grasp of the implications of that decision than a consenting patient. The law and commonsense demand that doctors verify the competence of patients who risk their lives by a refusal of treatment. There is a fine line, however, between sensible measures to ensure that the patient fully comprehends the consequences of a refusal and a reversal to paternalism, whereby patients' competence is unquestioned as long as they concur with the doctor.

### 1:1.4 *The autonomy of doctors*

Consent and autonomy are not the sole prerogatives of patients and it is not only the patient who has rights of consent and refusal. Doctors provide treatment, not simply because it is requested, but because in their view it is clinically appropriate. They recommend the treatment which is best for individual patients, having regard to that particular patient's needs and the treatments and resources available. Society thus places doctors in the role of gate-keeper of access to treatment. Difficult questions arise when a patient rejects a low-cost remedy in favour of a costly alternative which strips resources from others. The patient may then be in the position of consenting to a treatment which the doctor refuses. Yet if the patient is a Jehovah's Witness, for example, and the choice is an expensive alternative to blood products or allowing the patient to die, the doctor would make every effort to accommodate patient choice. This example highlights the difficult question of the comparative weight to be given to different value systems which underlie patient choices.

It is not only resource considerations which impose limitations on the patient. Doctors also refuse to give patients treatments which are "bad for them" or for others. Very different extreme examples are seen in patient requests for help to commit suicide or facilitate a surrogacy arrangement for inappropriate reasons. Everyday examples concern patient demand for amphetamine-type appetite suppressants or athletes' and body-builders' requests for steroids. The responsibilities and dilemmas involved in such issues are discussed in chapter 7 (section 7:5.1.4).

The effect of all such examples, however, is apparently to strip away some of the support for the vision of the doctor-patient relationship as an equal partnership. A "complementary" partnership may be a more realistic term since it functions best when the doctor's skills are tailored to meet the patient's requirements and the patient's requests do not exceed what the doctor is able legally, ethically and practically to provide. It must be conceded that doctors have responsibilities beyond their duty to individual patients, although individual patients must be the focus of attention. Doctors also have considerable power - not to decide the patient's treatment but effectively to influence the range of options from which the patient chooses.

### 1:1.4.1 Requests for a second opinion

An area where conflict may arise between the patient's desire to exercise choice and the doctor's clinical judgement concerns patients' requests for a second opinion. The Patient's Charter makes clear that, within the NHS, referral for a second opinion is dependent upon agreement between patient and doctor and is not an automatic patient right. Requests for a second opinion should, however, be handled sensitively by the patient's usual doctor and the patient should not be made to feel a "nuisance" or a "bad patient". The patient may feel unable to share the reasons behind the request with his usual doctor and such a request sometimes reflects a previous failure in communication. The doctor should attempt to assess objectively whether this is the case and, if so, whether anything can be done to rectify it.

### 1:1.4.2 Difficult or violent patients

The question of whether doctors are under a duty to provide treatment at all for some patients is unfortunately raised fairly often: the BMA receives, with some regularity, reports of violence or threats of violence against doctors and other health professionals. These problems occur both in hospital and general practice. Such patients cannot be left without treatment when they need it and various solutions can be considered, according to the circumstances. Sometimes the patient is not physically violent but is verbally abusive in a manner which upsets both staff and other patients. Hostility may be unfocused or it may be directed against particular health professionals, in which case it may be necessary to arrange for others to treat the patient. In some cases, violent or challenging behaviour may be a symptom of the patient's illness or a side-effect of treatment, beyond the patient's control. Therapeutic measures including sedation may be used. Great care is required, however, to ensure that any measures introduced are primarily designed to promote the patient's interest, or are used only when necessary to prevent damage to others. The routine use of behaviour-controlling measures, designed to facilitate ease of management rather than promoting the patient's interests, should be avoided. This is discussed further in 1:3.3 below on impaired capacity.

In extreme cases, for instance where a violent patient is brought, or comes voluntarily, to an accident and emergency department, the individual's behaviour may make treatment impossible or the patient may not actually need any treatment. Such individuals may have to be removed by the police and placed under the supervision of a police surgeon until such time as treatment, if appropriate, can be undertaken. It is not acceptable, however, to seek the removal of a patient who needs treatment solely because that person has behaved badly on a previous occasion. Patients can only be legitimately removed if a specific incident occurs on that particular occasion. Such patients cannot be banned from re-attending unless, as a result of an assault, bail conditions specify that the person should not return to the hospital. Senior staff should be involved in decisions about the treatment of such patients and should be aware of the possibilities of litigation if a person who needs treatment suffers harm as a result of not receiving it. Decisions should not be left to unsupported junior doctors and nurses. Doctors should inform the hospital management about violent patients who return persistently. Managers must ensure that a safe working environment is provided and failure to do so may leave them liable under the Health and Safety at Work etc. Act 1984. If the patient has been admitted for treatment, the minimum of restraint necessary to ensure the safety of staff and patients may be used. Restraining aggressive behaviour by use of physical restraints should be a measure of last resort. See also 1:3.3.1 below.

In less extreme circumstances, doctors may arrange for a colleague to take over the patient's treatment if the patient's behaviour is directed against one particular doctor or other health care worker. Counselling for the patient and talking to people close to the patient may prove helpful. Nevertheless some patients may have to be treated in a separate area from others and with adequate security for health staff. There are no easy solutions and it must be recognised that this problem often appears intractable. Such patients are treated at a cost of misery and inconvenience to those providing treatment.

In general practice, doctors have had little choice about accepting difficult or threatening patients although GPs have always been able to request that such patients be removed from their lists. GPs' representatives have discussed the problems with the Department of Health, requesting that abusive or violent patients be removed immediately and that responsibility for medical care for a temporary period should remain with the family health services authority (FHSA) or health board. Such bodies have, in the past, only been willing to arrange a transfer if the patient was not under active treatment at the time and so often there have been delays. Even after transferral, if the patient continues persistently to threaten all doctors a rota is organised between all the doctors in the area so that each practice treats the patient at some time. If an assault takes place, the doctor can take out an injunction to prevent the patient returning to that particular practice. Experience has shown that even in cases where the patient is subsequently re-allocated to the original practice, the act of removal may have helped to clear the air and to create a better relationship.

The BMA advises that an official complaint to the police should be made following any violent or threatening episode, while ensuring that confidentiality is preserved about the medical aspects of the consultation. A threatened or actual attack may contravene the Offences Against the Person Act 1861 and incidents which occur anywhere other than in a dwelling may constitute an offence under the Public Order Act 1986. In either case where an offence has been committed, the police or the doctor can prosecute.

Some GPs deal with the problem by seeing such patients outside normal surgery hours, ideally when the doctor has a colleague or another person at hand if necessary. Other patients of the practice are thus protected from abusive patients. Police officers will accompany doctors on home visits, if necessary, and the Association of Chief Police Officers issues a list of practical points on minimising risks of violence in the surgery and in the community. This includes advice about: the importance of training staff to identify and deal with the first signs of aggression; ensuring that the behaviour of doctors and surgery staff is above reproach; avoiding furniture which could be used as a weapon, and noting risk-patients in a patient register. This is a matter upon which support from colleagues is often valuable and any doctor who removes a violent or abusive patient from the practice list should inform the secretary of the local medical committee, without divulging any other information about the patient.

## 1:2 Seeking consent

### 1:2.1 *The nature and purpose of consent*

Consent may be implicit or explicit. It may be orally given, or written down in a formal way. For much of medicine, consent is assumed by, for example, the opening of the mouth for examination, the offering of an arm for taking blood pressure or by attending a doctor and giving information about an illness. Such implied consent can only be held to apply to the procedure in hand and not necessarily to subsequent treatments which flow from it.

Some people see the purpose of consent as chiefly being the provision of a defence for doctors against legal liabilities which come up for discussion when patients allege that their apparent agreement to treatment has been rendered invalid by the doctor's failure to give enough information for specific consent. In the BMA's view, respect for others and their rights lies at the heart of the issue of consent. A feature of our present society is the emphasis on the value and dignity of the individual. It is said that principles of inherent natural rights dictate that each person who is competent to do so should decide what happens to his or her own body. The patient exercises this autonomy by deciding which treatment option to accept. The decision is based on information given by the clinician. For consent to be valid, the patient must know what options are available and have the ability to choose.

In addition to the moral and symbolic importance of promoting patient self-determination, patient co-operation is a very practical requirement. Thus one of the main reasons for seeking patient consent has always been to ensure that the patient is properly prepared. In 1767, for example, before the use of anaesthesia, it was thought:

> "reasonable that a patient should be told what is about to be done to him, that he may take courage and put himself in such a situation as to enable him to undergo the operation".[3]

This perhaps foreshadows current thinking that most people fare best when they have a clear view of what is being proposed and its implications. In the past, concern to avoid worrying patients has been seen as a reason for not telling them the full implications of either their condition or different options for treatment. Sometimes only their relatives were given information of the likely outcome. Even nowadays, doctors are often reluctant to mention medicine's ubiquitous uncertainties and arguments are made for restricting information in certain circumstances on the grounds that autonomy is not the only ethical imperative. It is sometimes argued that an exaggerated regard for this single principle puts at risk the whole concept of the doctor-patient relationship.

Here, we take the opportunity to reaffirm that it is not the doctor's role just to provide a list of alternatives from which patients select options, according to their need and desires. Doctors must, indeed, bear in mind other ethical principles, such as the duty of acting in the patient's best interest by attempting to recognise what the patient wants. In most cases, patients can choose better for themselves than doctors can choose for them but occasionally the patient's final choice is to let the doctor choose. This is not an abnegation of choice and the patient who makes such a decision with regard to one aspect of treatment should not be seen as relinquishing choice on other issues. Nevertheless, whilst information and uncertainties should not be forced upon patients at a time when they are particularly vulnerable and clearly unready, most people do deal with very difficult choices despite their anxieties if given support to do so. Most doctors appreciate this and automatically take their cue from the patient as to the amount of information required by that individual at any stage of treatment. Patients are supported by doctors who clarify any misconceptions and who are, what has been described as, "caringly available".[4]

### 1:2.2 *Effective communication*

Information is only useful if it is provided in a manner intelligible to the hearer and at a pace at which the recipient can digest it. It is a cause of concern to the BMA that although all schools provide some form of communication-skills training for medical students, relatively few are committed to formal instruction and students are not bound to achieve any particular standards. This matter is considered further in chapter 5 on caring for the dying (section 5:2.1) but has implications for all branches of medical practice.

For non-English-speaking patients, provision of information in order to obtain effective consent may be a problem. Financial constraints may preclude the use of trained interpreters and family members may act as interpreters. In such situations, however, doctors must be aware of the possibility of the family influencing the patient's consent or refusal.

A small but important group of patients are those who come to Britain seeking political asylum after torture or maltreatment in their country of origin. It is vital that, where necessary, doctors treating or providing medical reports for such patients have access to experienced interpreters. The Medical Foundation for Care of Victims of Torture warns against the use of interpreters connected to the embassy or diplomatic services of the country in question as this can result in distortion of medical testimony and dangerous repercussions for the patient's relatives.

### 1:2.3 *Consent forms*

The documentation of consent was originally introduced to protect surgeons from allegations of assault by patients who came to regret the surgical intervention which had been carried out upon them. This is still seen by some as the function of consent. An eminent judge, for example, has recently said:

> "There seems to be some confusion in the minds of some as to the purpose of seeking consent from a patient... It has two purposes, the one clinical and the other legal. The clinical purpose stems from the fact that in many instances the co-operation of the patient and the patient's faith or at least confidence in the efficiency of the treatment is a major factor contributing to the treatment's success. Failure to obtain such consent will not only deprive the patient and medical staff of this advantage, but will usually make it much more difficult to administer the treatment. The legal purpose is quite different. It is to provide those concerned in the treatment with a defence to a criminal charge of assault or battery or a civil claim for damages for trespass to the person".[5]

Consent forms simply document that some discussion has taken place. The quality and clarity of the information which is given is what is paramount: that is more important than simply having a signature on a piece of paper. Consent forms are evidence of a process not the process itself.

Refusal forms, which are available in hospitals, are unambiguous in the sense that providing a legal defence is their sole function. They are similarly invalid if the patient has not been given adequate information to make a properly informed decision at the time of signing. Some groups, principally Jehovah's Witnesses, have drafted their own form, which specifies precisely what measures are unacceptable to them in all circumstances. In using such a form the signatory has undertaken in advance to consider fully the implications of the various choices. This question of anticipatory decision-making is discussed further in the section on advance directives in 1:3.4 below.

### 1:2.4 *Provision of information*

The World Medical Association's Declaration of Lisbon (1981) sets the tone for many statements of the rights of patients. It states the fundamental position that "the patient has the right to accept or to refuse treatment after receiving adequate information". As discussed previously, how much or how little is considered to be adequate will vary with each patient. It must also be a matter of clinical judgement and the standards set by other doctors. From an ethical viewpoint, the criteria should be as much information as the patient needs or desires. It is interesting to note that in the Bolam case the law set the level at the standard adopted by the medical profession and a doctor who gives as much detail as a recognised body of medical opinion considers appropriate would be unlikely to be held liable in law.[6]

Good practice, however, is not necessarily interchangeable with the legal minimum. Lord Scarman's comments in the Sidaway case,[7] while not necessarily indicative of all legal opinion, are held by many to encapsulate the true ethical position. His Lordship sets the standard for the amount of information to be given, not at what the medical profession thinks appropriate but ideally at what the individual patient requires and failing that, at what the average "prudent patient" would want to know:

> "If one considers the scope of the doctor's duty by beginning with the right of the patient to make his own decision whether he will or will not undergo the treatment proposed, the right to be informed of significant risk and the doctor's corresponding duty are easy to understand: for the proper implementation of the right requires that the doctor be under a duty to inform his patient of the material risks inherent in the treatment. And it is plainly right that a doctor may avoid liability for failure to warn of a material risk if he can show that he reasonably believed that communication to the patient of the existence of the risk would be detrimental to the health (including, of course, the mental health) of his patient.

> Ideally, the court should ask itself whether in the particular circumstances the risk was such that this particular patient would think it significant if he was told it existed. I would think that, as a matter of ethics, this is the test of the doctor's duty. The law, however, operates not in Utopia but in the world as it is: and such an

inquiry would prove in practice to be frustrated by the subjectivity of its aim and purpose. The law can, however, do the next best thing, and require the court to answer the question, what would a reasonably prudent patient think significant if in the situation of this patient. The "prudent patient" cannot, however, always provide the answer for the obvious reason that he is a norm, not a real person: and certainly not the patient himself."

Thus ideally, the doctor should inform the patient about any risks inherent in the treatment which might be particularly important to that patient as well as explaining the risks and benefits of alternatives and of non-treatment.

Information allows the patient to make a rational decision, but decision-making is not solely a rational activity. It involves intuition, personal values, preferences and emotion. Nor is it always just information that is sought but also the doctor's opinion. Details which are not wanted by the patient at one stage of treatment might be sought at another. The patient must be in control not only of the volume of information being given but also of the speed and flow of that information. Busy doctors sometimes point out the apparent impracticality of attempting to give information in stages to suit the patient. Sometimes written material or advice about specific patient support groups or voluntary organisations may help patients to inform themselves at their own speed; contact with group members will show how others in the same position have managed. Such solutions, however, should not be a substitute for appropriate discussion between the doctor and patient about particular aspects of each individual case.

This question of the amount of information to be given has particular resonance in relation to research on people who are ill and is discussed further in chapter 8 (section 8:6.3).

### 1:2.5 *The duration of consent*

Doctors often query the length of time for which patient consent can be considered valid. In usual practice, this is not at question since consent is an evolving matter and not a once-and-for-all decision. The patient's consent is clearly only valid until such time as the patient expresses a change of mind. In the provision of maternity services, for example, any special wishes which the woman expresses during the ante-natal period should be recorded in the notes but she may change her mind at any stage, including during labour. At that stage, decisions may have to be taken quickly. The woman's ability to consent may be affected by analgesics but she is still likely to be able to express a valid opinion, which should be respected.

Consent which cannot evolve and be confirmed because the patient has become incompetent is a different matter. While respecting the patient's previous decision, doctors must be cautious about acting on instructions

11

which can no longer be confirmed. It is for this reason that the BMA recommends to patients that full discussion of the provisions of any advance directive between patient and doctor forms a continuing dialogue. This is discussed further in 1:3.4 below and in chapter 6 (section 6:3.3).

Another common query regarding the duration of consent concerns the patient's authorisation to the release of medical data, whether for research or other purposes. The issue is discussed in chapter 2 on confidentiality (see particularly section 2:2.3.4).

### 1:2.6 *Exceeding consent*

As mentioned in the opening remarks, consent is valid insofar as it applies to the precise treatment in question, or at least to acts of a substantially similar nature. When a patient agrees to a particular operation, the surgeon is not justified to depart from instructions and perform a different one. The only time when doctors are justified in proceeding without prior authority is when it is necessary to do so to save the life or preserve the health of the patient and it is not possible to obtain that person's consent but the doctor has no convincing evidence that the patient would object.

## 1:3 When the patient cannot give consent

Consent is a necessary prerequisite to treatment but there are some exceptional circumstances, such as those described in Part IV of the Mental Health Act 1983[8] or emergencies. The Department of Health reminds doctors that under the Mental Health Act 1983, detained patients capable of giving consent can only be given medical treatment for mental disorder against their wishes in accordance with the provisions of Part IV of the Act. On rare occasions involving emergencies, where it is not possible immediately to apply the provisions of the Mental Health Act 1983, patients suffering from a mental disorder which is leading to behaviour that is an immediate serious danger to themselves or to other people may be given such treatment as represents the minimum necessary response to avert that danger. The administration of such treatment is not an alternative to giving treatment under the Mental Health Act 1983 nor should its administration delay the proper application of the Act to the patient at the earliest opportunity.

### 1:3.1 *Emergencies*

Doctors are sometimes faced with emergency situations where there is neither the time nor the possibility of gaining consent, for example, when an unconscious patient requiring urgent treatment is admitted to the accident and emergency department of a hospital. In such circumstances the doctor is not only entitled, but may be legally bound, to carry out such treatment as is necessary to safeguard the life and health of the patient until such time as the latter recovers and can be consulted about longer term measures. Consent to operate or act is properly assumed by the doctor unless there is convincing evidence that the patient would have withheld consent. Such evidence may take the form of an advance directive which addresses the particular situation which has arisen or the type of group consent form drafted by Jehovah's Witnesses to indicate a clear refusal of blood in all circumstances. Some query whether a patient's "suicide note" could be construed as a valid anticipatory refusal of treatment. The law and commonsense, however, require that a doctor provide necessary treatment unless absolutely convinced of the patient's competence and full appreciation of the facts at the time of drafting such a document. Since doctors are unlikely to have certain knowledge of this, it is assumed that instructions drafted immediately prior to a suicide attempt cannot be accorded the same respect as an informed advance directive. Similarly, patients who refuse life-saving treatment at a time when their judgement might be seriously impaired, by drugs or alcohol, for example, would probably fail to meet the test of competence required for such grave decisions to be persuasive. Impaired capacity is discussed further in 1:3.3 below.

Thus, in cases of doubt as to the patient's real intention, the law and the public interest urge doctors to take all necessary measures to sustain life rather than to speculate about what the patient intended.[9] In an emergency, however, the doctor should not exceed the treatments necessary to sustain life and health. For example, elective measures or procedures such as the use of blood samples for forensic rather than diagnostic purposes are not condoned. This latter point is discussed further in chapter 9 (section 9:6.4).

### 1:3.2 *Minors*

Adults make decisions for children until children acquire enough understanding to decide for themselves. As they grow towards adulthood, young people take increasingly more responsibility. For almost 25 years, the law and medical practice has been moving towards empowering young people, even quite young children, in health care decision-making. In 1985, it was stated that "parental responsibility diminishes as the child acquires sufficient understanding to make his own decisions" and "at Common Law a child of sufficient intelligence and understanding could consent to treatment".[10] Subsequent legislation, such as the Children Act 1989 and the Access to Health Records Act 1990,[11] reflected the increased attention that society seemed prepared to pay to children's views. Even when children do not have sufficient understanding to make a valid decision, involving them in an appropriate way, so as to gain their co-operation, is seen as valuable. Doctors are thus accustomed to seeking the participation and consent of even very young children. This is good practice even if the

13

tender age or immaturity of the child makes it necessary to have supporting parental consent. Where children or young people are mature enough to understand the purpose and effects of the treatment proposed, their consent is considered sufficient to allow treatment to take place.

Several legal cases[12] have established, however, a difference between the minor's ability to consent and to refuse treatment. This can be summarised by saying that although the young person may be able to consent to the measures proposed, that does not automatically imply an equally valid right to refuse them. Treatment can be given if consent is forthcoming from any person authorised to give it: either the young person, a parent or guardian or the courts. Parents or guardians who withhold consent for necessary treatment for a child may be considered guilty of child neglect. If valid consent is provided by someone entitled to do so on the minor's behalf, the fact that the minor refuses is not determinative legally. It has been shown that the views of those under 18 can be overridden by the courts in wardship if the health care decisions of the young people conflict with what are perceived to be their best interests. In the BMA's view, the tendency to regard mature young people as autonomous in their own right is a very welcome trend which should not be undermined. The moral implications of these legal decisions are explored in chapter 3 on children and young people (sections 3:3.2 and 3:3.3).

### 1:3.3 *Impaired capacity*

The fact that a person acts in a way that an ordinary prudent person would not act, is not in itself evidence of impaired capacity. The capacity to consent in a valid way may be affected by many factors, including pain or fatigue. In addition, some patients suffer from mental disorder or impairment. None of these conditions necessarily prevents the patient from giving valid consent. A very wide spectrum of ability is found within the group of patients whose competence to decide rationally is permanently or temporarily affected. Competency may also be variable over time and doctors may have to be more selective about timing in order to raise the issues with the patient in a meaningful way. Pending the English Law Commission's review of measures for making decisions for people who cannot decide for themselves, the BMA has issued interim guidelines for the medical profession on the treatment of such patients. These are available from the BMA's Ethics Division.

Although recognising that in some instances doctors may have a professional predisposition to recommend treatment over non-treatment, society takes the view that whatever measures doctors propose will be in the best interests of patients. Thus a low threshold of understanding is required in order for a patient to consent effectively to a necessary therapeutic procedure: it is sufficient for the patient to understand in broad terms why the treatment is proposed and its effects. Patients are encouraged to exercise to its limits the decision-making capacity they possess. On the same premise that any treatment proposed is designed to benefit the patient, a higher level of capacity is required in order for patients to refuse necessary therapeutic treatment. Treatments which are elective, including health screening or preventive measures are not usually proposed if the patient cannot understand and co-operate with them. Mentally incapacitated patients, however, should not be deprived of the benefits of such measures if they demonstrate no overt objection to them. The participation in research of people with impaired capacity is discussed in chapter 8 (section 8:8.1.3).

### 1:3.3.1 *Physical restraints and other measures of control*

As has been discussed above in 1:1.4.2, restraining measures may be required to prevent violent patients from hurting themselves or other people but the restraint used should always be the minimum possible in the circumstances. Restraints or physical support may also be used, with the patient's consent, in connection with provision of treatment. For example, an anorexic patient had her arms encased in plaster, with her consent, to prevent her pulling out feeding tubes.[13] This section is concerned primarily with patients who cannot consent but it must be noted that competent adults who may need such measures, but who do not endanger others, must understand the purpose and give consent.

The routine use of measures to restrain people, particularly elderly people or those with learning disabilities, may give cause for concern. A wide range of measures may be used including locking people in, placing them in special chairs which restrict movement, treating them with inappropriate sedation or simply arranging seating at a height or angle which makes it difficult for the sitter to rise unaided. Measures which are sometimes put forward as alternatives to such restraints are electronic tagging or surveillance cameras. The purpose of these measures should be to allow people the maximum amount of freedom and privacy compatible with their own safety. They should also respect patients' dignity.

Particular concerns have been expressed that in residential care, generally, the main reason for restraint is to forestall behaviour which might be potentially disruptive to the smooth running of the home, so that the objective is institutional compliance rather than protection of individuals.[14] The Mental Health Act Commission is frequently asked to give guidance on the use of restraint in relation to mentally incapacitated older people with dementia or adults with learning disabilities. The Commission advises that physical restraints should be used as little as possible. Where any form of restraint is proposed to protect mentally incapacitated people from hurting themselves, restraint should be used only to the extent of preventing risk beyond that which would normally be taken by a similarly frail, mentally alert person. Restraint which involves

15

either tying or attaching a patient to some part of a building or to its fixtures or fittings should not be used. Staff must make a balanced judgement between the need to promote individuals' autonomy by allowing them to move around at will and the duty to protect them from likely harm. In every case where the physical freedom of an individual is curtailed, staff should record the decision and the reasons for it and state explicitly in a care plan under what circumstances restraint will be used, what form the restraint will take and how it will be reviewed. Every episode of restraint should be fully documented and reviewed. Restraint should not be routinely used as a substitute for sufficient staff or as a punishment and can only be justified when it contributes to the individual's quality of life or prevents risk to others.

A controversial issue raised in recent years has concerned the use of anti-psychotic drugs, without consent, to modify the behaviour of disturbed adolescents or young people classified as having profound learning difficulties. In 1991, for example, an image projected by the media of young people being "repeatedly and sometimes forcibly drugged"[15] caused a brief spate of public outrage and a Department of Health investigation. In some cases, it was said, these drugs were prescribed primarily to deal with unwanted behaviour - an implication being that society would not have tolerated similar treatment to deal with challenging behaviour by "normal" individuals. While it is generally recognised that such measures may be acceptable in the short term, many would object to them on a long term basis. The issue raised here, however, is not particular to doctors or to this one form of treatment but might exemplify the wider problem of how society sometimes fails to accord members of all groups the same respect for their physical integrity. Such issues highlight the particular duty owed by doctors to safeguard the interests of people with serious learning difficulties, who can neither give nor withhold their consent. Prescribing issues are fully discussed in chapter 7 (see particularly section 7:4.1).

### 1:3.3.2 Consulting those close to the patient

At present nobody can give consent to treatment on behalf of another adult (except in Scotland if a "tutor dative" has been appointed, see 1:3.5 below), although possibilities for a change in the law are being explored by the Law Commission. It is clear that patients suffering severe mental impairment cannot act autonomously, although they may be able to express preferences on some matters. In these circumstances, ethical principles require doctors to act in patients' best interests. Wherever possible, the doctor should involve those close to the patient in the decision-making process. If the patient has previously been autonomous, decisions should be based on the patient's known views and preferences. People close to the patient can reflect these. Treatment which is contrary to the known wishes of the patient when competent cannot be justified.[16] If it is believed that the patient's prior views were opposed to life-prolonging treatment, doctors should seek substantial evidence of this before considering curtailment of treatment. Such evidence may be in the form of an advance directive or "living will" or a specialised form drawn up by Jehovah's Witnesses with regard to blood products.

### 1:3.4 *Advance directives*

The BMA supports the principle of the advance directive. This is a mechanism whereby competent people give instructions about what they wish to be done if they should subsequently lose the capacity to decide for themselves. Its purpose is to provide a means for patients to continue to exercise autonomy and shape the end of their lives by pre-selecting or refusing treatments which are likely to be proposed for them. The principle is not new and embodies advantages for the openness of the doctor-patient relationship. Patients who are aware of approaching death often discuss with their doctors how they wish to be treated. The advance directive registers these views in a more formal way and can be seen as part of a broader willingness to discuss death openly and to deal with the anxieties patients have about what might happen to them if they become mentally incapacitated.

Advance directives are likely to be particularly useful to those who have some form of advance warning by age or illness of approaching death or of impending mental incapacity. Commentators have envisaged that the most common condition for which an advance directive would be appropriate would be senile dementia of the Alzheimer type or dementia related to arterial disease. The later stages of dementia always lead to mental incompetence but by means of an advance directive, the individual would be able to control the provision of treatment as far as this could be foreseen.

It has been indicated in the Appeal Court[17] that when a patient has made an anticipatory choice which is "clearly established and applicable in the circumstances" doctors would be bound by it. This implies that advance directives are legally binding if they fulfil these two conditions. A clear and informed statement by a Jehovah's Witness would be binding in the same way.

In case of doubt, however, as to the patient's true intention or if it is considered that the individual was not fully apprised of the implications when drafting an advance directive or that medical advances have substantially changed the circumstances, the courts would be unlikely to support it. The general approach of the law in this country has been based on a bias in favour of preserving life in cases of doubt. The BMA has issued guidance on advance directives (obtainable from the Ethics Division) and these are discussed further in chapter 6 (section 6:3.3).

### 1:3.5 *Other relevant decision-making mechanisms*

Although no person can consent on behalf of another adult in England, Wales and Northern Ireland, Scottish law makes provision for courts to appoint a "tutor dative" who can be given powers to act on behalf of an incapacitated adult in all respects.[18] The extent of the authority of the "tutor dative" is determined by the court decree but if appointed to act as a virtual health care proxy, the tutor dative must assess where the patient's best interests lie and therefore must have access to all the relevant information that patients would seek for themselves.

In England, Wales and Northern Ireland patients who are aware that they are likely to become incompetent can hope to make their views known at that later stage by appointing, in advance, another person to speak for them. Decisions expressed by such a proxy would not have any greater legal force than an advance directive but unlike a written document, a proxy decision-maker would have been primed to reflect the known views of the patient in the particular circumstances which might arise. The precise role, powers and title of a proxy decision-maker are not defined by either custom or law. The English Law Commission is considering such issues, including extending the role of guardians or the powers of attorney into health matters. (A BMA proposal for a decision-making procedure on behalf of incompetent patients is available from the BMA's Ethics Division).

### 1:3.6 *Community treatment orders*

In early 1993 the Department of Health considered proposals to amend the Mental Health Act 1983 to permit compulsory treatment of mentally ill people living in the community, following concerns about the lack of medical supervision of such people after their release from hospital. So-called community treatment orders were first suggested in 1987 by a working party of the Royal College of Psychiatrists and the BMA gave its support to the idea in 1989.

It is not yet clear whether the proposals will be implemented. The Royal College has now effectively abandoned the idea of compulsory treatment in favour of community supervision orders which would require patients to re-enter hospital if they defaulted on treatment in the community. In the Association's view community treatment orders would only be acceptable if safeguards were included which would ensure that competent patients' decisions about treatment were not overruled. The implications of the orders have not yet been fully considered and will be the subject of on-going debate.

## 1:4 Pressures on consent

In some circumstances doctors provide care in full recognition that the consent of the competent patient may not be entirely voluntary and free from pressure. The medical treatment provided to prisoners is an example. Pressure to conform and inability to give independent consent can also arise in relation to individuals who are in some way dependent upon others, such as young or elderly people or, for example, the homeless. Pressure can be exercised on elderly people, especially those apparently inclined to self-neglect, to accept hospital treatment, transfer from home to nursing home or other measures contrary to the individual's desire, in order to satisfy the community's wish for order. This issue is discussed further in chapter 9 on the ethical duties of doctors with dual obligations (section 9:5.2).

Even in the absence of pressure as such, doctors should be alert to the susceptibility of some patients either to give or withhold consent to please others and contrary to their own interests. For example, adult patients may be strongly influenced by the religious views of family members, particularly on issues such as abortion. It has also been suggested that relatives of Jehovah's Witnesses, for example, might be influenced to reject life-prolonging treatments.[19] In such cases, it is important that patients have the opportunity to receive independent counselling and access to pastoral advice if they wish it. Sociodemographic factors may also play a role in the susceptibility of some groups to agree in an almost automatic way to what is proposed. This has been shown, for example, in studies regarding how certain groups of parents are more inclined than others to volunteer their children for clinical research.

### 1:4.1 Consent in the context of teaching

It has been assumed sometimes that, by seeking treatment in a teaching hospital, patients are implicitly consenting to a variety of measures which are commonly associated with teaching. It is evident, however, that patients are not always aware of teaching practices and cannot be assumed to have implicitly agreed to them. It is important to inform patients about such measures and to seek their explicit consent.

#### 1:4.1.1 Presence of students

Such measures may include the presence of medical students in consultations. The system of the doctor introducing the patient to a student who is already seated in the consulting room seems to assume consent in advance. It is important that patients feel they have a genuine option in this matter. The implications of changing practice in busy clinics are substantial but this is an area in which the Patient's Charter has set the tone in the United Kingdom by, for example, emphasising patient choice in such matters.

### 1:4.1.2 Recording of consultations

Consultations with GPs or other doctors may be recorded by visual or auditory means as a teaching aid for doctors. Clearly patients must consent and have the opportunity to refuse. If patients agree to video-recording, they should be asked to give signed consent. This appears a valid teaching strategy but requires pre-planning and careful thought. Even when the patient agrees, some people have reservations about how this practice might alter the fundamental nature of the consultation. It may be felt that some patients who have sensitive matters to raise and do not have fore-knowledge of the practice may feel pressured into ill-considered agreement. How the patient will be approached for consent, and the amount of time available for the patient to reflect, are important considerations, as is the information given to the patient about who will see or hear the material, whether it will leave the hospital unit or GP surgery and the length of time for which it will be preserved. This is especially important now that the development of technology allows students in many parts of the country to have access to material which previously was only shown to very limited audiences. Some have suggested that the information should be given to the patient in writing. The BMA stresses, however, that written information should supplement, but not replace, verbal discussion.

In the accident and emergency departments of hospitals, video-recording of patients undergoing resuscitation is sometimes carried out for teaching or audit purposes. This is obviously done without patient consent, even though patients will be identifiable in the recording. The BMA recognises society's interest in thorough training for doctors in resuscitation techniques but emphasises that patient confidentiality must be respected. Upon recovery, the patient's permission for the keeping and use of such material should be sought unless the film is subsequently digitized to obliterate patient identifiers. The video-taping of patients for clinical and teaching purposes is further considered in chapter 2 (section 2:1.6.1). Photographs may also be taken of patients, with their permission, for clinical purposes, for legal reasons, for teaching or to illustrate research. Patients must be informed of the reason. If it is considered later that a photograph obtained for one purpose would be valuable for another purpose which would involve the patient being identifiable, the patient's consent must be sought anew. The visual recording of minors and incapacitated people should only be carried out with the agreement of carers or parents (except in cases of suspected abuse) and with the proviso that subjects can withdraw permission for the use of the material when they attain the capacity to do so. This matter is also considered further in chapter 2 (section 2:1.6.1) and chapter 3 in relation to minors (section 3:4.2).

### 1:4.1.3 Use of excised tissue

Complex issues arise in connection with the use of tissue from living patients for research, teaching or commercial development. Such tissue is obtained in the course of therapeutic operations and most is used in research or teaching projects which do not involve important commercial considerations. Cases of large financial profits arising from the manipulation of discarded patient tissue are extremely rare. An American legal case[20] arising from a patient's claim to share the potential profits accrued from the development of his cell line concluded that use of tissue must be subject to the patient's informed consent. The issues have not been tested under British law but the BMA has taken a similar stance in that it believes patient consent should be sought in advance when there is an intention to use the tissue.[21]

Patient consent to therapeutic investigation or treatment should be separate from consent to the possible use of excised tissue or organs. Whenever discarded material is not for incineration, patients should be informed in general terms that tissue may be used for one of several purposes. There is often little knowledge at the time the tissue is stored of how it will be ultimately used and therefore patient consent can only be given in general terms. Where a specific purpose is intended, patients should be so informed. Patients who object for religious or other reasons, should be assured that their tissue will be incinerated.

Women who donate fetal tissue (see 1:7.1.6 below) must consent to the use of that tissue in transplantation or research. They relinquish property rights over it and are prohibited from receiving any payment.

### 1:4.1.4 Pelvic examination under anaesthesia

In the past, the practice arose of allowing medical students to gain experience of carrying out intimate examinations by practising on unconscious patients. Such a practice is unacceptable unless the specific consent of the patient has previously been obtained. Hospitals that teach medical students should seek prior written consent for vaginal examinations on anaesthetised patients who are to undergo gynaecological procedures.

### 1:4.2 Prisoners

Imprisonment deprives the individual of autonomy. A detained person is less free to give consent and may be restricted in terms of privacy but nevertheless retains a right to medical care of a proper ethical standard. A convicted prisoner has no choice of doctor, but the prison medical officer has the same obligation as other doctors to obtain consent to treatment. It is BMA policy that doctors should not carry out procedures such as intimate body searches without the subject's consent. The ethical duties of doctors who treat prisoners are discussed in chapter 9 (section 9:7).

The BMA also provides advice for doctors practising in countries where corporal and capital punishment is carried out. Many doctors seek guidance from the Association when asked to participate in executions and judicial punishments. Doctors may be asked to take a number of roles, including verifying mental competence for execution, fitness for flogging or supervising judicial amputations or mutilations. In the BMA's view, doctors should not participate in such procedures. The Association believes that medical participation gives a spurious humanity and respectability to corporal punishment.

On the question of the artificial feeding of prisoners on hunger strike, the BMA supports the World Medical Association's Declaration of Tokyo, which states that when prisoners refuse nourishment and are considered by the doctor to be capable of forming an unimpaired judgement, they shall not be fed artificially. The Association recommends that prisoners be clearly informed in advance of the doctor's policy regarding resuscitation during hunger strike. A doctor who has any doubts about a prisoner's intention, or who is asked to treat an unconscious prisoner whose wishes the doctor cannot ascertain, must strive to do the best for that prisoner. This might involve resuscitating the prisoner and providing artificial feeding.[22]

Doctors in an increasing number of countries may also be asked to participate in operations to remove organs from prisoners following execution. Even though a form of prior consent is obtained from such prisoners, the BMA does not believe that this can be truly considered as valid and voluntary consent. It has condemned such practices.

### 1:4.3 *Members of the armed forces*

Members of the armed forces tacitly consent to give up some of the freedoms of civilian life in the interests of the unit as a whole. Confidentiality and the right to decline treatment are areas where servicemen and their families are likely to experience constraints or pressures. Although doctors in the armed forces have a duty to obey any lawful command, they also have the same ethical duties as other doctors to ensure that patient autonomy is not improperly compromised. This issue is discussed further in chapter 9 (section 9:9).

## 1:5 Treating without consent

As is mentioned in section 1:3 above, there are circumstances which justify treatment or diagnostic procedures even though the patient cannot consent.

It is sometimes argued that doctors should be able to carry out procedures they consider to be appropriate without specifically informing the patient, thus sparing the patient anxiety. As is stressed throughout this book, however, the BMA favours frankness between doctor and patient whenever possible. It considers that doctors should generally be prepared to discuss their uncertainty where appropriate. The Association does not consider it appropriate to carry out HIV-testing, for example, without patient consent.

### 1:5.1 *HIV-testing*

Ethically and legally, no treatment or diagnostic procedures should be undertaken without the valid consent of the competent patient. Some diagnostic procedures, particularly HIV-testing, have such profound implications for the patient that specific patient consent is deemed indispensable. Counselling is an essential prerequisite to HIV-testing.

The BMA is opposed to the compulsory testing of either patients or doctors.[23] It has long been committed to the view that testing must only take place with consent unless very exceptional circumstances justify other action. The General Medical Council has also firmly rejected HIV-testing without specific consent, save in the most exceptional circumstances. It requires doctors to be prepared to justify decisions to test in the absence of patient consent.

It is often suggested that wide testing should be encouraged in the population. Some evidence implies benefits for the HIV-infected individual in early establishment of HIV-status since, with treatment, the onset of AIDS might be delayed. Pre-test counselling should include mention of both the potential advantages and disadvantages of testing. The BMA supports the opportunity for all pregnant women to undergo screening for HIV-antibodies. When testing is routinely offered, it must still be accompanied by thorough counselling so patients can make an informed choice and have the time to discuss the matter with partners or people close to them, if they wish.

## 1:6 Refusal of treatment

Competent adult patients have a clear right to refuse treatment for reasons which are "rational, irrational or for no reason".[24] In such cases, the doctor should seek to explore the patient's motive for refusal and correct any misunderstanding, advise the patient of the increased risks of non-treatment and, if appropriate, other treatment options. No pressure should be brought to bear but the patient should be allowed time to consider the information.

Patients are sometimes asked to sign a declaration stating they have refused a particular treatment and that they accept responsibility for declining medical advice (see 1:2.3 above). The legal validity of such a document would partly depend on how much information had been given to the patient. It may prove an adequate legal defence if the doctor records in the patient's notes that testing or treatment has been refused. It may not be so, if the doctor has not given the patient sufficient information or help.

In some cases, refusal of the treatment recommended by the doctor may indicate that the doctor-patient relationship has broken down and the patient may require a transfer to another doctor. If this is not the case, the doctor should not give the impression of abandoning the patient who has refused a specific treatment.

### 1:6.1 *Refusal of life-saving treatments*

The doctor's legal duties in relation to a patient's refusal of treatment have been recently discussed by a former Master of the Rolls, who stated:

> "Doctors faced with a refusal of consent have to give very careful and detailed consideration to the patient's capacity to decide at the time when the decision was made. It may not be the simple case of the patient having no capacity because, for example, at that time he had hallucinations. It may be the more difficult case of a temporarily reduced capacity at the time when his decision was made. What matters is that the doctors should consider at that time he had a capacity which was commensurate with the gravity of the decision which he purported to make. The more serious the decision, the greater the capacity required. If the patient had the requisite capacity, they are bound by his decision. If not, they are free to treat him in what they believe to be his best interests".[25]

The judge went on to recommend that in case of uncertainty doctors seek a declaration from the courts as to the lawfulness of treatment. This summary of a legal view does not, however, fully reflect the profound moral difficulties which doctors experience when faced with a patient who declines life-saving treatment. Clearly this is the most difficult area for doctors in connection with patient autonomy.

Particular problems arise with Jehovah's Witnesses if treatment requires a blood transfusion. Nevertheless, from an ethical viewpoint, if a rational adult who has been fully apprised of the consequences of not receiving this treatment persists in a refusal, the decision should be respected. In practice, the dilemma seldom has a simple answer and doctors faced with such a problem are urged to explore fully with the patient any alternative measures which both doctor and patient might find acceptable.

When a parent is making this decision on behalf of a child the courts should be involved and will override the parents' decision in the interests of preserving the child's life. The issues surrounding refusal of treatment are further discussed in relation to minors in chapter 3 (section 3:3.6), and adults in chapter 6 (section 6:3.2).

## 1:7 Consent to special treatments – treatment not in the patient's interest

### 1:7.1 *Treatment not in the individual's interest*

Most treatment is proposed in the interests of the person who will undergo it. In some circumstances, treatment is designed to benefit another rather than the subject. An example of such treatment is the practice of intubating newly deceased patients so that the technique of intubation can be mastered by inexperienced doctors in the interests of the general public without risk to living patients. The practice is common in most accident and emergency departments and some obstetric units. Some staff have expressed concern that the procedure is performed without consent and is not generally subject to a framework of ethical guidelines. Some doctors believe that adequate experience could be obtained by practising intubation techniques under supervision on live patients who require the procedure and with their prior permission. Others consider that the experience of perfecting the technique of intubation on a recently deceased patient cannot be adequately duplicated by other means and in particular prepares practitioners for the difficulties of intubating patients who do not conform to standard models because, for example, they have suffered mutilation or physical distortions in accidents. Many also consider it essential to train paediatricians in emergency resuscitation techniques of neonates. The practice has been to obtain training on recently deceased babies without parental consent, given the difficulties of approaching parents at such a traumatic time for them.

The BMA has concluded that the procedure is ethical if done responsibly as part of a training programme and if subject to appropriate guidelines which avoid secrecy and ensure a proper respect for the deceased person. This might involve a campaign of public education to make people aware of the fact that such training is currently carried out in some circumstances and the reasons for it. Thus the present air of secrecy would be dispelled. The Association requested that representatives of all groups of health staff involved in such procedures consider whether such guidelines could be produced. Wide consultation, however, appeared to indicate variable support for the practice, and this led to difficulties in devising acceptable guidelines. This is an issue upon which the BMA would like to encourage further debate.[26]

Other well known examples of treatments designed to benefit someone other than the patient are organ and tissue donation and the emerging practice of ventilating moribund patients in order to facilitate organ donation after their death.

### 1:7.1.1 Organ and tissue donation from live donors

Most live donors are genetically related to the proposed organ or tissue recipient.[27] Doctors must be aware of the possibilities of pressure on donors which might compromise the voluntariness of their consent. Since donation is not in the individual's interest, doctors are advised to give careful thought to providing counselling and information to the donor about possible risks of the procedure. Clearly, a high degree of understanding will be necessary, in keeping with the seriousness of the intended procedure.

25

Awareness of a potential conflict of interest between donors and recipients has influenced the development of organ transplantation. The medical response to this in the conventional adult donor situation is to have two quite separate health care teams: one responsible for the care of the donor, the other responsible for the care of the recipient.

### 1:7.1.2 Children as tissue donors

Although pressure may be brought to bear by families on potential adult donors, they cannot oblige them to donate tissue. Since parents are responsible, however, for making health care decisions for children, donation involving minors is a particularly difficult issue. It raises questions of the degree to which parents can give valid consent to a procedure which is not in the child's interest and involves pain and suffering to the child. There are no clear legal guidelines specifically relating to tissue donation by minors but general arguments raised in cases such as Re F,[28] concerning people who cannot give consent, established the principle that the treatment must be necessary for the person undergoing it and the doctor must act in the best interests of that person.

The type of argument usually put forward in favour of donation by minors is that it is in the child's emotional interests that the life of a sibling, for example, be saved. Similar arguments may be put forward to support the idea of donation from a mentally incapacitated person. Some object, however, to the possibility of regarding those who have not attained full autonomy, for one reason or another, as available tissue providers. The same can be said of pregnancies generated with the express purpose of providing a new potential live tissue donor.[29] Such practices raise fears that non-autonomous people are being used as a means to promote another person's interests.

The argument that donation is in the donor's emotional interests does not always reflect reality. The donor child may resent the attention constantly given to the sick brother or sister and manifest fear and bitterness at being subjected to treatment. Cases must be decided on an individual basis. There are no simple solutions, given the conflicting imperatives of saving life and protecting the developing autonomy of the potential child donor.

In the BMA's opinion, the views of the potential child donor must be sought if he or she has sufficient maturity to understand the situation. Weight must be placed on a competent child's refusal to consent to tissue donation. In order to be ethically justifiable, the procedures proposed for potential child donors should only involve minimal risk and suffering and should not be contrary to the child's health interests. The BMA does not consider it appropriate for live, non-autonomous individuals to donate non-regenerative tissue or organs. In some cases, the long-term risks to the donor cannot be adequately predicted. This issue is discussed further in chapter 3 (section 3:6).

### 1:7.1.3 Neonates as donors

In general, the ethical problems relating to neonatal transplant therapy are the same as those which arise in consideration of other donor groups. Some procedures may be regarded as experimental and, whereas adults can consent to undertake dangerous options, some question whether parents can reasonably consent to the treatment of a child which involves unnecessary risk. The problems in separating such research from acceptable innovative treatments are discussed in chapter 8 (section 8:2.3).

Even more problematic is the issue of anencephalic neonates as organ donors. It is estimated that approximately 40 anencephalic babies are born alive each year in the United Kingdom but few donate organs because of the special ethical and legal problems they pose. Since there is no time limit on abortions performed for fetal abnormality, such infants are born to women who object to termination in principle or who wish to allow the fetus to mature in order to provide organs. Many would regard the latter view as immoral and compromising to the individual value of handicapped people in its implications.

A major difficulty in the proposal to use organs from anencephalics is the impossibility of defining brainstem death. The royal colleges take the view that "organs for transplantation can be removed from anencephalic infants when two doctors who are not members of the transplant team agree that spontaneous respiration has ceased".[30] Many[31] support this view, seeing it as no more than a restatement of a diagnostic test for death which has long been the norm. They consider attempts to introduce a brainstem death standard as unnecessary and impractical in this context. Other legal experts,[32] however, have raised doubts about the use of anencephalic babies as heart donors, pointing out that the anencephalic child's heart may spontaneously continue to beat for some hours after respiration has ceased and, in the absence of clear brainstem death criteria, no death certificate can be issued. Very few anencephalic donors are used but for the few cases that are presently considered suitable, clarification of the law would be welcomed by doctors.

### 1:7.1.4 Ventilation of moribund patients for organ donation

Usually organ donors have been chosen on the basis of irreversible brain damage which has resulted in "brain death". When death is clearly inevitable, any attempts at resuscitation have been seen as unhelpful intrusions. Practice now, however, includes applying resuscitative procedures to the prospective organ donor, without hope of benefit for that person but with the objective of maintaining the quality of the organs to be removed for transplantation.

The BMA has considered the legal and ethical implications of the elective ventilation of moribund patients, without their prior consent, for the purposes of organ donation. In such cases, patients such as those dying of intracranial cerebrovascular catastrophes in general wards are transferred to intensive care units although it is recognised that they are very unlikely to derive any benefit. The patients are not in a condition to be able to express consent or refusal. The purpose is to maximise the possibilities of organ donation from those patients on their death. No patient can be considered as a potential donor until all treatments for the benefit of that patient have been exhausted. The BMA recognised that respect for individual autonomy could be compromised by instituting procedures not to benefit the donor but to maintain organ quality, and that this must be weighed against the potential for benefiting many organ recipients and saving lives. Patient autonomy could be preserved if patients were able to express their views on this practice in advance, either through some form of advance directive or re-worded donor card but public knowledge about this practice is not yet widespread. Current practice is for the people close to the patient to be asked to agree to the procedure. The possibility of causing symbolic harm by accepting relatives' views, as if the dying patient were already legally dead, is recognised. Nevertheless, elective ventilation and the intensive nursing care accompanying it, although not undertaken with the purpose of benefiting a potential donor, are not clinically deleterious to the patient.

The BMA considers that this practice is not unethical of itself but that it must be subject to a strict ethical framework and safeguards. It has recommended that a protocol be agreed nationally between interested bodies. Criteria for identifying potential organ donors; criteria for exclusion from consideration for organ donation; procedures to be followed in approaching consultants and in approaching those close to the patient, and management of the patient in the intensive care unit, are all matters which should be agreed by discussion between all members of the health care team, including the chaplain.

Much discussion has concentrated on the attitude of those close to the patient. Consent by those in close relationships with a living patient is not legally valid but they may be best placed to reflect how the patient would have viewed such procedures. Current practice is to keep the potential donor's partner or relatives fully informed of all procedures, and to obtain their consent to those procedures. Some have seen this as a franker way of treating dying patients and their relatives, as it allows the relatives to realise that there is no hope of recovery. This approach includes explaining to relatives, in advance, that the dying patient may eventually prove to be an unsuitable donor and may be removed from ITU and returned to a general ward for a number of reasons, especially if another patient requires intensive care for his or her own benefit. There has been concern that patients without a partner or relatives to speak for them might be accorded less consideration than those who have representatives to speak for them and the BMA has recommended that they should be excluded from the potential pool of donors.

The Association's views have been transmitted to interested bodies such as the British Transplantation Society, which has been asked to co-ordinate discussions for a nationally agreed protocol.

### 1:7.1.5 Dead donors

Individuals can consent during their lifetime to the donation of organs after death. Consent given orally and witnessed by two people is sufficient, although many people carry donor cards or make a written statement. Even if the subject has not expressed consent, tissue or any part of the body may be removed on the authorisation of the person lawfully in possession of the body, (either an institution such as a hospital or a nursing home or the family) as long as no relative of the deceased objects.[33] Schemes have been proposed whereby consent to donate is assumed automatically unless the individual has actively registered a refusal prior to death. In such schemes, the consent or refusal of relatives carries no weight. The BMA's view is that the potential donor's known views should be determinative. In cases where it is shown by relatives that the deceased was opposed to donation on religious, cultural or other grounds, these views should be respected in the same way that any other expression of the patient's wish, such as an advance directive, would be respected.

### 1:7.1.6 Use of fetal tissue

Tissue from aborted fetuses has been used for therapeutic and research purposes. Fetal brain tissue, for example, has been used in treatment of Parkinsonism, and clinical use of fetal thymus and liver cells continues in some centres abroad. In the early stages of such treatment moral qualms were expressed about the information given to, and the consent obtained from, the women whose aborted fetuses are so used and the potential for conflict of interest between the donor and the recipient of tissue. The original consent forms signed by women disclaimed their having any views on the disposal of the fetus. Many people maintained that such women should be told if there was a possibility that the fetal tissues would be used for transplantation or research, and their specific, unpressured consent obtained. The Polkinghorne Report,[34] which codifies the views of Government and the profession, recommends that any fetal tissues used in therapy or research should be subject to the "positive explicit consent" of the mother but states that the information given to her will be general and "embrace all uses to which the fetus may be put". Thus the mother will not be informed of the actual purpose for which her fetus is used. This is consistent with the BMA's general views about the use of other tissue taken from live patients during therapeutic operations (see 1:4.1.3 above).

Importance is given in the Polkinghorne Report to the timing of consent. In the case of spontaneous abortion, consent is necessarily obtained after fetal death and timing of the request should be dictated by the need to minimise distress. In the case of therapeutic abortion, consent to the use of the fetus should not be sought until the mother has consented to the termination of pregnancy; and the doctors dealing with the termination should be entirely separated from those using the tissue.

HIV- or hepatitis-testing of the fetus is carried out if the tissue is to be used for transplantation. Such testing is required in the interests of the tissue recipient but the results may have grave implications for the mother and her consent to this is necessary. Issues arising in other cases where treatment for the benefit of one patient has profound implications for others are discussed below in 1:9.

The method of termination of pregnancy is dependent upon a number of factors, including the gestational age of the fetus. The technique selected to produce the abortion also affects the usefulness of any fetal tissue made available for transplantation, since the interval between fetal death and tissue collection may be significant. Fetal organs deprived of oxygen and blood supply, at maternal body temperature, deteriorate very quickly. Fetal pancreatic islet survival, for example, has been shown to be much more impaired by prostaglandin-induced abortion than by hysterectomy. Use of tissue from prostaglandin- induced termination is thus said to have contributed significantly to the failure of fetal pancreatic islet transplantation to gain acceptance in the treatment of diabetes. The abortion technique selected also affects the possibility of identifying particular types of tissue. Suction evacuation of the uterus while avoiding the problems of warm ischaemia (oxygen deprivation at body temperature) results in soft tissue being delivered in disrupted form, making isolation of brain tissue a difficult procedure.

It has thus been suggested that, given that tissues produced by some types of abortion are unsuitable for transplantation, trends in relative popularity of different techniques may gradually come to reflect transplantation requirements.[35] Modification of abortion technique solely in order to improve collection of fetal tissue is ethically unacceptable. The importance of separating the obstetricians from the experimental therapists was also recognised by the Polkinghorne Committee, which proposed the use of an intermediary.

Although there is no evidence suggesting that such practices occur, some still fear that pregnancies might be generated for the express purpose of providing fetal cells for the treatment of a relative, and call for comprehensive legislation covering the whole spectrum of transplantation therapy. Two decades ago the BMA categorised as unethical the generation or termination of a pregnancy solely to produce suitable material; and any financial reward, for the donation of fetal material. It recommended that there should be no link between donor and recipient and that nervous tissue should only be used as isolated neurones or tissue fragments. In 1989, the Polkinghorne Committee codified such recommendations but did not consider "that legislation would allow the flexibility which may be needed in the light of developing knowledge and experience" but "that it is best to proceed, where possible, by means of ethical guidelines and a Code of Practice".

## 1:8 Consent to special treatments – irreversible procedures

The voluntariness and well informed nature of consent is clearly of particular importance if the treatment carries permanent consequences or effects which prudence dictates should be regarded as irreversible. Psychosurgery and sterilisation are examples of such procedures. Irreversible procedures are particularly controversial when the autonomy of the patient is in any way impaired or under pressure, either because of mental incapacity or imprisonment, for example.

### 1:8.1 Psychosurgery

Part IV of the Mental Health Act 1983 deals with treatment for mental disorder of patients detained without their consent. Psychosurgery (any surgical operation for destroying brain tissue or the functioning of brain tissue) and the surgical implantation of hormones for the purposes of reducing male sexual drive require both the patient's consent and a second opinion (section 57 of the Mental Health Act 1983). As the Mental Health Act Code of Practice makes clear, section 57 reflects public and professional concerns about the voluntariness and validity of patients' agreement to such procedures and the possible long term effects. The facts and results of such irreversible treatments must be notified to the Mental Health Act Commission. Prior to psychosurgery, the Commission will usually visit the patient.[36]

In 1992 there was an international outcry when an American judge offered a prisoner convicted of sexual offences surgical castration, as an alternative to a very lengthy sentence. Although initially consenting, the prisoner subsequently withdrew consent to the procedure. "Chemical castration" or the administration of drugs to reduce male libido has been used in efforts to rehabilitate sex offenders in the United States but there has been little support for it in Britain, even in cases where patients have sought it. The issue is discussed further in chapter 4 (section 4:4.3) and the medical treatment of prisoners in general is explored in chapter 9 (section 9:7.4).

31

### 1:8.2 *Non-therapeutic procedures*

As regards minors and patients who are mentally incapacitated, some procedures are regarded as so serious and controversial that doctors are required to seek judicial approval before carrying them out. Non-therapeutic sterilisation, for instance, requires authorisation from the courts. Thus, if sterilisation is advised because of a fear that the incapacitated woman may become pregnant, but would be unable to cope with pregnancy or childbirth, court approval should be sought. Sterilisation for therapeutic reasons, such as treating a disease of the reproductive organs, does not require court authorisation (see also chapter 4, section 4:4.2). The patient's interests must come first. Public policy or the convenience and concerns of those who care for the patient are not determinative factors in the decision to authorise sterilisation.

## 1:9 Consent to special treatments – implications for others

### 1:9.1 *Treatments affecting fertility*

Any treatment affecting an individual's reproductive capacity has potential implications for that person's spouse or partner. In the past, consent to treatments such as sterilisation was sought routinely from the patient's spouse. This is now acknowledged to be unacceptable although it is good practice to encourage patients to discuss sterilisation with their partners.

### 1:9.2 *Genetic screening*

Genetic screening helps individuals or couples to make decisions about their own lives and those of their future children. Information obtained, however, about one family member in relation to genetic disease may have profound implications for other family members who have not sought or consented to screening.

Such screening is prompted usually by the awareness of a history of the disease within the family. Thus, family members are likely to be aware of the implications of screening and the importance of sharing information. Such co-operation, however, cannot be assumed and careful counselling may be required. Any refusal by relatives to be involved in detection of genetic markers must be respected. Other aspects of genetic screening are discussed in chapter 4 (section 4:9.2).

### 1:9.3 *HIV-testing*

Investigation of some conditions has implications for those close to the patient. Many of these implications involve issues of confidentiality and are discussed in chapter 2 (section 2:4.4.1). Some also raise difficult questions of consent, such as pre-adoption HIV-testing of babies. In such cases, the test result will plainly have implications for both the birth mother and the adoptive parents. If the child is in local authority care, it may be sufficient in law for the authority to give consent but many people would recognise a moral obligation to trace and counsel the natural mother in the event of a positive result in the child.

### 1:9.4 *Paternity testing*

The BMA receives enquiries from time to time about consent to paternity testing, which many patients believe can be carried out on a routine basis with the consent of a parent or assumed parent. Paternity testing, however, clearly carries important implications for the child whose genetic background it seeks to clarify. In very many cases, it is extremely dubious as to whether such testing would be in the child's interest, since it could irrevocably affect the attitudes of those caring for the child. As the most vulnerable party, the child's interests are generally owed greater consideration than those of others. Procedures for obtaining consent for blood samples for paternity tests may also have implications for the presumed father, who is sometimes unaware that the child's paternity is in doubt.

Such testing cannot be carried out simply at the request of the adult parties involved but is subject to strict regulation. The Home Office issues guidance on this subject and regularly nominates a very limited list of practitioners authorised to carry out paternity testing. Decisions about paternity tests must usually be made by the courts.

## 1:10 Summary

1   Doctor-patient relationships should be founded on mutual respect. The importance accorded to patient consent reflects the respect with which doctors regard their patients. The recognition by doctors that patients usually know better than any one else what is best for them imposes a duty upon doctors to empower patients to make their own decisions, based on information and support.

2   Decisions about health care should be made by the individual, with advice and information from the doctor. In order to be valid, patient consent must be informed, voluntary and competent. Apart from legal provisions in Scotland for the nomination of "tutors dative", no one can consent to treatment on behalf of another adult (although this is under legal review).

3   Doctors should attempt to enter into continuing dialogue with patients about decisions which affect their wellbeing. Trust will only grow from frankness. Patients should control the amount and timing of information. In exceptional circumstances, distressing or harmful information may be withheld from the patient for a time. Decisions to withhold information should never be routine or taken casually.

Such decisions must be subject to continuing review and efforts made to prepare the patient for full disclosure.

4   In emergencies, life-saving treatment should be provided if it is impossible to gain consent. Unconscious patients and those suffering very severe mental impairment cannot act autonomously but may have made an anticipatory decision. In other circumstances, ethical principles require doctors to make a judgement as to the patient's best interest.

5   Consent is a process, not an event, and it is important that there be continuing discussion.

6   The opportunity to consent to treatment is counterbalanced by a right to refuse it. If a rational adult who has been fully apprised of the consequences of not receiving this treatment persists in refusing it, the decision should be respected.

7   Implied consent can only be held to apply to the procedure in hand and not necessarily to subsequent treatments which flow from it.

8   Consent and refusal forms simply document that some discussion has taken place.

9   Ideally, the doctor should inform the patient about any risks inherent in the treatment which might be particularly important to that patient, as well as explaining the risks and benefits of alternatives and of non-treatment.

10  The concept of advance directives is supported by the BMA. They are useful to those who have some form of advance warning by age or illness of approaching death or of impending mental incapacity.

11  Doctors should be alert to the susceptibility of some patients either to give or withhold consent to please others and contrary to their own interests.

12  There is no legal minimum age at which young people can consent to treatment. Competence, not age, is the key but there are limits on the scope for competent minors to refuse necessary treatments.

13  Patients are not always aware of teaching practices and cannot be assumed to have implicitly agreed to them. It is important to inform patients about such measures and to seek their explicit consent.

14  Patient consent to investigation or treatment should be distinct from consent to the possible use of excised tissue or organs. Patient consent can only be based on the knowledge available at the time consent is sought. In any instance where discarded material is not for incineration, patients should be informed in general terms that tissue may be used for one of several purposes.

15  In order to be ethically justifiable, the procedures proposed for potential child donors should only involve minimal risk and should clearly not be contrary to the child's health interests. The BMA does not consider it appropriate for non-autonomous donors, such as

children, to donate non-regenerative tissue or organs.

16 Fetal tissues used in therapy or research should be subject to the consent of the mother, who should be informed in general terms about the procedures in which the tissue may be used.

17 Irreversible procedures are particularly controversial when the autonomy of the patient is in any way impaired or under pressure. Doctors should be aware of and alert to the possibility of such pressure.

# 2 Confidentiality and Medical Records

*Introductory remarks including the traditional emphasis on confidentiality and the contradictory demands on doctors; definition of the scope of confidentiality and the type of materials covered by it. The concept of ownership of medical records and those who can claim access to them; arrangements for access to other people's records, including the records of children, young people, mentally incapacitated people and the deceased; access by employers and access for audit purposes; aspects of security, use, storage and disposal of medical records. Instances where patients can only expect restricted confidentiality, including members of the armed forces and prisoners. Rules governing disclosure, including with patient consent, in the patient's interest, disclosure required by law, the overriding duty to society, research and teaching. The need for legislation on medical confidentiality. Summary of points.*

## 2:1 Introduction

### 2:1.1 *The issues*

This chapter deals with two separate issues. Medical confidentiality is a traditional principle and a practical requirement of the relationship between doctors and patients. The management and security of medical records is one facet of that duty of confidentiality. Society's efforts to empower the individual to control information about him/herself has resulted in a series of measures, following on from the Data Protection Act 1984, which permit subject access. What is worrying for doctors, however, is the extent to which access by patients themselves has brought about wider, third-party disclosure.

### 2:1.2 *Privacy and public interest considerations*

Privacy is a fundamental right which allows individuals to decide the manner and extent to which information about themselves is shared with others. Such personal control is at the core of legislation enabling patient access to health records and reports. Self-determination in this respect is also central to the preservation of the dignity and integrity of the individual. On occasions, however, public interest may be seen to override the privacy of an individual, but in such instances the facts must be subject to close scrutiny as to whether there is a genuine necessity for disclosure. It has been aptly said that "there is a wide difference between what is interesting to the public and what is in the public interest".[37]

In the case of medical information, there are likely to be both private and public interests active in any claim for confidentiality and it may be difficult to differentiate between the two. Where patients have individual interests that their medical details should not be disclosed to others, there is likely to be some public interest present. Good medical practice depends upon patients being able to discuss openly with the doctor wide-ranging aspects of their health on the understanding that such details will be kept secret. It follows that any disclosure contrary to the individual's interest is also potentially very detrimental to the public interest since it may discourage frank exchanges in future. This is discussed further in 2:4.6.1 below on HIV infection.

### 2:1.3 *The ethos of confidentiality*

Long before the relatively modern emphasis on privacy, the principle of confidentiality was germane to the ethics of medical practice. The function of the confidentiality principle is to protect the doctor-patient relationship, although it is not shielded by legal privilege as are communications between lawyers and their clients. The concept goes back to the time of Hippocrates and beyond, and is continually re-stated in various codes, including the International Code of Medical Ethics[38] which says that a doctor must preserve "absolute confidentiality on all he knows about his patient" even after the patient's death. "All he knows about the patient" goes far beyond the usual formulation of "all that the doctor learns in the course of his professional practice" and is a counsel of perfection rather than practical guidance. Furthermore, the injunction to maintain strict confidentiality "even after the patient's death" contradicts the provisions of British legislation[39] intended to support patient interests.

### 2:1.4 *Changing practices*

#### 2:1.4.1 NHS changes

It is no surprise to doctors that issues of medical confidentiality are beset by contradictions. The BMA, in all its ethical guidance, sets a high value on medical confidentiality but it recognises that new pressures, largely outside the control of doctors, are being brought to bear on the confidentiality rule. These come from changing patterns of health care delivery, the increasing emphasis on health promotion and preventive measures, and the commercial demand for health-related information. In 1992, the Association was so concerned by changes in practice within the NHS, which it saw as threatening confidentiality, that it established a working party to look into the issues in depth. The BMA, however, has frequently found it difficult to convince both the government and society at large that apparently small compromises in confidentiality made in the name of efficiency or convenience gradually erode patients' rights.

There is, nevertheless, a strong public interest in enforcing the medical duty of confidentiality. In the absence of guarantees that their secrets will be protected, patients may withhold information important to their health care and possibly to the wellbeing of others, including health professionals. Many consider that this holding back by patients of important facts is already common, not because patients no longer trust their doctors but because some of the same measures designed to put control into the patient's hands also left them vulnerable to pressure to permit almost indiscriminate disclosure.

### 2:1.4.2 Social changes

Health information has always been given to doctors with the intention of providing the basis for appropriate medical care. Increasingly, details about life-style and family history are also sought as part of health promotion but health data is, in fact, also used routinely for a wide range of other purposes. Patients needing life insurance, loans, mortgages, employment, access to sheltered and council housing, state benefits and private pension schemes, often need a medical report from their general practitioner to support their application. Reports to third parties can only be provided with specific patient consent but patients who decline to authorise the release of information can dismiss the possibility of success in whatever application they are pursuing. Thus health records play an increasingly important social function and doctors frequently object that, instead of preserving the secrecy of identifiable medical data, they spend much effort in circulating it, with patient consent, to batteries of different recipients who sometimes have ill-defined obligations regarding its confidentiality.

Nor is it patients alone who open the way to disclosure. Personal health information is sought by a variety of interests claiming "a right to know". Such information has a commercial value and there is a market demand for data. A great risk to confidentiality arises out of the multiplicity of repositories of health information where it is controlled by a number of different health professionals, administrators and social workers - all of whose records are subject to different criteria for disclosure, to a range of possible others from trainees to town councillors. Increased risks appear with the introduction of widespread computerisation and the use of systems which can easily be penetrated by those with an interest in so doing.

### 2:1.4.3 "Tele-medicine"

Advances in medical technology mean that some patients with serious conditions do not necessarily require hospital in-patient care but can be monitored elsewhere, either at home or in convalescent clinics or modest medical centres. Telecommunication technology allows doctors to manage the medical needs of such patients at a distance if necessary. A range of medical information can be transmitted by telephone and fax, including electrocardiograms, encephalograms, x-rays, photographs and medical documents of all kinds. Patients with pacemakers, for example, can transmit an electrocardiographic rhythm strip by telephone from home to a doctor in a distant monitoring centre. It is envisaged that, in the future, such central stations may receive and respond to information fed in from a variety of bio-televigilance systems and "tele-medicine" will assume an increasingly important role, not only in geographically isolated areas, but in the everyday care of a growing population of sick and disabled people worldwide.

Other communication systems such as television and satellite contacts permit visual contact and co-operation between doctors in different countries. Such measures facilitate good collaborative care when, for example, patients resident in one country fall ill in another. Trans-border transmission of patient histories and other identifiable material such as scans and biological analyses can be problematic from the point of view of confidentiality since not all countries have developed systems of data protection.

Such systems do, therefore, raise difficult problems for ensuring patient confidentiality. There are also problems associated with making sure the equipment itself is always working efficiently, such efficiency being essential if patients are to have safe care. Some of the problems to do with ensuring confidentiality will be addressed by efforts within the European Community aimed at providing common standards for all processing of manual and electronic data. (This is discussed further in 2:5.3 below.) It is clear that ethical considerations require the implementation of full safeguards for patient confidentiality prior to the introduction of new technology on a routine basis.

### 2:1.5 Scope of confidentiality

There are different perceptions of confidentiality and of the information to which it relates. Information which doctors acquire outside the sphere of their professional practice is arguably unconstrained by their duty of confidentiality. In respect of this information, doctors are subject to the same conventions as any other citizens. Whether or not doctors are engaging in their professional practice depends to some extent on the perception of the person giving the information. If any doubt exists, the higher (professional) standard of confidentiality should prevail.

#### 2:1.5.1 Sharing information with other health professionals

In the BMA's view, all information that doctors acquire as part of their professional practice is subject to the duty of confidentiality. This does not mean that it can never be revealed but that doctors must be able to show just grounds for its disclosure. Such grounds are usually that the patient has given consent. Patient consent should be sought, for example, for the sharing with other health professionals of information necessary for the effective care of the patient. Increasingly, care is provided by inter-disciplinary teams and it is important that patients are aware of this and explicitly agree to information being given to those who need to know it. The criteria governing such disclosure is that the receiving health professional has a demonstrable "need to know" that particular piece of information in the interests of patient care. The sharing of identifiable information for the convenience or interests of health workers or administrators cannot be so justified. Managers, including those with a medical or nursing qualification, do not have a right of access to identifiable patient information simply by fact of their managerial responsibilities.

Some health information is so sensitive that legislation has been introduced to cover the sharing of it with other health professionals. Initially, under the Human Fertilisation and Embryology Act 1990, doctors providing fertility treatment in licensed centres were restricted from transmitting clinical information to medical colleagues who were not covered by a licence, even with the patient's consent. To disclose information direct to medical colleagues was an offence. Such restrictions caused enormous practical difficulties in relation to communicating a patient's necessary follow-up care with a GP. It also introduced unintended dangers for the patient, for example in situations when the fertility specialist and another doctor prescribed conflicting treatments unaware of each other's activities. The restriction on disclosure of information also meant fertility specialists were unable to defend themselves in law because they were not allowed to discuss the details of the case with solicitors.

In July 1992, amending legislation in the form of the Human Fertilisation and Embryology (Disclosure of Information) Act passed into law. This Act relaxed some of the restrictions on liaison between clinicians but at the same time retained the safeguards which give patients control over who has access to personal health information. The Act allows direct communication between doctors on a need to know basis, with the patient's consent, and without the patient's consent in emergency situations where disclosure is necessary to avert an imminent danger to the health of the patient. Disclosure without consent is also permitted for the purposes of legal proceedings or formal complaints procedures.

### 2:1.5.2 Disclosure to other people

Other justifiable grounds for disclosure arise with notifiable diseases, which doctors have a statutory obligation[40] to report to the authorities, or situations where the doctor believes other people would be put at grave risk by non-disclosure. Thus, the right to privacy is considered an essential element of human rights but it is not absolute. When rights collide some mechanism must be available to permit an objective determination of which of the conflicting interests is most important. In the matter of confidentiality of health information, a judgement will often fall to doctors, who may even be considered negligent in some circumstances if they fail to breach confidentiality to the authorities or the police when there is a public interest in doing so. The grounds for disclosure are discussed further in 2:4 below.

### 2:1.6 *Definition of patient information*

Doctors often enquire which particular pieces of information are classified as confidential patient information. Common questions concern whether the fact that a patient is registered with one doctor rather than another colleague is confidential, or whether a list of patients who have attended surgery can be given to the police, for example, after a petty theft has taken place. In the BMA's view, all information collected in the context of health care is confidential and the activator of its release is patient consent. Only in exceptional cases, such as when there is a serious risk to other people (or in the case of some research when a local research ethics committee has specifically approved disclosure), can the doctor dispense with the need for the patient's consent.

Patient information covers not only the written record but all patient-identifiable material, including that which is not recorded at all but held in the doctor's head. In addition to the traditional written record, health data can also be held in computerised form, on x-rays and in audio-visual form. Different forms of records pose different risks to confidentiality.

### 2:1.6.1 *Types of records*

Whatever type of record is under discussion, the basic principle is that a record, whether written or visual, which is undertaken for one purpose, should not be used for any other purpose without the subject's consent.

Written records, photographs or video films compiled for the provision of health care to an individual patient should not be used in an identifiable form for teaching without that patient's consent, or the consent of the parent(s) of children.

This has led some people to support staged consent forms, so that patients clearly give or refuse consent for each of the separate stages that might arise. Such forms would generally be applicable to video-taped as well as other records. The consent forms currently used by many family therapy units enable patients to authorise review of the tape to help the team and the family and to give separate authorisation of the material to be used for teaching. It has sometimes been suggested that similarly staged consent forms might be used in connection with other types of record allowing, for example, patients to say whether information about them

41

could be used for research. The BMA emphasises that forms alone are not important. It is the discussion which accompanies the signing of a form which is important.

*Computer records* are replacing manual records within the NHS. Such records are subject to the Data Protection Act 1984, which gives legal protection to individuals against the misuse of personal information.[41] Questions of confidentiality arise when computer systems require repair or servicing by external contractors, who must be subject to confidentiality agreements.[42] Increasingly, patient data can be transmitted from computer to computer. Doctors should bear in mind the principle that only necessary information should be shared and they should ensure that recipients of patient data have access only to relevant parts, and not to the whole, of the patient's file.

*Photographic records* are used in some specialties, such as paediatric and accident and emergency departments, more than others. Whenever feasible the taking of photographs should be subject to the patient's consent or with the consent of parents of children. Many health authorities have introduced their own guidelines on the subject of consent and confidentiality, in particular circumstances. Documenting suspected cases of child abuse, for example, may involve photographic records. When such clinical illustration is required for legal purposes, it may be obtained without parental consent, although this should be sought. There is a clear duty to seek the co-operation of the child if this is feasible and to explain the purpose of the record. Whenever possible, the photography or video-recording of children should be undertaken by an appropriately accredited professional.

If identifiable visual material is recorded for teaching purposes, it is necessary to get the patient's consent. Minors must be able to withdraw consent upon attaining maturity. Still-births and neonates on the point of death are sometimes photographed at the request of parents but photographs should not be used for any other purposes, unless the parent indicates that this would be acceptable. Great sensitivity is required regarding this issue.

The Mental Health Act 1983 makes no provision for visually recording mentally disordered patients. In practice, such records are sometimes made with the consent of those close to the patient if the patient is unable to consent. When patients regain competency, such material is subject to their control and should be destroyed if consent is refused.

Except where patients have given specific consent to other arrangements, patient-identifiable photographs should remain part of the patient's confidential medical record, subject to the same safeguards as other data. No identifying material may be published in textbooks, journals or for teaching without express patient consent. In this context,

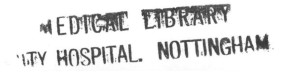

the BMA takes the view that consent is not blanket permission but should be periodically renewed, at intervals of five years for example, if identifiable material continues to be used. The patient has the right to withdraw consent at any time. When consent is withdrawn all copies and the master material should be destroyed.

*Video-taped records* are becoming increasingly common in clinical use, especially in the field of paediatric psychiatry, and as a teaching tool. A particular area of concern, mentioned in chapter 1 (section 1:4.1.2), involves the video-recording in accident and emergency units of patients undergoing resuscitation, since this practice is not subject to consent by the patient or the agreement of any person close to the patient. Professional bodies, such as the Royal College of Psychiatry, give guidance on such matters. In the past, however, the confidentiality of such records has been dubiously observed. They should be subject to the same general safeguards as other confidential, patient-identifiable material. Patient consent should be required for inclusion of illustrative material in the patient's record; further consent should be required for the use of patient-identifiable material for teaching, and additional consent should be required for its wider dissemination to, for instance, medical video-libraries. Some bodies, including the BMA, have been concerned that doctors are not able to exercise adequate control over such visual teaching material, which could be illegally copied. The BMA considers it difficult, if not impossible, to police provisions that all material must be withdrawn if the patient withdraws consent to its use. Video-taped records which cannot be made secure should be destroyed or anonymised.

The validity of minors' consent to video-taping is sometimes questioned. As is discussed in chapter 3 (section 3:4.2), such consent is valid if the child or young person understands the reason for the procedure and it implications.

One solution is that video-taped records can be edited and anonymised by obscuring or "digitizing" identifying features. Although this is not universally possible, it is recommended that this procedure is followed wherever feasible for teaching. Patients' facial expressions, however, are important for some teaching material, such as that dealing with neurological and neuropsychological conditions. Unfortunately this usually concerns patients incapable of giving consent. Again, in practice, relatives authorise the use of such material for teaching and in some instances hospital administrators give temporary authorisation for recordings to be made in exceptional circumstances. There is a danger that patient confidentiality may be under-valued in such circumstances, particularly when hospital administrators may be looking for income generating proposals. All those involved in such procedures must ensure that due regard is given to confidentiality.

43

## 2:2 Ownership, access and control of records

There are both legal and ethical considerations to be borne in mind when discussing ownership, access and control. The BMA considers it ethically appropriate for patients to exercise control over how information about themselves is used. For this, they need access to it. Exceptionally, such access may be considered detrimental to the health interests of the patient. The Association considers that such cases would be rare. In most respects, the BMA's ethical views about control of information and access to it coincide with the legal provisions for control and access.

Ownership, however, remains a disputed area, and the legal opinion quoted by Government does not coincide with the BMA's ethical views. These are expressed below.

### 2:2.1 *Ownership*

Questions of access to and control of medical records by patients themselves turn on the fact of ownership. In law, the concept of ownership of information is very underdeveloped.[43] Many differentiate the "information" which belongs to the patient, the opinion which the doctor brings to that raw information, and the documentation of this process. At common law, the person who "controls" the records is the person who writes them. Private doctors are considered to "own" the records which they write (subject to statutory rights of access) and NHS records, made on materials supplied by the family health service authority (FHSA) are expressly stated to be its property, ultimately belonging to the Secretary of State.

In 1990, the Secretary of State sought legal opinion on confidentiality and the use of GPs' medical records. The opinion given was that FHSAs are the legal owners of all data obtained by GPs in the course of carrying out their NHS contractual duties and that FHSAs can authorise disclosure of such information "within the NHS family circle" without the consent of either the patient or the GP. The BMA has expressed grave anxiety about this. The Association deplores the notion that information held by doctors about their patients should be deemed to belong to the Secretary of State and considers that this endangers confidentiality. The BMA is also opposed to the transfer of patient registration information from FHSAs to other bodies, including health authorities, without the express permission of patients.[44]

Despite its opposition to any routine disclosure without patient consent, the BMA has not been able to challenge effectively the concept of ownership of records by the Secretary of State but has sought to draw public attention to the issues. In August 1990, the BMA issued a press statement, reiterating its view that:

- when a patient registers with a GP, personal information is imparted to the doctor in confidence and by the doctor to the FHSA for the sole purpose of administering the GP's NHS contract;

- this information should be controlled by the patient, as it belongs to neither the GP, the FHSA, the NHS nor the Department of Health;

- the patient is registering with the GP specifically for NHS general medical services, not with the NHS as a whole;

- it is recognised that both patients and the NHS may benefit from the sharing of registration data with health authorities, but because this information remains the property of the patient, this change should not have been introduced without a full and informed public and parliamentary debate.

### 2:2.2 Access by patients

In the past, the concept of confidentiality meant that health records were kept secret from patients themselves. Nowadays, there is broad support for openness and frankness between doctor and patient. Patients' right of access to information about themselves is enshrined in law in the Access to Medical Reports Act 1988 (see also chapter 9, section 9:3) and the Access to Health Records Act 1990.[45] The Access to Health Records Act 1990 gives patients access to health records made after 1 November 1991 and to information recorded earlier when this is necessary in order for the patient to understand what was written later. The Act does not prevent doctors from giving the patient wider access to the whole record, including that made before November 1991, nor does it mean that doctors can only give access upon formal application. Patient access outside the scope of the Act is at the doctor's discretion. The BMA encourages doctors to give patients access to all health information held about them, unless the doctor believes it deleterious to the patient's health to do so or unless the confidentiality of other people might be compromised. These are also the two grounds for withholding information specified in the legislation. Withholding access solely because disclosure would be embarrassing for doctors or might give rise to legal claims against them is not acceptable.

Refusing the patient access because the doctor believes the information would be harmful to the patient should be rare. Sometimes, however, the doctor will have to hold back information which identifies or relates to someone else. No information which identifies any other person (unless that person is a health professional) can be revealed to the patient without the consent of the person so identified. Their NHS contract requires general practitioners to include in the patient's record information about some diseases suffered by the patient's blood relatives. This may be an area where doctors would have to consider the interests of other parties in allowing the patient access.

## 2:2.3 *Access on behalf of others*

### 2:2.3.1 Children

Since the needs of children and young people are different, access by children to their records is considered separately from that by young people. In law, patients who are capable of understanding what is entailed have a right of access to their own health records. The age of the patient is not relevant to such access. If patients are minors and capable of giving consent, parents[46] can apply to have access to their records only with the minor's consent. As discussed in chapter 3 (section 3:5.1), ideally parents should help young people to make medical decisions and should be aware of information in the minor's record. In some cases, however, minors may wish to keep secret from their parents some of the matters they have raised with their doctor. It is possible that parents may place pressure on children to authorise access to their records. Contraceptive advice, examination for sexually transmitted diseases, assistance in stopping smoking or drug abuse are examples of matters which minors may wish to conceal from parents. Sometimes children seek advice from the doctor on such matters, not because their behaviour puts them at some health risk, but rather because they are worried about other family members or have a mistaken view of what is actually involved. Consultations on such issues may be recorded in the patient's file and doctors may believe that the minor is under pressure to grant disclosure. When parental access is authorised by the minor in such circumstances, the doctor may wish to talk to the patient separately from the parents to ensure that consent is voluntary. In all cases, doctors should encourage minors to share information with their parents.

In cases where a child cannot understand the nature of the application but parental access would be in his or her interests, the law allows such access. Parental access to a minor's medical record should not be allowed where it conflicts with the minor's interest. The Children Act 1989 emphasises the principle of consulting children and young people about any matter which concerns them closely. Any information which the child previously gave in the expectation that it would not be revealed, cannot be disclosed to any other person, although it must be noted that a doctor can exceptionally breach the confidentiality of any patient if the doctor considers that there are sufficiently serious grounds to justify it (see 2:4.2 below on disclosure without consent).

There may be a conflict between the duty of confidentiality the doctor owes to the child and the parents' claim to exercise parental rights. This is of particular relevance in cases of suspected child abuse. Doctors must put the child's interests first but do all they can to avoid compromising the interests of other parties. Current emphasis is on working with parents, whenever possible. This often gives rise to difficulties, some of which are discussed in 2:4.2.3 below and in chapter 3 (section 3:5.1.2). Once a guardian ad litem has been appointed by the court, his or her views and consent can be sought.

Parents' responsibility for children does not cease when married parents separate. In such cases either parent can apply for access to information about the child, subject to the previously stated limitations, unless specific prohibitions have been imposed by the courts. Where parents are not married, the mother alone has parental responsibility in law unless the unmarried father acquires it by a court order or a parental agreement. In chapter 3, the interests of children and young people are discussed further.

### 2:2.3.2 Young people

Young people are not "children" but the transition between the two stages varies from one individual to the next. The legal provisions for access to records reflect this variability, turning as they do upon the individual's understanding of the application. Young people are seen as developing in autonomy as they acquire the attributes of adulthood and accordingly become able to take more control of the information about themselves. Young people should make decisions on their own behalf if they are sufficiently mature to understand the implications.

Young people can authorise access to their records if they understand the concept of access. A problem which arises often is that of the minor who has been prescribed contraception and who then refuses to allow her doctor to grant parental access to her medical record, even though the doctor believes this to be in her best interests. Since the decision to prescribe in such cases turns on the capacity and understanding of the patient, it would follow that a patient capable of making up her mind about contraception should also be able to control access to her health record. More difficult perhaps is the case of a minor whose record shows she requested contraception which the doctor declined to prescribe on grounds of her lack of comprehension of what was involved. Such decisions are subject to the doctor's clinical judgement in each individual case. As a general principle, the BMA considers that doctors' duty of confidentiality is not dependent upon the capacity of the patient. Unless there are very convincing reasons to the contrary, the doctor should keep secret a minor's request for treatment such as contraception even if the doctor believes the minor to be insufficiently mature for the request to be complied with. This is further discussed in 2:4.2.5 below.

### 2:2.3.3 Mentally disordered patients

Mental health legislation allows patients access to reports about them prepared for the courts. In practice, this poses little problem. When patients are incapable of managing their own affairs, the person appointed to do this on the patient's behalf may exercise a right of access to the patient's notes under the Access to Health Records Act 1990. Very generalised statements and categorising may not be helpful since individual ability varies and patients may display altered ability at different times. Information given by patients at a time when they were competent and believed it would be kept confidential, cannot be disclosed subsequently to other people. The BMA's interim guidelines on consent to treatment on behalf of mentally incapacitated adults[47] draw attention to the rights of the mentally incapacitated to confidentiality, as well as recommending their treatment be discussed with those who have their interests at heart.

### 2:2.3.4 Deceased patients

Patients' rights to confidentiality extend beyond their death. Information about deceased patients cannot be disclosed without proper justification. The law, however, now gives anyone with a claim, such as an insurance claim, arising out of a patient's death, a limited right of access to medical information about the deceased person in order to settle the claim. This undercuts a long held BMA policy on "duration certificates".

"Duration" or "interval" certificates are requests for medical information about a deceased patient. Such requests usually come from life assurance companies, who having failed to seek medical information with the individual's consent at the time a life policy was issued, seek such information after the person's death. Requests for duration certificates commonly arise when a patient dies soon after taking out a policy. Companies may suspect that the patient withheld relevant medical information when applying for insurance cover and they often approach the deceased patient's doctor for confirmation of the facts.

Traditionally, BMA policy was that doctors should not issue duration certificates, since to do so would breach the duty of confidentiality owed to the deceased patient. The consent of relatives was not seen as ethical justification. BMA policy had to be reviewed when the Access to Health Records Act 1990 came into force in November 1991 since the Act gives legal right of access to people who have a claim related to the patient's death. The BMA considered the provisions of the Act and modified its policy to concur with the law but reiterated a general commitment to patient confidentiality after the patient's death. Present BMA ethical advice is that medical information which is not covered by the Access to Health Records Act 1990 and which was recorded prior to the implementation of the insurance contract, may be released to an insurance company if the patient had agreed to its disclosure at the time of the original contract and if the information is not of such a sensitive nature that, in the doctor's opinion, the patient would have wished it to remain confidential.

In law, doctors must still refuse to disclose information where they are of the opinion that the patient provided it, or underwent the relevant medical procedures, in the expectation that the information would not be disclosed. Clearly it may be difficult for a doctor, after the patient's death, to determine whether the patient would have permitted the release of certain pieces of information and to whom. It follows that, wherever possible, doctors should advise a patient on such matters in advance and seek his or her views about eventual disclosure if it is obvious that there could be some sensitivity about the matter. Eventually, as awareness of the Act becomes widespread, patients are likely to give clear instructions in advance.

### 2:2.4 *Access to information about donors*

The confidentiality of people who donate sperm or eggs in order to enable other people to have children has been much debated. Under the provisions of the Human Fertilisation and Embryology Act 1990, information must be recorded about gamete donors as well as about recipients of fertility treatment, and about any child born following treatment. The Human Fertilisation and Embryology Authority keeps a register of such information, from which applicants over the age of 18 (or earlier, if marrying, with the consent of parents) can seek specific details. Precisely what details are yet to be determined. It will be possible, however, for people born following fertility treatments to find out, when they reach 18, whether they are genetically related to their proposed spouse. Also, people born with disabilities will be able to identify, on a court order, the donor(s) of their genetic material. There is much debate on whether provisions should be wider to allow applicants more details on a routine basis, possibly including donor identity. Those involved in provision of treatment for infertility fear disclosure of donor identity would significantly reduce the numbers of donors although one preliminary survey indicated strong opposition to identification in only one third of donors, while two thirds were either in favour or reserved their opinion.[48] Counselling agencies are in favour of discarding anonymity and report that lack of information about donors is a cause of much disquiet among couples receiving infertility treatments. If this is the path chosen, donors will need to be counselled about the implications of being traced by future genetic descendants.

### 2:2.5 *Access by employers*

Access by employers to information contained in occupational health records is outlined in chapter 9 (section 9:4.3). Basically, the sharing of information with the employer cannot go ahead without the subject's consent but the implications of findings must be made known to employers in cases where there may be a risk for others. Employees with conditions like epilepsy, for example, may possibly put others at risk. When asked to disclose medical information to an employer without the employee's consent, the doctor must weigh up how genuine is the risk to other employees. A poor working environment may also adversely affect the health of workers and must be made known to employers.

### 2:2.6 *Access for audit or verification*

Within the NHS, access for the purposes of audit or verification of GP payments must be carried out by a medical officer who is allowed to see relevant parts, but not the whole, of the patient's file.

### 2:2.7 *Security of use, storage, transferral and disposal*

#### 2:2.7.1 *Use and storage*

Doctors have obligations relating to the storage and use of health information and are held responsible for any breaches of confidentiality resulting from insecure handling. The Data Protection Registrar has warned, for example, that doctors could face criminal charges as well as private actions by patients if they fail to provide adequate protection for computers and software in surgery premises, which are sometimes targeted by burglars. Doctors are also advised to take only necessary information with them when they leave the surgery to visit patients, because occasionally records have been stolen from doctors' cars. In many cases, the danger of possible loss or theft is outweighed by the improved quality of care which can be provided when the health records are available but all reasonable precautions must be taken to ensure that identifiable information is not left unattended in risky situations.

#### 2:2.7.2 *Fax machines*

Frequently doctors ask about the implications of using technology such as fax machines to communicate patient details. The Association recognises that this is a common and convenient medium but reminds doctors that they are responsible for ensuring that identifiable information does not arrive in the wrong hands. The Eighth Principle of the Data Protection Act 1984 also requires data users to take "appropriate" security measures when handling computer generated information. Obvious measures, such as using the patient's NHS number or another means of identification instead of the name, may be useful. It would also be sensible to enquire whether the receiving machine is in a publicly accessible area, such as a waiting room, or in a private office. The BMA recommends that patient-identifiable information should only be faxed when the receiving machine is known to be secure both during, and out of, working hours.

#### 2:2.7.3 *Transfer of records*

When NHS patients transfer from one doctor to another, arrangements to transfer their records are made through the FHSA. The BMA has received complaints that after such transfers, or when partners dissolve their partnership agreement, patients' former doctors continue to hold patient data or to send unsolicited letters to people who are no longer their patients. The Data Protection Registrar has reminded such doctors that in holding information about previous patients they are contravening the Fourth, Fifth and Sixth Data Protection Principles. These state that data held must be relevant and not excessive for the purpose for which it is held; personal data must be accurate and up to date; personal data held for any purpose cannot be kept longer than is necessary for that purpose.

### 2:2.7.4 Disposal

Within the NHS, manual or computerised records can be returned to the FHSA on the death of the patient, or of the doctor, or if the patient changes doctors. Private GPs (or their heirs) are advised to ensure that private health records are stored securely either until they may be transferred to another doctor or until the expiration of the recommended period of retention of records.[49] It goes without saying, that manually held data which are no longer required should be destroyed efficiently, either by incineration, shredding or the like.

### 2:2.7.5 Occupational health records

Occupational physicians may encounter problems in ensuring records pass to the control of other health professionals when they leave, or when a company is disbanded and the possibility of future employment-related litigation on the part of employees remains. Occupational health records should normally be retained for at least 10 years after the termination of service and records of significant accidents should be preserved for 30 years. The BMA is sometimes approached about disputes of ownership of records where no new doctor has been appointed and records are left in the hands of an employer. The Association advises that arrangements for records should be clearly defined in the occupational doctor's contract of employment. Where no new occupational doctor is appointed, records must be kept locked or given to an independent doctor to hold. Access to locked records, in the absence of any medical control of them, should be restricted to a doctor appointed to look into them for a specific purpose (ie a doctor appointed by a solicitor in case of litigation against the employer, or a doctor appointed by the patient or a doctor acting under the Control of Substances Hazardous to Health (COSHH) Regulations 1988). If the patient claims a right of access under the Access to Medical Reports Act 1988, a doctor must be involved to determine whether access is not detrimental to the patient or any other person. Occupational health records could also be supervised by a suitably qualified nurse who took responsibility for the unit. Where confidentiality cannot be preserved, the records should be destroyed. Occupational health issues are discussed further in chapter 9 (section 9:4.6).

## 2:3 Restricted confidentiality

### 2:3.1 *Armed forces*

Although armed forces and prison doctors are generally subject to the same ethical rules as other doctors, this is not the case in relation to confidentiality. The health of members of the forces (and their families) has a bearing on the wellbeing of the unit. Regulations for each of the forces specify that the medical officer shall submit a daily sick-book and a weekly return of sick to the captain. The duties of medical officers can in theory be enforced as a matter of discipline but in practice the position is understood and accepted in the forces. Aspects of medical treatment in the armed forces are considered further in chapter 9 (section 9:9).

### 2:3.2 *Prisoners*

Prisoners forfeit many rights but are entitled to medical confidentiality unless the doctor considers that a serious risk to other people justifies breaching confidentiality in an individual case. All obvious measures should be taken to ensure the security of medical information. The BMA recommends,[50] for example, that when prisoners are moved the transfer of their medical details from one doctor to another should be in sealed envelopes. Prison doctors have an obligation to give the prison governor enough medical information to allow proper order to be maintained. This often has the effect of according convicted prisoners reduced rights of confidentiality, particularly since the manner in which prisoners have access to treatment is seldom conducive to privacy. Doctors should insist on being able to conduct private consultations with prisoners whenever this is possible. In this context, prison doctors may experience conflicts of interest between their duty to their patients and to their employers in a more acute form than those experienced by occupational physicians, and particularly so in relation to sensitive issues such as HIV infection among prisoners. It is unacceptable and unnecessary, however, to have information such as the HIV status of the prisoner (or about any other infection) publicly displayed outside the cell. Medical treatment of prisoners (and the role of occupational health doctors) is discussed further in chapter 9 (section 9:7).

## 2:4 Disclosure

### 2:4.1 *Circumstances which permit disclosure*

The doctor is responsible to the patient for the confidentiality and security of any information obtained in a medical consultation. There must be no use or disclosure of any confidential information gained in the course of professional work for any purpose other than the clinical care of the patient to whom it relates. The only exceptions to this standard are:

- If the patient consents. Patients can only give valid consent if they know exactly what information is to be disclosed;

- Rare exceptions when it is considered to be in the patient's interest that information should be disclosed, but it is either impossible, or medically undesirable to seek the patient's consent;

- If the law requires (and does not merely permit) the doctor to disclose the information, such as the law requiring notification of certain diseases;

- If the doctor has an overriding duty to society to disclose the information, for instance, when a serious crime, such as murder or assault, has been, or is very likely to be, committed;

- If the doctor agrees that disclosure is necessary to safeguard national security, for example, when a doctor discovers information about terrorist activity;

- If the disclosure is necessary to prevent a serious risk to public health, for example, if a patient suffering from a serious infectious disease refuses to take precautions to prevent others being infected or the condition of one worker indicates that others may be exposed to a serious health hazard in the workplace;[51]

- In certain circumstances, for the purposes of medical research, appropriately approved by a local research ethics committee.

Each of these provisions is discussed below.

### 2:4.1.1 Consent to disclosure

Patients may authorise disclosure of information to third parties when, for example, they are requesting a medical report for employment or insurance. Consent to disclosure is only valid if the patient understands the nature and consequences of the disclosure. In practical terms, it is unworkable and undesirable for doctors to catechise their patients about every such decision. Doctors should, however, make efforts to verify that patients recognise the implications when disclosure of information is foreseeably detrimental to them. Patients may not realise the nature of the information to be made available and may - and frequently do - authorise disclosure without requesting sight of the report. In such cases, they should be encouraged, if possible, to exercise their statutory rights of access to it.

### 2:4.1.2 Disclosure for purposes of litigation

Doctors approached by lawyers seeking the release of patient notes for court proceedings often turn to the BMA for guidance. They are advised:

i) to obtain the patient's written permission for the records to be released, and ii) to ensure that the patient understands the extent of the disclosure. Some patients, for example, presume that only information relevant to the current litigation will be disclosed, whereas common practice is for the patient's full record to be requested. Nor do patients always realise that the rules governing pre-trial disclosure of documents[52] may mean that their personal health information will also be made available to the representatives of the other parties to the litigation.

Disclosure of hospital records will be handled usually by health authority staff nominated to discharge this function in liaison with the consultant(s) concerned with the patient's care. GPs should handle requests for release of records carefully and promptly once patient consent has been verified. If the GP holding the record is the potential subject of litigation, the relevant defence society should be consulted immediately but doctors cannot withhold records simply from fear or embarrassment about such procedures. Since the doctor is responsible for the safekeeping of patient records, which the Department of Health deems to belong to the Secretary of State, it is preferable that certified photocopies rather than original documents be made available.

There is no obligation for doctors to seek the consent of colleagues who have previously contributed to the patient's record before releasing it and it would be impractical to contact all contributors to a large record. It is, however, an accepted courtesy to inform colleagues that the record is to be released, if this can feasibly be done without causing delay. It is clearly more important to let colleagues know about disclosure if they are the subject of litigation and may be unaware of the request. The BMA has general guidelines for doctors receiving requests from solicitors to release notes for litigation purposes and these are available from the BMA's Ethics Division.

### 2:4.2 *Disclosure without specific consent*

#### 2:4.2.1 *When the patient is incapable of receiving information or is unwilling to know details*

Confidential information may be disclosed to people close to patients in order for carers to help patients manage their condition. In most cases such disclosure is dependent upon the patient's consent but his or her condition may itself preclude the patient from understanding what is involved. When the patient cannot consent, because of incapacity, to information being shared with carers, it is most important that respect is paid to the "need to know" principle. The BMA occasionally receives reports of almost haphazard disclosure; many of these are to do with mentally disordered patients resident in hostels. Aspects of patients' health, such as their HIV and Hepatitis B status, have sometimes been widely divulged with little apparent forethought. While doctors must take the necessary steps to protect other residents and carers in such situations, as well as guiding the latter in supporting the patient, it is preferable to give careful thought to the setting up of routine preventive measures against infection for all residents rather than to label some as posing a risk. It is regrettable that in some cases insufficient resources have been channelled into training staff in safe practices and routine precautions. Obviously, doctors have to take decisions to share information in some circumstances but they should always have clear grounds for disclosure and a good idea of what they expect the recipient to do with the information revealed.

There may be special circumstances; for instance, when competent patients make it clear that they are not ready to know the full prognosis. The BMA believes candour to be the best approach but considers it misguided to force information on the sick person in the interests of ethical rectitude. In such cases, it may be appropriate to share information with those people close to the patient rather than with the patient. This is discussed further in chapter 5 (section 5:4.1).

### 2:4.2.2 Social security "special rules" for the dying

It is with such cases in mind that the Government instituted the "special rules" procedure. This procedure comes into play when a social security benefit which requires a medical report is sought and the patient in question is terminally ill and thought to have less than six months of life left. Information is passed from the patient's GP to the doctor who is assessing the patient's financial need, without the patient necessarily being aware of the prognosis. When the patient is not the initiator, carers are inevitably involved in such measures. In some cases, the doctor dealing with the claim may need to seek further information from the GP but should not approach the patient or question the family. The BMA has registered strong protests when such an unauthorised approach has been made to a terminally ill patient, contrary to the advice of the general practitioner. Clearly such errors can be profoundly distressing to those involved.

Just as these procedures allow doctors to ensure that state benefits are paid immediately, without the patient necessarily being aware of the full prognosis, so in other similar circumstances doctors may feel justified in breaching confidentiality in the patient's interests.

### 2:4.2.3 Abuse of children and the elderly

More difficult are those cases in which the patient does not wish confidential information to be disclosed although it would be in the interests of the patient, and possibly others, if the information were acted upon. Abuse of dependent elderly or young people may fall into such categories. In the United States, laws requiring the reporting of cases of suspected abuse of children and elderly people have not resolved the dilemma for doctors but have rather compounded it, since victims often plead that the matter be kept confidential. In this country, there is growing awareness of the physical maltreatment of the elderly and many bodies have issued local guidelines for combating the problem. As mature adults, the validity of the refusal of elderly people to permit disclosure cannot be impugned, as it may be in the case of very young people. Victims may be concerned that disclosure of what has occurred might lead to further maltreatment. There are no easy solutions but doctors must bear in mind such factors as whether other people in institutions or in the family are also at risk and the possibility of continued or more severe abuse resulting in permanent damage. The mature patient may need time to come to a firm decision about disclosure. Counselling and support in the interim may help the patient decide. In the case of minors, doctors should not make promises to the patient about maintaining confidentiality which they may not be able to keep but in the case of any patient, trust in the doctor is best maintained if disclosure is not made without prior discussion between doctor and patient. Since doctors cannot protect children from further abuse, they should ensure that statutory bodies with such powers are involved (see chapter 3, section 3:5.1.1).

The question of sharing information at child protection case conferences causes misgivings amongst doctors. Frequently doctors are intensely sceptical of the possibility of limiting the wide dissemination of information given, even though it is stated that for "reasons of efficiency and confidentiality the number of people involved in a conference should be limited to those who need to know and to those who have a contribution to make".[53] Given the need to maintain medical confidentiality, doctors will sometimes have to request that certain information be given in a limited forum or in writing to the chairman of the conference. The child's interests must be regarded as paramount and must override the interests of other parties in cases of conflicting interests. The consent of parents or carers should be sought for disclosure of information concerning possible child abuse, although if permission is not obtained from them, disclosure may still be justified in the child's interest.

### 2:4.2.4 *Abuse of incapacitated people*

An issue which has been brought to the forefront of attention by the Law Commission's deliberations in the early 1990s on possible changes to the law relating to mentally incapacitated adults, has been the need for a protective mechanism enabling intervention when vulnerable adults are subjected to neglect or abuse. The Commission clearly identified that "the problem of maintaining the balance between protection from harm and abuse and respect for individual rights is particularly acute in this area".[54] It is also an area in which it is difficult to provide unequivocal advice for doctors because of the immense variation in individual circumstances and the present lacuna in the law regarding any intervention on behalf of an adult without that person's consent.

The General Medical Council has made a general statement about abusive situations, which is applicable to children and to incapacitated people:

"Deciding whether or not to disclose information is particularly difficult in cases where a patient cannot be judged capable of giving or withholding consent to disclosure. One such situation may arise where a doctor believes that a patient may be the victim of physical or sexual abuse. In such circumstances the patient's medical interests are paramount and may require the doctor to disclose information to an appropriate person or authority".[55]

In resolving such issues, the doctor may need assistance in confidence from other health professionals in the community and other agencies such as social work departments.

### 2:4.2.5 *Young people*

The BMA upholds the principles established by the Gillick judgement that young people who are mature can consent to treatments without parental involvement, if necessary. Sometimes the treatments involved may be controversial or indicative of an unsafe lifestyle. A doctor might sometimes consider it to be in the best interests of a young person to disclose such information to parents contrary to the patient's wish. The BMA's general approach, however, is to support the autonomy of the patient unless it seems clear that: i) serious harm may well result from the parents not being involved and, ii) that the patient is unlikely to be mature enough to avert such harm. When the young person is adamant about refusing to allow a parent to be given information, he or she may consent to another responsible relative being involved. Doctors must form a clinical judgement in the individual case after taking appropriate advice and they must be prepared to justify their decision.

### 2:4.3 *Disclosure required by law*

Doctors are required by law to disclose certain information, regardless of patient consent. The principle subjects of such regulations are potential dangers to society from serious diseases, control of illegal substances sought by addicts and the interests of order and justice, which oblige the reporting of abortions, births, deaths and accidents.[56]

As discussed in section 2:4.1.2 above, patients may request doctors to release records for the purposes of litigation. At this stage, the doctor is under no legal duty to comply but will usually do so in the patient's interests. A doctor may also be summoned to court to give evidence or be obliged to release medical records at pre-trial disclosure of documents if litigation has begun.[57] If asked by a court to disclose information in breach of confidentiality, the doctor should explain why such disclosure should not be made. It may, for example, reveal sensitive information about third parties unconnected with the action. The court may take this into consideration and hear evidence in camera, but if the judge or magistrate orders the doctor to answer questions, the doctor must do so or be held in contempt of court. A former Master of the Rolls, Lord Denning, summarised the situation, thus:

> "Take the clergyman, the banker or the medical man. None of these is entitled to refuse to answer when directed to by a judge. Let me not be mistaken. The judge will respect the confidences which each member of these honourable professions receives in the course of it, and will not direct him to answer unless not only is it relevant but also it is a proper and, indeed, necessary question in the course of justice to be put and answered. A judge is the person entrusted, on behalf of the community, to weigh these conflicting interests - to weigh on the one hand the respect due to confidence in the profession and on the other hand, the ultimate interest of the community to justice being done".[58]

### 2:4.4 *A duty to society*

It may be considered an offence to conceal information about a serious crime and doctors have little problem in judging whether to co-operate with police or other authorities when information clearly concerns lives being put at risk. There are some legal arguments, which appear persuasive, that doctors may have a positive duty to disclose in such circumstances. It has been suggested, for example, that a doctor who knew that a patient was driving incompetently but failed to take any action, might be liable in damages for negligence to anyone harmed by the patient on the road.[59] Some legal experts have considered such a scenario improbable although the BMA was informed of a civil action on precisely this issue in 1992. The Association, however, would hesitate ever to tell doctors that they had a "duty" to breach confidentiality in any particular circumstance. Ultimately, this must be a matter for the doctor's clinical decision, since it is the doctor who must defend it if called upon to do so.

It is argued that when some foreseeable harm is in view, people who have a special relationship either with the dangerous person or potential victim(s) have a duty to take some action to avoid it. The doctor-patient relationship is a special one in this sense. The full extent of the doctor's duty, and legal liability if the doctor fails to act, is unclear. In one case,[60] the appeal court ruled that, although there is a public interest in maintaining confidentiality, this is rightly overridden by the need to protect the public against a real risk of danger. Even when the risk of danger is indisputable, the doctor must ensure that information is only given to an appropriate person and not disclosed indiscriminately. It follows that doctors may be justified in disclosing information about patients who are dangerous drivers to the medical officers of the Driver and Vehicle Licensing Authority but not to the Sunday newspapers. Fitness to drive is discussed in more detail in 2:4.4.2 below.

The decision about disclosure is most problematic when the degree of risk is ill-defined or not immediate. Some doctors, for example, refuse to disclose information to the police about past activity by paedophiles if the patient is undergoing active or residential treatment, on the grounds that no individual is actually at risk. Issues concerning disclosure without consent are a matter for clinical judgement and doctors must be prepared to defend whichever decision they make.

### 2:4.4.1 HIV infection

An increasing preoccupation as regards confidentiality concerns HIV infection. Fear associated with its fatal prognosis, together with its connotations of drug addiction and homosexual orientation, despite the fact that sufferers increasingly defy such facile labelling, leads to considerable stigmatisation. In addition, HIV-positive patients are vulnerable to practical disadvantages in numerous ways which leads them to particular anxiety about the confidentiality of their status.

Some see HIV as a flashpoint, where public and private interests clash. It is sometimes said that the individual's interest in privacy may be superseded by a public interest in protecting health workers or patients and others who might be at risk to exposure to body fluids. This is not an argument which the BMA supports. Public debate on the issues occurred in 1988 when health authority employees sought to divulge to the media information about two practising doctors who were being treated for AIDS. The court did not accept that disclosure was in the public interest since it might deter others from seeking treatment. The judge maintained that "in the long run, preservation of confidentiality is the only way of securing public health; otherwise doctors will be discredited as a source of education".[61]

HIV infection also gives rise to dilemmas concerning the sharing of such information between doctors. It is usual to infer that in cases where necessary medical information is exchanged between doctors responsible for the patient's care the original consent covers this transaction. In respect of HIV infection, patients sometimes prohibit the passing on of such information to other doctors. Some doctors have consequently been accused of being over-protective of confidentiality by respecting the patient's instruction. Clearly, such restrictions are likely to hinder the provision of optimum treatment to the patients, who must be made aware of that fact. Nevertheless, the competent patient must retain the right to make such decisions even if they entail therapeutic disadvantages.

It is sometimes predicted that doctors will be confronted by mounting dilemmas about patients who refuse to disclose their HIV status to their sexual partners or, in the case of drug abusers, to people who share needles with the patient. How much this reflects a genuine problem is difficult to ascertain, although at least one case, sensationalised by the media in 1992, of a young man who apparently knowingly risked infecting several women, indicates that the problem is not a theoretical one for doctors. Such cases, however, appear to be exceptional. If the patient understands the implications of behaviour which endangers others but refuses to modify it or to share information with sexual partners, so depriving them of the opportunity to make an informed choice, there is a strong case for the doctor breaching confidentiality after warning the patient of this intention. Doctors must first seek to persuade the patient to either discontinue all behaviour which puts others at risk, to disclose the information voluntarily or to consent to the doctor so doing. The doctor may be considered to have a duty in very exceptional circumstances to disclose information to a particular individual or to a responsible authority, capable of restraining the patient's behaviour. Magistrates have powers under the Public Health (Infectious Diseases) Regulations 1985 to order compulsory treatment and examination of people who have, or are suspected of having AIDS or to be HIV-positive, if such individuals pose a real risk to others. Doctors would need to think very carefully about the genuineness of the risk. These powers appear to have been invoked only once in the case of a patient with AIDS.[62]

As stated previously, the BMA does not seek to lay down "blanket" rulings in such situations and recognises that there may be scope for negotiation with patients which allows them to make the disclosure at their own pace, without exposing others to risk. However, if the patient does not admit to such behaviour the doctor is faced with the difficult problem of assessing the extent of the risk of the patient infecting someone else. It is to be hoped there will be few such cases that cannot be resolved by education and counselling. Doctors must bear in mind that they may have to justify the decisions they take: where there is any doubt, advice should be sought in confidence from professional bodies.

### 2:4.4.2 *Fitness to drive*

Much attention has been paid to assessing medical fitness to drive, particularly in relation to assessment of patients with diabetes, epilepsy, defective eyesight or cardiac conditions. In 1992 some avoidable fatalities were drawn to the BMA's attention by coroners who sought specific ethical advice about doctors' duties in relation to patients who are dangerous drivers. In this and all other cases of dangerous behaviour, the BMA emphasises that the principal onus to take action must fall on the individual who knowingly puts others at risk. Doctors, however, have a duty to inform patients that they should not drive when, in the doctor's opinion, it would be dangerous to do so. If there is disagreement or uncertainty as to the extent of the patient's impairment, doctors should draw to patients' attention the importance of obtaining an objective view from a driving examiner. Individuals with suspected impairment can obtain independent evaluation of their driving skills at specialised driving assessment centres.

Having informed the patient of the danger of driving, doctors must actively encourage the patient to inform the licensing authorities and must indicate that they will do so themselves if the patient continues to drive. This may require further follow-up. Doctors should ask patients to return after considering the matter and inform them of the action they have taken. Patients should be aware that withdrawal of licence is not necessarily automatic, since options exist for a second medical opinion and an independent assessment of driving competence. In exceptional circumstances doctors may consider breaching confidentiality in the public interest, if they deem this appropriate. A separate question concerns the liability of doctors who fail to take action to protect members of the public. As noted above this is not, as yet, clear in law.

Elderly drivers are a group which might be expected to represent an increasing risk to other road-users for health reasons and yet there are no standard procedures for assessing their competence. The DVLC does not request a driver to undergo a medical examination unless it has received a report questioning that driver's ability. It requires drivers over the age of 70 to indicate that they consider themselves fit to drive but there is no requirement that this statement be supported by a medical opinion. Problems of failing vision and cataracts in elderly drivers might be thought to be obvious hazards about which eye specialists would counsel patients. In practice, this does not seem to be the case and the Association considers it necessary to draw this matter to the attention of such eye specialists.

Furthermore, many patients with dementia continue to drive despite significant deterioration in ability. This raises problems about defining the onset of dementia. Whilst the Association considers it would be entirely inappropriate to expect doctors accurately to judge a person's competence to drive in the absence of any clear medical condition, it feels they should take the opportunity to raise the question with patients if it seems appropriate. Clearly, doctors may be placed in an invidious position since they do not have the advantage of seeing the person actually drive, but in some cases the patient's incompetence to drive because of a medical condition would be patently obvious.

Doctors have a duty to raise the issue of ability to drive when they know that a patient suffers from a visual impairment or medical condition which makes driving hazardous. Some assume that such a duty applies only to general practitioners, who can be seen to have a continuing duty of care, rather than to ophthalmic specialists and other consultants, who have only a transitory relationship with the patient. The BMA's opinion is that this duty extends to all doctors and particularly to those treating impaired vision.

### 2:4.5 *Research and teaching*

Many argue that doctors ought to permit and facilitate the collection and use of data for purposes other than the health care of the individual, such as research or teaching. Generally speaking the feeling of the profession is that research should be supported and that access to medical data by a researcher, bound to observe rules of confidentiality, poses little risk to the individual patient. Nevertheless, in general, identifiable information should be disclosed only with the patient's consent. In its advice on confidentiality, the General Medical Council says:

"Medical teaching, research and medical audit necessarily involve the disclosure of information about individuals, often in the form of medical records, for purposes other than their own health care. Where such information is used in a form which does not enable individuals to be identified, no question of breach of confidentiality will usually arise. Where the disclosure would enable one or more individuals to be identified, the patients concerned, or those who may properly give permission on their behalf, must wherever possible be made aware of that possibility and be advised that it is open to them, at any stage, to withhold their consent to disclosure."[63] (See also chapter 8, section 8:9.2).

The BMA supports this emphasis on patient consent but considers that this may be impracticable or insensitive in the case of some kinds of research, such as childhood cancer or mortality rates. It has also supported the provision of limited information by doctors about incidence of cancer to Cancer Registries which operate under strict codes of confidentiality. It believes that decisions about disclosure for research and the requirement for specific patient consent for each protocol should be made by a local research ethics committee or a similarly approved and independent ethics committee. Although obtaining consent is not practicable in all cases, in most it is feasible.

It has been suggested that all patients be asked to indicate whether they are content for their health details to be used for research purposes. The question could be put to new patients registering with a GP or at the beginning of an episode of hospital treatment in the form of a staged consent form, as discussed in 2:1.6.1 above. The proposers of such schemes envisage that once confirmed by the patient, the duration of consent would be indefinite. The BMA, however, has tended to the view that in this, as in all aspects of patient consent, the seeking and obtaining of that consent should not be a once-and-for-all matter but should be subject to review by the patient. Thus, while seeing a value in any schemes which facilitate patient agreement to use of data for research purposes, the Association considers there should be recognised limits to the duration of such consent, after which patients should be asked to reconfirm their consent.

Efforts should also be made to make the general public aware of the uses to which medical information is put and the protection given to information acquired for research purposes. Such information is likely to encourage public support. It should include the following points: i) that the researchers will proceed properly; ii) that they will adequately secure the data against unauthorised access; iii) that no patient will be identifiable from the published results without consent, and, iv) that all the data will be destroyed when they are no longer required for the research.

As stated above, anonymised cases may also be useful for research and teaching purposes: this poses no ethical problem. Issues involving research are discussed further in chapter 8.

In teaching settings it is crucial that students realise the significance of confidentiality and are encouraged in the proper handling of such information. Prospective medical students, sixth-formers and individuals carrying out medically-related projects sometimes request access to GP surgeries or hospitals with a view to observing procedures. The GP or senior clinician who arranges such visits is responsible for ensuring that a strict undertaking is given to observe confidentiality. If breaches occur as a result of such access, the doctor may be held liable.

## 2:5 Need for legislation on confidentiality

During the last ten years the BMA has been deeply concerned with the effects changes in the health service might have on patient confidentiality. The Association's aim has been to protect the professional ethos of respect for patient autonomy and to allow individuals to decide how information about themselves is used. Present arrangements for confidentiality depend upon a patchwork of contractual terms and professional duties. The Association has sought the establishment in law of principles which will govern confidentiality and clarify the exceptional circumstances in which identifiable information might be disclosed to third parties without specific patient consent. It has considered that legislation should draw upon a number of fundamental principles, some of which have been explored in this chapter. These include the following:

a)   Personal health information is held for the purpose of health care. Patients have a right to expect that such information will be kept confidential and used only for the purpose of providing health care (except in some exceptional cases which are listed in (d) below). The patient must understand both the extent and the nature of the information that is to be disclosed.

b) Health professionals have a duty to keep personal health information confidential. Health professionals entrust information to health authorities on the understanding that the right to confidentiality of the person to whom it relates, and the corresponding obligations of the health professional, will be respected. Health authorities have a duty to ensure this is the case.

c) Access to information should be confined to those authorised to have it for the purpose for which it was supplied. Personal health information is disclosed with the patient's consent to those who need to know in order to provide health care to that patient.

In addition, personal health information may be disclosed where it is essential to enable those close to patients to look after them when they are unable to consent. Similarly, when the patient cannot consent, information may be disclosed to a social worker or other person recognised as responsible for some aspect of the patient's wellbeing. These provisions are subject to the qualifications that the information is limited to what is essential and there is no reason to believe that the patient would object; and that the recipient of the information understands and respects its confidentiality.

d) Information may also be disclosed:

- to prevent serious injury or damage to any person;

- to prevent a serious risk to public health;

- as part of the training of health professionals when the patient has agreed to take part in training;

- where disclosure is approved by a research ethics committee and there are safeguards to ensure no distress or damage to the subject of the information;

- where disclosure is essential for the health authority to carry out functions imposed by the Mental Health Act 1983;

- where disclosure is essential for health authority functions such as investigation of a complaint or an untoward incident, disciplinary proceedings, and monitoring the effectiveness of health care services;

- where disclosure is required by statute or a court of law.

The particular health professional with overall responsibility for the relevant aspect of the patient's care should be the person to decide whether or not disclosure can be made in the individual circumstances. In relation to doctors, this would involve hospital consultants supervising disclosure in relation to specialist or hospital care and general practitioners supervising aspects of confidentiality in relation to the care they provide.

e)  Before deciding to disclose personal health information to any person, the health professional must be satisfied that there are appropriate safeguards against the information being used for any purpose than that for which it is disclosed.

f)  Health authorities should establish, with the agreement of all relevant health professionals, detailed procedures which ensure that all disclosures comply with the agreed principles. Health authorities should ensure that its management arrangements are formally adopted at meetings open to the public and that they are regularly reviewed.

The Data Protection Registrar has also seen a need for statutory strengthening of the Data Protection Principles in respect of medical confidentiality. He is "unconvinced that the common law provides as good a constraint on the use and disclosure of personal health information as could be provided were there to be appropriate statutory provisions".[64]

Nevertheless, the Department of Health has not supported the introduction of a statutory code based on a comprehensive document drawn up over a decade and completed in 1988 by an inter-professional working group which included representatives of all health professions and the Department itself.

### 2:5.1 *Handling of information by non-medical employees*

Some of the concerns about the use of patient data arise from the expansion of information systems within the NHS and the handling of data by non-medical administrative staff. Doctors have a professional obligation to preserve the secrecy of information provided by patients but are increasingly confronted by demands for disclosure which conflict with this duty. The data they collect is provided for the purposes of patient health care. Such information is demanded by health administrators for convenient handling of administrative tasks. In the past administrative control of records by non-doctors has resulted in decisions further to disseminate information to other third parties as the holder sees fit. The introduction of designated "safe havens" is intended to reduce the likelihood of this happening by establishing "a set of management procedures and physical security to ensure that only those who are authorised to do so can have access to specified personal health information". This begs the question of who "authorises". A statutory definition of circumstances in which passing information to third parties might be justified, would clarify the duties of all people coming into contact with identifiable health information.

Some opposition has been expressed to the concept of a statutory code on the grounds that it would be inflexible and superfluous, since breaches of confidentiality by doctors are heard by the GMC. Anxiety remains, however, about breaches by non-doctors. A statutory code would leave all sections of the health service in a much clearer position. Individuals would know which colleagues were covered by the code and could feel confident about sharing information, whereas a voluntary code will necessarily give rise to uncertainty. It can be argued that flexibility is not hindered by an unambiguous code which can be amended in the light of experience.

The BMA believes that individual contracts of employment may be insufficient to safeguard confidentiality since there is nothing to be done about misdemeanours discovered after the employee has left. The plurality of employers within the NHS is likely to hinder disciplinary procedures against administrators who transfer to other posts and the powers of the Department of Health over self-governing trusts may be questioned.

### 2:5.2 *Collection of health information outside the health service*

The position of health information held by non-doctors outside the NHS is also a major concern. Any provision for confidentiality within the NHS does not cover outside organisations. In this context some believe that a non-statutory code would lack credibility and be ignored.

### 2:5.3 *European developments*

Developments in the UK are being overshadowed by the progress in Europe of a draft directive on privacy and the protection of the individual's rights in relation to the processing of personal data. In 1990, the Commission of the European Community proposed a package of measures relating to data protection, among which was a draft directive to harmonise substantially data protection laws within the Community. These proposals include arrangements for data crossing national borders and extensive application of data protection rules to manual records. It also provides additional protection in its requirement that people be given information about the intended use of data when it is collected from them. This may be seen as an extension of the current UK Act which requires that information be obtained fairly. At the time of writing, an approval date for the directive is envisaged as late 1993, with possible UK adoption by late 1995. It seems that legislation covering all the European Community is likely in the next decade.

## 2:6 Summary

1 Individuals should control information about themselves and how it is used. Children, young people and the mentally incapacitated all have the same right to confidentiality as other patients.

2 Patient consent should be sought to the sharing with other health professionals of information necessary for the effective care of the patient. It should only be shared on a "need to know" basis. The sharing of identifiable information for the convenience or interests of health workers or administrators cannot be so justified.

3 All information that doctors acquire as part of their professional practice is subject to the duty of confidentiality. This does not mean that it can never be revealed but that the doctor must be able to show just grounds for its disclosure.

4 Identifiable information disclosed for purposes other than treatment should have patient consent for disclosure. Reports to third parties can only be provided with specific patient consent.

5 There may be exceptional circumstances where it is in the patient's interest for the doctor to disclose data without patient consent. Doctors may also need to breach confidentiality to protect other people but, if possible, should first discuss their intention to do so with the patient. When a patient's medical condition poses a risk to others, doctors must, wherever possible, seek to persuade the patient either to discontinue all behaviour which puts others at risk, to disclose the information or to consent to the doctor so doing.

6 A very cautious approach must be taken in cases where it appears in the patient's interest to breach confidentiality but the patient specifically forbids this. The doctor is advised to seek counsel in confidence from colleagues and professional bodies.

7 If identifiable visual material is recorded for teaching purposes, the consent of the patient is necessary. Except where patients have given specific consent to other arrangements, patient-identifiable photographs should remain part of the patient's confidential medical record, subject to the same safeguards as other data. The patient has the right to withdraw consent to the use of identifiable material at any time.

8 Separate patient consent should be required for inclusion of illustrative material, such as videoed material or photographs of parts of the patient's body, in the patient's record. Further consent is required for the use of patient-identifiable material for teaching purposes and additional consent to its wider dissemination.

9 When a patient registers with a GP, personal information is imparted to the doctor in confidence and by the doctor to the FHSA for the sole purpose of administering the GP's NHS contract.

10   The BMA encourages doctors to give patients wider access than statute prescribes to health information held about them, unless the doctor believes it deleterious to the patient's health to do so, or unless the confidentiality of other people might be compromised.

11   Parents can have access to the record but can only apply with the child's consent, if the child is capable of giving consent. Any information which the child previously gave in the expectation that it would not be revealed, should not be disclosed.

12   The BMA considers that doctors should generally keep confidential a minor's request for treatment such as contraception, even if the doctor believes the minor to be insufficiently mature for the request to be complied with.

13   Issues concerning exceptional disclosure without consent are a matter for clinical judgement and doctors must be prepared to defend the decision they make.

14   The approval of a local research ethics committee must be obtained for the use of medical information in research. Efforts should also be made to make the general public aware of the uses to which medical information is put and the protection given to the information so acquired.

15   The confidentiality of personal health information should be subject to agreed guidelines which are clear to all and binding on all those who handle such information. The guidelines should be agreed and reviewed in public with the involvement of all relevant health professionals and patient representatives.

# 3 Children and Young People

*This chapter discusses the rights and vulnerabilities of children and young people. It brings together themes of respect for the individual, maintaining trust and competence to make valid decisions, all of which are discussed at greater length in other parts of the book, particularly chapters 1 and 2. It also echoes discussion of conflicting rights and duties touched upon in chapters 4, 8 and 13 and mentions legal as well as ethical views about consent and refusal of treatment. It looks at the criteria for "best interests" judgements. Some of the advice in this section will also be relevant to treatment of other vulnerable groups such as people with learning difficulties, whose rights may be unclear or overlooked. Also, the role of the doctor is considered in regard to the whole family.*

## 3:1 Introduction

During childhood and adolescence most people attain the maturity which eventually allows them to take responsibility for their own lives. In this phase of development, young people sometimes seek to exercise their growing autonomy in a way which conflicts with other people's views of their best interests. Doctors, parents and others who care for young people are torn between respecting the values of developing individuals and protecting those same individuals from the possibly adverse effects of their inexperience. This raises questions of who is best able to judge what is in an individual's interests. In other sections of this book, while recognising that autonomy has some limits, we have strongly supported the view that the valid judgement is that made by any competent patient about his or her own situation. From an ethical viewpoint, therefore, a decision by a competent young person which is based on an informed appreciation of the facts demands respect. Both law and ethics stress that the views of children and young people must be heard. In some cases, however, their views alone will not determine what eventually happens. In this chapter we briefly examine some of the ethical arguments which arise in relation to the treatment of children and young people. Reference is also made to legal opinions since doctors may find awareness of both legal and ethical standards helpful.

We have not attempted to define a "child" or "young person" but have tended to use the term "children" for people who are probably not mature enough to make important decisions for themselves, whereas "young people" may be.

### 3:1.1 *Guiding principles*

Basic principles have been established regarding the manner in which treatment of children and young people should be approached. These reflect standards of good practice, which find an echo in statute and international declarations.

a)  Children and young people should be kept as fully informed as possible about their care and treatment.

b)  The views and wishes of children and young people should always be sought and taken into account. The individual's overall welfare should be the paramount consideration and listening to minors' views is conducive to promoting their welfare in the widest sense.

c)  There should be a presumption that young people have a right to make their own treatment decisions when they have sufficient "understanding and intelligence".

d)  Although minors should be treated in such a way as to promote their personal responsibility consistent with their needs, they should also be encouraged to take decisions in collaboration with other family members, especially parents, if this is feasible.

### 3:1.1.1 *The reasoning behind the principles*

Various strands of thought have contributed to the changing perception of minors' rights in the last 25 years. The main trends have been classified[65] as libertarian, protectionist and parentalist. Libertarians have set the pace in recent times, arguing that children and young people should be able to exercise rights of autonomy as fully as they are individually able to. Protectionists, as the name implies, support intervention to defend the child's interests on the grounds that children are inexperienced and vulnerable. Parentalists would like to see decisions made on behalf of the child by the adult person who is most closely involved with the child. This need not be a family member but has been described as a "psychological parent", someone who would exercise decision-making powers until the young person attained legal maturity. Each of these attitudes, however, appears flawed if it is the only option. Libertarians may be criticised as too absolutist, the parentalists as over-protective, and the role of the protectionists is ill defined. The BMA sees value in an approach which combines elements of all three.

70

### 3:1.1.2 Combining respect for autonomy with support for minors

In such a combined approach, children and young people are encouraged to make all those decisions which they feel comfortable and able to make. This is the message of the Children Act 1989,[66] which states that children's views should be heard in all decisions which affect them. Children sometimes refuse medical treatment because their anxieties are focused on the short-term effects, such as fear of injections, in which case they are not expressing a considered choice in favour of non-treatment. A child's refusal of treatment which is based on awareness, is consistent over time and compatible with the child's view of his or her best interests beyond the short-term: such a refusal is a valid expression of choice. Adults responsible for providing care retain a duty to intervene if the child appears to be exploited and/or abused, or if decision-making seems seriously awry by the usual standards of what a reasonably prudent person in the patient's position would choose. In cases of decision-making for immature children, there must be a reasonable presumption that the parents have the child's best interests most at heart. Such a presumption cannot be taken for granted, however, and where there seems grounds for doubt it should be contested.

In many cases at present, such a combination of the roles we have described reflects the reality of decision-making. Medical decisions are made in partnership between the patient, the family and the health team, with the parental role gradually fading as the child develops in maturity.

### 3:1.1.3 The independent arbiter

In exceptional cases conflict arises, particularly where the patient lacks family support, but it may also be that a conflict of opinion arises between parents and doctors with the child caught in the middle. Such cases are sometimes resolved on an individual basis by the courts but in some circumstances, reference to the courts seems an extreme measure. Some people would prefer to see the intervention of an independent arbiter, who would represent the child's interests and ensure that these are given precedence. The Children Act 1989 requires that the opinions of minors be heard. Young people can exercise this right by instructing their legal representatives to speak for them on matters such as where they live and with whom. Younger children, however, are unlikely to be able to take the initiative.

The Children Act also makes provision for a guardian ad litem to be appointed in public law cases to advise the court on the child's welfare and to instruct a solicitor to represent the child. In private law cases, the court welfare officer may be asked to advise the court. Various other suggestions which have been discussed but not implemented, include the establishment of a children's ombudsman or advocate. This suggestion has been criticised in that it would perhaps represent only a procedural right rather than a substantive right as far as the minor is concerned. The BMA tends to agree that while another formal mechanism may be unnecessary, the concept of an independent arbiter need not necessarily be formal, or confined to legal issues. In the case of disputes about medical treatment, for example, another doctor or health professional unconnected with the care team might be helpful in giving fresh consideration to the views of all parties. In some cases, this might be a useful way of achieving a negotiated settlement between the young person, parents and the care team without involving the courts.

### 3:1.2 *Background*

Over recent decades, society has paid increasing attention to the rights of groups of individuals who have been previously rather ignored. For example, societal attitudes towards the civil liberties of the mentally disordered and the elderly have changed, with a consequent emphasis on the rights of individuals to self-determination and to receive assistance or services to maximise their liberty. The rights of children and young people have also been the focus of reappraisal. In 1989, the UN General Assembly adopted the Convention on the Rights of the Child, which was ratified by the UK in 1992. This set internationally accepted minimum standards on issues such as freedom from discrimination on grounds of disability (article 2), privacy (article 16) and the child's right to have his or her views accorded due weight in relation to the child's maturity (article 12).

### 3:1.2.1 *Consent to treatment*

In Britain, the legal ability of 16-year-olds to give valid consent to surgical, medical and dental treatment has been recognised for over twenty years. Thus, the medical treatment, including voluntary treatment in a mental hospital,[67] of mentally competent 16-year-olds does not require reference to the patient's parents. Even prior to the Family Law Reform Act 1969,[68] the general assumption was that consent by any minor who was sufficiently mature to understand the implications of treatment, would be valid.[69] Many saw the 1969 Act, therefore, as freeing doctors from any doubt about the legal validity of consent in the over-16s and preserving the status quo for under-16s, for whom doctors would continue to make an assessment of maturity. This assumption was challenged in the early 1980s, by the Gillick[70] case (see 3:3.1.1 below) which eventually confirmed the legal position as being that minors, who are able fully to understand what is proposed and have "sufficient discretion to be able to make a wise choice in their best interests" are competent to consent to medical treatment regardless of age. The BMA has welcomed the recognition of young people's autonomy, seeing it as productive of better relationships between doctors and young patients. Trust in the doctor-patient relationship is a matter upon which the Association lays great emphasis and such trust should be established as early as possible.

In England and Wales, the Children Act 1989 radically reformed the law relating to children and young people. It confirmed the rights of minors to refuse physical or psychiatric examination or assessment. The Act emphasised the participation of children and young people at every level of decision-making and encouraged doctors to develop techniques for consulting them about their views. Similar reviews of the law in Scotland and Northern Ireland followed. In the review of the law in Scotland, the Scottish Law Commission agreed that a rigid adherence to age limits for decision-making was undesirable but interestingly suggested that there should be a presumption of maturity at the age of 12. All recognise, however, the risks of specifying certain ages as an appropriate marker of autonomy, since individuals vary and the impression is given that the views of young people under that age can be disregarded.

### 3:1.3 *Who is the patient?*

This chapter considers the examination and treatment of people under the age of 18 - the point at which English and Welsh law defines the beginning of full adult status. In Scotland, young people attain legal capacity at 16. Either age represents an arbitrary definition of adulthood. Many people under the age of 18 live independently. Some are married and are parents. As mentioned above (see 3:1.2.1), valid decision-making, particularly on questions of medical treatment, has been based in recent years on individual maturity rather than age. The capacity to understand choices and their consequences is what determines individuals' legal and moral right to decide for themselves about medical treatment.

Minors are not a homogeneous group but people with varying needs and capacities. Like any other patients, all children and young people are individuals but this fact can be overlooked, since others often make decisions for them. Ideally, decision-making involves the family and parents can give consent on behalf of children who are too immature to decide for themselves. This situation, however, sometimes leads to ambiguity about who is the real patient. In providing treatment doctors must focus on the patient. Parents might choose options for their children which help alleviate parental anxiety but which are not necessarily in the children's best interests. Examples are discussed below, in the section on best interests (see 3:2.3).

## 3:2 Autonomy and competence

### 3:2.1 *Defining autonomy*

What we understand by the principle of autonomy is also discussed in chapter 13 (section 13:2.2). It may be summarised as the capacity to think and decide independently (competence), the capacity to act on the basis of that decision, and the ability to communicate in some way with other people. Minors as a group have often been regarded as lacking competence and therefore as having no right of autonomy. The libertarian J S Mill,[71] for example, who saw a moral obligation to respect individual autonomy except where it compromised the rights of others, set out three categories of people unable to exercise such self-determination - children, lunatics and barbarians. This reflects the "status" or "category" approach, which judges people's capacity according to factors such as their age or diagnosis, but without enquiry as to how membership of that category affects the individual's competence. Few nowadays would see this as the correct approach.

In the BMA's view, respect for autonomy must be commensurate with the ability of the individual to decide. This is discussed further in chapter 1 (section 1:3.3), where we stress that all individuals should be encouraged to exercise to the full, the decision-making capacity that they possess. Whether any person, adult or minor, has or lacks the capacity to make autonomous decisions must be a question of clinical judgement in each case.

### 3:2.2 *Assessing competence/capacity*

Capacity is a legal concept but invariably medical or psychiatric tests are involved in its assessment. The English Law Commission[72] has examined the various tests of capacity and agreed that there is no magical definition, no right method, but that the "function" approach has the greatest support. This approach relates the individual ability of the patient to the particular decision to be made and the subjective processes followed by the patient in making it. It takes into account the fluctuating nature of capacity and allows most people to make some valid decisions even if they are unable, perhaps to make others. Using this approach, apart from people who are unconscious, absolute incapacity is rare. The BMA supports this approach where the young person's competence to decide is judged in terms of the actual matter to be decided. (See also 3:3.1 below on prerequisites for valid consent).

Some have found it helpful to draw an analogy between children's sharing of decision-making with their parents and their right to a place at the adult table. Young children are accorded a place at the table but are closely supervised and have decisions made for them. As children develop, they have their own place at the table, shared with others, such as their parents or guardians, who take precedence in certain situations. As children mature into competent young people, their views assume increasingly greater importance with the others at the table. On reaching adulthood, they move to a table of their own and from then on, no one can make decisions on their behalf.

Such development is a continuous but uneven process. Research[73] in the 1970s and 80s has indicated that children's cognitive development is not inexorably fixed. The competence of children and young people is increasingly coming to be seen in individual terms, but as being influenced by the child's own experience as well as society's expectations. Recent studies[74] appear to show also that when entrusted with responsibilities, children and young people often respond well but when perceived by others as immature, respond accordingly. Such studies have contributed to the increasing empowerment of children and young people.

Health professionals who work with seriously ill children often comment that those who have undergone suffering and discomfort develop wisdom at an earlier stage than other children. In this sense, wisdom is not simply the acquisition of knowledge but involves an ability to understand the implications of present decisions in the light of past experiences. Children who have already undergone treatment have greater imaginative perception of what is being proposed when treatment options are put forward. Where preventive treatment is being offered, the child has less clearly defined perceptions of the consequences of non-treatment.

Children should not simply be considered incompetent to decide if they are unwilling to agree. In practical terms, although small children might not be given major decisions such as whether to undergo surgery, they should be given a voice on all the lesser points, such as whether parents accompany them to the anaesthetic room. In this way, many of the child's decisions can be respected and it can be feasible to offer even young children alternatives.

### 3:2.3 *"Best interests"*

In accordance with views expressed in the Gillick judgement (see 3:3.1.1 below), the decisions of children and young people should be consistent with their best interests in order to be valid. The minor's best interests will be seen as favouring medical treatment if the benefits of treatment outweigh the burdens of it. Assessment of the child's quality of life during and after the treatment, separation from the family, the risks and side-effects of the procedures involved and the degree of improvement anticipated may modify the presumption that treatment is the best choice. In some situations, the patient's suffering cannot justify the expected benefits of specific treatment and a judgement based on the child's best interests will favour non-treatment. This was the conclusion of the courts and the medical profession in the case of Baby J, discussed below (see 3:3.6.3).

If, however, other people consider children have chosen inappropriately according to the best interests standard, they may be deemed incompetent. Others will decide for them according to the adult's view of the child's best interests. In the absence of very clearly defined criteria for what constitutes an individual's best interests, vulnerable people may be at the mercy of carers as to how their interests are weighed. In brief, adult views of best interests will usually prevail. This entails obvious risks. One danger is that adults can make bad choices, based on their own priorities rather than on the interests of the child, and this is discussed below in 3:2.3.1. A further risk is that of confrontation, with young people and health professionals taking polarised positions or even going to court. The BMA view is not that minors who refuse treatment should be permitted to die or damage their health but rather that there is often scope for negotiation and compromise, which may be lost in the adversarial legal system. The opinion of an independent outsider (see 3:1.1.3 above) could be helpful in throwing light on where the minor's overall best interests lie.

### 3:2.3.1 Whose interests?

The extent to which society will intervene when parents make what appear to be bad choices for their children is unclear. It is notable, for example, that health authorities are generally prepared to act contrary to parental choice if parents seek to deprive the young person of some treatment - Jehovah's Witnesses and Christian Scientists are the paradigm - but not necessarily to prevent parents submitting their children to painful treatments, whose benefit for the child is dubious. Participation in research, tissue donation, sterilisation and some forms of cosmetic surgery (for example on Down's syndrome children) are procedures which might reflect the priorities of other people rather than the patient. In the BMA's view, irreversible treatments of questionable necessity carried out on people who cannot give valid consent, must be subject to review by the courts. These issues are discussed further in 3:3.5. (Tissue donation and research involving minors are discussed in 3:6 and 3:7 below).

It is also suggested that for desperate parents to expose fatally ill children to all manner of painful, unproven or essentially futile treatments breaches the child's right to be free from intrusion. Assessment of the child's best interests in such cases is complicated and reliant upon many factors, including possibly the child's wish to please and show confidence in the parents. Thus it is seen as being an area where parental views often prevail even at the cost of additional suffering to the patient. The bias appears to favour any treatment over non-treatment partly because of the psychological comfort parents derive from knowing that they have tried everything. But this is to put the interests of the carer before those of the patient. As is discussed in chapter 5 (section 5:3.4.1) the doctor's first duty is to the patient and in such cases the main task may involve helping the family face reality. Family pressure to provide aggressive intervention of dubious clinical value should be resisted.

### 3:2.4 *Preventing harm*

The best clinical outcome may not be synonymous with an individual's best overall interests since these also depend upon factors such as congruence with personal values and respect for autonomy. The law, however, makes clear that it is not prepared to countenance non-treatment decisions by young people which would lead them to suffer harm. Parents or courts will overrule the views of minors in such cases. Ethically, too, doctors feel a positive duty to benefit young patients and avoid harm.

This raises the potential conflict between the principles of respect for autonomy and avoiding harm which runs through many areas of our discussion and is mentioned further in chapter 13. It also means that we must question what is "harm" and whether there is a duty to avoid harm, even if by so doing we wrong the patient in some other sense. Harm is often seen as being an actual injury or impairment, whereas patients are wronged if their own values are denied, regardless of whether they are physically or psychologically damaged by that denial. Arguably, by imposing treatment contrary to the will of a competent young person, we prevent harm but nevertheless wrong the individual. The degree to which this is acceptable is dependent upon the scale of the potential harm in comparison with that of the wrong.

Most people would agree, for example, that it would be ethically justifiable to provide treatment contrary to the minor's wishes if this has a very good chance of saving the individual's life or preventing serious deterioration in health and does not involve a degree of suffering which would generally be considered unacceptable in relation to the net benefit. Prevention of suicide and treatment for drug addiction, depression or anorexia nervosa exemplify circumstances where denying the wishes of an apparently competent minor do not usually raise profound ethical dilemmas. Also in these cases, patients may appear competent but the nature of the underlying condition raises questions about the validity of refusal. Chemotherapy for leukaemia is an example of a treatment which carries particularly unpleasant side-effects. Children who have previously undergone the treatment and therefore understand what is involved may be reluctant to accept further treatment. Nevertheless, the chances of successfully treating the condition in children are generally such that some pressure on the child to agree would be justifiable, with the parents' consent, and the child's opinion may be overruled if the anticipated benefits in the individual case are good.

On the other hand, imposition of treatments which either are likely to bring only minimal improvement or which involve distressing side-effects and have only a dubious chance of success cannot be easily justified if refused by a minor who understands the implications. The treatment proposed may not involve a question of life and death but gradations of foreseeable improvement. Children with chronic illnesses who have undergone a lot of medical and surgical interventions may be able to weigh for themselves whether the anticipated improvement is worth another period in hospital and it may be appropriate to defer to their opinions.

## 3:3 Consent to examination and treatment

### 3:3.1 *Prerequisites for valid consent*

In order for the consent of any person to be valid it must be based on competence, information and voluntariness. In our view, this can be broken down into several fundamental points:

a)   the ability to understand that there is a choice and that choices have consequences;

b)   a willingness to make a choice (including the choice that someone else choose the treatment);

c)   an understanding of the nature and purpose of the proposed procedure;

d)   an understanding of the proposed procedure's risks and side effects;

e)   an understanding of the alternatives to the proposed procedure and the risks attached to them, and the consequences of no treatment;

f)   freedom from pressure.


*3:3.1.1 Gillick and the legal position on minors' consent*

The general legal position has been briefly mentioned in 3:1.2.1. This was challenged in 1982, when Mrs Gillick went to court seeking a declaration that the advice issued by the DHSS, which said that under-16s could be treated without parental consent, was wrong and did not reflect the true legal position. After recourse to the Court of Appeal (which ruled in favour of Mrs Gillick) and House of Lords (which ruled against her), the final judgement confirmed that people under 16, who understand what is at stake, can legally consent to therapeutic treatment without reference to their parents. This continues to be the legal position. If the minor has enough maturity to understand the implications of what is being proposed and the treatment is in his or her interests, the treating doctor is not at risk of civil action or criminal prosecution. If the proposed treatment is not in the interests of the person under-16 because, for example, it involves donation of tissue to another patient or participation in non-therapeutic research, parents should be involved and even their consent may not be sufficient, either legally or ethically, if the procedure involves risk or suffering (see 3:3.5, and 3:6 and 3:7 below).

### 3:3.1.2 Consent to contraception and abortion

The focus of Mrs Gillick's case was the provision of contraceptive advice or treatment. She wanted the health authority to instruct doctors not to give contraceptive or abortion advice or treatment to any of her daughters without parental consent. The Lords were divided on the issue, although the majority (three to two) took the view mentioned above, that a mature minor could decide for herself. The conflicting legal views stated at the various levels of the appeal may be thought to reflect a general disquiet about the issues involved. Medical evidence shows that early sexual intercourse increases the risks of sexually transmitted disease and cervical cancer. There may also be a danger of psychological or emotional damage. Many people, however, believe that some under-16-year-olds will have sexual intercourse regardless of the doctor's opinion and that they are better protected if they have at least been advised, in confidence, of the risks and if they have access to measures which minimise those risks. The BMA has tended towards the stance that establishing a trusting relationship between the patient and doctor at this stage will do more to promote health than if doctors refuse to see young patients without parental consent.

All agree, however, that a request for contraception by a girl under 16 who refuses to allow her parents to be informed poses problems for doctors. In considering such cases, there are a number of issues which doctors should consider:[75]

i) the doctor should assess whether the patient understands his or her advice;

ii) the doctor should discuss and encourage parental involvement and explore the reasons if the patient is unwilling to inform her parents;

iii) the doctor should take into account whether the patient is likely to have sexual intercourse without contraceptive treatment;

iv) the doctor should assess whether the patient's physical or mental health or both are likely to suffer if she does not receive contraceptive advice or treatment;

v) the doctor must consider whether the patient's best interests require him or her to provide contraceptive advice or treatment or both without parental consent.

Some object that this is a counsel of perfection, impossible for a busy doctor to carry out. In general practice and family planning clinics, however, experienced nurses are often able to provide appropriate counselling and to discuss the medical and emotional implications with the patient. The BMA and a number of other bodies (RCGP, FPA and Brook Advisory Centres) have been alarmed by the rising pregnancy rate in the 13–15 age group[76] and evidence that many young people are reluctant to approach their own GP for contraceptive services. These agencies issued a joint statement on teenage contraception in 1993 and this is available from the BMA's Ethics Division.

Few patients are aware that they have the option of registering with another GP for contraceptive services only[77] either because the patient is unwilling to consult her own GP or because that GP does not provide contraceptive treatment to a competent minor in such circumstances. This may provide a valuable opportunity to reassure the patient about confidentiality issues in general. It must, however, be explained to the patient that it is in her medical interests for her GP to be informed if contraception has been prescribed and of any medical condition discovered, which requires investigation or treatment. This is particularly important if the patient is at the same time under the active clinical care of her own GP or that of another doctor. Providing that young people trust that their confidentiality will be respected by their GP, they are unlikely to refuse a request that information be passed to their usual doctor.

### 3:3.2 *Can an unwise choice be valid?*

In contrast with adults' decisions, discussion in the Gillick case led to other criteria for decision-making by children in that the case appeared to specify they must be capable of choosing wisely as well as in their own best interests. Competent adults are not obliged to choose wisely and both the law and ethical principles confirm that adult choices may be "rational, irrational or for no reason"[78] and still remain valid.

This is clearly a dilemma of some magnitude, since if we define valid choice by minors as that which is wise and in the best interests of the patient, consent will effectively only be valid when it concurs with the views of the proposer - the doctor, who is also the person entrusted to assess the patient's competence. This is essentially the message of some recent legal cases in which the courts have said that children and young people have a right to consent to what is proposed but not to refuse it if this would put their health in jeopardy. Such advice appears irreconcilable with the basic tenets of autonomy which we have sought to emphasise and leads us to examine what are the requirements for valid refusal of treatment by a minor.

### 3:3.3 *Requirements for valid refusal*

One might expect the requirements for refusal of treatment to be identical to those for consent. As we have seen in chapter 1 (section 1:6), this is not the case. Society assumes that treatment is proposed because it will bring benefit to the patient. Ethically and legally, to give valid consent to a therapeutic procedure, the patient need only understand in broad terms what is involved.[79] To refuse (or to undergo non-therapeutic procedures such as tissue donation) the individual must demonstrate understanding "commensurate with the gravity of the decision which he purport(s) to make. The more serious the decision, the greater the capacity required".[80] In recent legal cases, the courts have indicated that refusal of treatment by a competent person under 18 can be overridden in law by parents or the High Court. This is discussed further in 3:3.7 below.

### 3:3.4 *Where children and young people are competent*

Where children are competent to understand the nature and implications of medical treatment, their consent is sufficient. It is desirable for parents to be involved if the procedure under consideration has serious implications and doctors should try and persuade the young person to agree to parental involvement. If the patient refuses, however, that decision must be respected and should not affect the young person's right to receive treatment. As explained above, the validity of a refusal of treatment by competent minors is more open to question than their consent (see 3:3.7).

### 3:3.5 *Consent by parents/guardians*

Children have variable capacity. When children lack the requisite competence, consent by a person with parental responsibillity permits treatment to take place. Both parents have parental rights and duties if they are married to each other. Where mothers are unmarried, they alone have parental responsibility but the natural father may acquire it by formal agreement with the mother or by court order. Others may acquire parental responsibility by court order. Local authorities may acquire it by a care order or emergency protection order.

#### 3:3.5.1 *Cultural practices*

Parents sometimes ask doctors to carry out procedures which are not medically necessary but are traditional cultural practices. The circumcision of male infants and female children (infibulation) are examples. Medical opinion on the possible benefits of male circumcision is divided, although the procedure appears to confer some benefits in later life to the partners of circumcised men by way of protection against sexually transmitted diseases.

Doctors sometimes question whether male circumcision should be available within the NHS or only privately. In practice, some doctors and hospitals are willing to provide it routinely on demand and, in cases where parents are unable to pay, would prefer to do it without charge rather than risk the procedure being carried out in unhygienic conditions. Doctors must ensure that they have obtained appropriate consent, especially where the child's parents do not both follow the same cultural tradition. For example, a case raised with the BMA concerned a GP who circumcised, without any enquiry, a baby unknown to him but whose parents were, in fact, unmarried and estranged. The child's father had taken the baby without the mother's permission, fully aware that the procedure would be completely contrary to her wishes. The mother made a formal complaint about the doctor concerned.

Female circumcision involves suffering and mutilation. It can give rise to very serious health risks in later life. The BMA strongly opposes female circumcision and, in the early 1980s, sought to have the procedure banned in Britain.[81] In 1985, it was made illegal by the Prohibition of Female Circumcision Act. The Association is also opposed to the training of doctors in this cultural practice. The BMA takes the view that participation by doctors in such practices appears to lend respectability to an unacceptable procedure. The Department of Health has funded the production of a video and a guidance booklet on female genital mutilation and advises local authorities to consider exercising their investigative powers under Section 47 of the Children Act 1989 where there is reason to believe that a child is at risk of female circumcision.[82]

### 3:3.6 *Refusal of treatment by parents/guardians*

There are other, more common, cases where the parents' wishes are not determinative even though the child is incompetent. Such cases usually occur when parents refuse treatment which is clearly compatible with the child's best interests. Parental objection to life-saving treatment on religious grounds, for example, can be contested. In such contexts, it is hoped that an independent person might be able to mediate and avoid court proceedings.

Nevertheless, if after discussion parents refuse to authorise a procedure which is in the child's best interests doctors can ethically and legally give treatment to the child. Decisions about how to manage the condition of severely malformed infants sometimes pose dilemmas for both parents and doctors.

#### 3:3.6.1 *Severely malformed infants*

A malformed infant has the same rights as any other infant. It follows that ordinary non-medical care which is necessary for the maintenance of the life of a normal infant should not be withheld from a malformed child. Treatment which involves possible suffering or distress to the child must be weighed against the anticipated benefit (see 3:3.6.3).

Where medical or surgical procedures might be needed to preserve the life of a severely malformed infant every opportunity should be taken for deliberation and discussion as time permits. The closest possible co-operation between the doctor in charge, the parents of the child and any colleague whose opinions are felt to be helpful is essential. The doctor has a particular duty to ensure that parents have as full an understanding as possible of the options and the likely outcome, with or without surgery, or other means of intervention.

The parents of an infant born severely malformed must never be left with the feeling that they are having to exercise their responsibility to make decisions regarding consent to the management of their child without help and understanding. They should be encouraged to seek advice from anyone in whose judgement they have faith. The doctor in charge is responsible for the initiation or the withholding of treatment in the best interests of the child. Doctors must attend primarily to the needs and rights of the child but they must also have concern for the family as a whole. If doubt persists in the minds either of the parents or the doctor in charge as to the best interests of the infant, another independent opinion should be sought.

### 3:3.6.2 Time for decision-making

It is important to emphasise that, if possible, decisions should be taken at a slow pace. Generally a gentle process is better for parents, who may require lengthy discussion on more than one occasion. Parents may change their initial decision upon further reflection and thus need time to get accustomed to the situation. The health team must stress that withdrawing treatment is not withdrawing love and care. Good liaison between all staff is required when non-treatment decisions have been made and ensuring this happens is the responsibility of the doctor in charge, who should put the emphasis on a positive plan of care rather than convey a negative view of non-treatment.

In emergencies there may be no time for consultation with parents or anyone else and the doctor in charge must exercise his or her clinical judgement. Difficulties arise when the benefits of treatment are in doubt and must be weighed against the pain or distress of the procedure. The courts have given some guidance on how the child's interests in such cases can be judged.

### 3:3.6.3 Quality of life

In the case of Baby J,[83] the Court of Appeal ruled that the benefits of treatment must be balanced against its burdens because "to preserve life at all costs, whatever the quality of life, and however distressing to the (child) .. may not be in the interests of the (child)". In deciding to recommend non-treatment, the Appeal Court considered that the baby's existence would be painful and the benefits of the treatment continuing this painful existence would be minimal. The court distinguished between a foreseeably poor quality of life for J and an earlier case,[84] where surgery on a newborn baby with Down's syndrome was the issue. In the earlier case, the parents opposed treatment but the court authorised it, believing that the baby's subsequent quality of life would be such as to justify the treatment. Thus parents do not have a right to refuse treatments for children who have the potential for some quality of life. In tragic cases where there is little prospect of that or in cases where the benefits of treatment fail to outweigh the burdens, parents may want to restrict treatment to loving care and keeping the child as comfortable as possible. In such cases, their views should be respected.

It was made clear in Re J that the court's decision should not be seen as sanctioning widespread non-treatment of handicapped neonates (or older children). The judges emphasised a generally strong presumption in favour of life and the need for substantial proof that the child faced a very poor quality of life before non-treatment could be considered. The criteria for quality-of-life judgements, it was said in Re J, should be what the child would choose "if he were in the position to make a sound judgement".

### 3:3.7 *Intervention by the law*

Where the views of competent young people come into conflict with those of doctors and other people responsible for the minor, the law may intervene as a last resort. In the 1991 case of R,[85] for example, the refusal of anti-psychotic treatment by a 15-year-old ward of court was overruled. R was deemed incompetent but the judge went on effectively to deny the right of minors to refuse treatment which others considered in their best interests and said that, even if she had been competent, R could still have been overruled. At the time of refusing medication, R appeared lucid and rational. The local authority which had previously consented on the girl's behalf to medication being administered to her, withdrew its consent in the face of her refusal. By so doing, the authority was acting in accordance with the principle established in Gillick that young people under 16, with sufficient understanding to comprehend the treatment proposed and sufficient maturity to make up their own minds could themselves legally consent to medical treatment. At the subsequent Appeal Court hearing of R's case, it was confirmed that the court acting in wardship could overrule the decisions of a Gillick competent child as well as those of the child's parents or guardians.

The R case raised some uncertainty because of the interpretation offered by the Master of the Rolls, Lord Donaldson, of the principles established by Gillick. Lord Donaldson differentiated between powers to consent and powers to refuse treatment. He stated that both minors and their parents have the power to consent. A consent given by either is sufficient for treatment but only refusal of treatment by both the parent and the minor would create a veto. This appeared to contradict previous opinion, which assumed the refusal of a competent child would be equally valid as his or her consent and that the relevance of the parents' consent decreased in proportion to the increasing competence of the child. The Children Act 1989 gives a competent child the right to refuse medical or psychiatric examination or other assessment which seems to conflict with the principles stated in Re R.

Following R, a further case was awaited to clarify the importance of Donaldson's remarks but the liberal perception of the rights of young people was further damaged by the subsequent case of W[86] (also known as J), where a 16-year-old anorexic patient was deemed competent but was overruled in her refusal of treatment. In this case, the patient's age might have been thought more persuasive as to the validity of her consent than in Re R, since the Family Law Reform Act 1969, establishes that a 16-year-old may consent as effectively as a person of adult years. (The Act does not, however, address refusal of treatment.) J was considered competent[87] but her refusal of treatment for anorexia nervosa was overruled by the court, building upon the remarks of Lord Donaldson in the case of R.

Since W was acknowledged to have sufficient understanding to make a decision the effect is to diminish the importance of refusal given by any person under 18. Both judgements take the "status" approach, which we have tended to reject (see 3:2.1 above), rather than the "functional" approach to the competence of young people, and use the status argument to justify intervention in the minor's best interests. The cases illustrate the great difficulty society has in dealing with the emerging autonomy of young people. The law is clear that, in the last resort, medical treatment can be imposed upon minors who refuse it. Is this also the most ethical response? Doctors are unlikely to be very happy with such a view and, as mentioned earlier in 3:1.1.3, the BMA would hope that all possibilities of a compromise solution would be explored first, including bringing in independent people to work out measures that the young person might feel able to accept, without losing face or having to argue through the courts. In our view, minors who are clearly competent to agree to treatment must be acknowledged as also having an option to refuse treatment if they understand the implications of so doing. Refusal of treatment in some cases, however, may raise questions of competence.

## 3:4 Consent for other procedures

### 3:4.1 *Photographs*

Doctors may need to seek a minor's consent for procedures other than treatment, such as the taking of photographic records, particularly in relation to documenting child abuse. In the case of young people and children capable of understanding, doctors should explain the reasons why photographs need to be taken. Under the Children Act 1989 a minor may make an informed refusal of examination for forensic purposes. Photographs may be taken for clinical reasons and repeated photographs in different lighting conditions may be required. In this situation the doctor has control of the procedure, which should be at a pace acceptable to the subject. If they are taken for evidential reasons, the police will take them and the doctor will have no control over the process.

If a child or young person refuses examination or photography for treatment purposes, the doctor must make a careful judgement of how critical the need is for such procedures. Usually, they should not be performed contrary to the patient's wishes as this may cause further trauma. In a minority of cases, there may be an urgent imperative such as the assessment of the future safety of the child or siblings and in the face of the patient's informed refusal, the matter should be referred to the local authority who may need to seek a court order urgently. Gaining consent in such contexts may be a slow process and will require the doctor to talk the situation through with the patient and provide reassurance.

Patient-identifiable photographs, taken for diagnostic purposes, must be subject to strict arrangements as to their confidentiality. Doctors should bear in mind also that competent minors can exercise a statutory right of access to their own medical records (see chapter 2, sections 2:2.3.1 and 2:2.3.2) although material which the doctor considers damaging to the patient may be withheld.

### 3:4.2 Video-taped material

Similar rules concerning consent and confidentiality must apply to video-taped material. These are discussed in chapters 1 (section 1:4.1.2) and 2 (section 2:1.6.1) but may be summarised in the following points:

- Where two-way screens are used either to monitor or film interviews, all individuals so monitored should be informed in advance and should know precisely who is observing them.

- Doctors must be sure of the purposes for which videos or photos are taken and decide whether such purposes are valid.[88]

- Identifiable material should be treated with the same confidentiality as other medical records.

- Valid patient consent should be sought. If a child/young person is recorded on film, video or photograph, that person's consent for retention or use of the material must be re-confirmed at a later date when the patient is mature.

- Consent should be specifically sought for each and every purpose to which the illustrative record is put; this includes specific consent for use in teaching.

- Ideally such records should be made by registered medical illustrators, subject to a strict code of practice. Such people are usually aware of the potential difficulties involved and can help minimise the unease of the child or young person.

- If a third party is featured (other than a health professional) the same rules of consent and confidentiality as for that person's other records apply.

- Videoed interviews should not be over-long and must be carefully managed. In efforts to capture film of inter-action, interviews have sometimes been unnecessarily protracted.

- When a medical interpretation of filmed behaviour or clinical examination is to be discussed, such interpretation must be left to doctors.

## 3:5 Confidentiality

The duty of confidentiality owed to a minor is as great as the duty owed to any other person. The General Medical Council states:

"Patients are entitled to expect that the information about themselves or others which a doctor learns during the course of a medical consultation, investigation or treatment, will remain confidential.

An explicit request by a patient that information should not be disclosed to particular people, or indeed to any third party, must be respected save in the most exceptional circumstances, for example where the health, safety or welfare of someone other than the patient would otherwise be at serious risk".

In exceptional circumstances, the doctor may believe that the young person seeking medical advice on sexual matters is being exploited or abused. It is important for the doctor to provide counselling with a view to preparing the patient to agree, when ready, to confidentiality being relaxed. This task assumes greater urgency if the patient, siblings or other minors continue to be in a situation of risk so that in some cases, the doctor will have to tell the patient that confidentiality cannot be preserved. Disclosure should not be made without first discussing it with the patient whose co-operation is sought. To breach confidentiality without informing the patient and in contradiction of patient refusal may irreparably damage the trust between doctor and patient (see 3:5.1.1 below).

### 3:5.1 *Involving parents*

Ideally, treatment decisions involve people close to the patient and for an immature child, the parents, or parents and child together, will decide. In all cases involving competent young people, a doctor should try to persuade the patient to allow parents to be informed of the consultation but should not override the patient's refusal to do so. In the BMA's view, even when the doctor considers the young person is too immature to consent to the treatment requested, confidentiality should still generally be maintained concerning the consultation. The BMA considers that doctors' duty of confidentiality is not dependent upon the capacity of the patient and, unless there are very convincing reasons to the contrary, the doctor should keep secret a minor's request for treatment such as contraception, even if the doctor believes the minor to be insufficiently mature for the request to be complied with.

### 3:5.1.1 Confidentiality and suspected abuse

A child or young person who comes to a doctor with a suspicious injury should be the focus of the doctor's concern - not the family. Some doctors say that they feel a divided loyalty when they have as patients other members of the family, including the alleged abuser. As stated earlier in 3:1.1.2, adults responsible for providing care, including doctors, retain a duty to intervene if a child or young person appears to be exploited or abused. When such cases arise, the child or young person who seeks help must be the priority, although the doctor must also bear in mind the safety of siblings who might also be at risk. Doctors must also be alert to the possibility of abuse of children in institutions.

Children often try and elicit a promise of confidentiality from adults to whom they disclose information about abuse when, in fact, they really want something to be done, rather than their plight to be kept secret. This is a common situation, which teachers, in particular, encounter, since they are often the first recipients of such information. Like teachers, doctors should not promise to keep the information confidential if the child's safety is in any way threatened. Doctors may find it helpful to call upon the skills and expertise of other members of the health team but neither doctors[89] nor other health-workers have any statutory powers to intervene and so are unable to protect a child or young person from continuing abuse. If there are safety protection issues to be considered, the matter should be passed to an agency with statutory powers - social services or the police but, wherever possible, this option should first be discussed with the patient (see 3:5 above).

In most cases, children disclose to adults the facts of their abuse because they want the abuse to stop but doctors alone do not have the power to do this. Doctors should familiarise themselves with relevant guidelines[90] and be aware, for example, of the work of Area Child Protection Committees. The overall welfare of the child or young person must be the paramount consideration but, as stated earlier, the minor's own views are not necessarily the final arbiter in making ethical decisions.

### 3:5.1.2 Child protection case conferences

The question of sharing information at child protection case conferences also raises dilemmas for doctors. The role of the doctor in such fora is seen as pivotal but frequently doctors are intensely sceptical of the possibility of limiting the dissemination of information. Only information which is relevant to the purpose of the case conference and in the best interests of the child should be disclosed. Doctors will occasionally have to request that certain information is given in a limited forum or in writing to the chairman of the conference. Such measures should be used selectively for highly sensitive information and be avoided as regular practice.

The child's interests must be regarded as paramount and, if possible, the child's consent to disclosure obtained. The consent of parents or carers to disclosure should also be sought as appropriate and their consent is particularly important if disclosure relates directly to them such as information about their physical or mental health.

### 3:5.2 *Access and control of medical records*

Access by children and young people to their own medical records is discussed in chapter 2 (sections 2:2.3.1 and 2:2.3.2). In brief, patients who can understand what is entailed have rights of access, regardless of age, and also have a right to veto access by third parties, including parents.

## 3:6 Transplantation and children

Organ donation by live donors[91] raises very difficult questions as to the degree to which parents, or the child, can give valid consent to a procedure which is not in the child's interest and which involves suffering for the child. Some question whether parental consent in such cases might constitute an abuse of parental power[92] and many legal experts maintain that a parent can only give legally valid consent to a procedure which brings some benefit for the child and is, therefore, in the child's interests.[93] Many believe that ethical requirements, too, rule out procedures which are clearly contrary to a minor's interests and this tends to be the BMA view. This is contested by some analysts, who consider it impossible, and perhaps even unethical, to require parents to make the best interests of one child (ie the potential donor child) assume greater importance than the life of another child. Some argue that "the family is thought of as an intimate arrangement with its own goals and purposes ... it is inappropriate to impose upon that arrangement ... abstract liberal principles".[94] Others, however, see it as very dangerous to depart from the best interests principle as a guidance principle in decision-making for children, but recognise that there can be conflicts of individuals' interests within the family which are difficult to resolve.[95] In 1992, the then Master of the Rolls, Lord Donaldson, briefly mentioned the problems regarding consent to organ donation by minors in the course of a case concerning a young person's consent to treatment.[96] He made clear that even if a minor is "Gillick competent", both parental and potential donor's consent would be required and that doctors would also be well advised to seek guidance from the courts as well.

As is discussed in chapter 1 (section 1:7.1.2) the usual argument put forward to justify donation is that it is in the child's emotional interests that the life of a sibling, for example, be saved and that the potential donor is likely to suffer psychologically if a close family member dies. It can also be argued that such donation is in the public interest, since most people would feel appalled if children needing transplantation were allowed to die when the means to save them were at hand. Caution must be exercised, however, since there may be harm in regarding those who have not attained full autonomy as available tissue-providers. In general, people should not be seen as means to an end. Similarly, many doctors would feel unhappy about providing treatment to generate a pregnancy with the express purpose of providing a new potential tissue donor. Others feel justified in doing so in order to help parents save an existing child (see also chapter 4, section 4:5.3).

Many believe that to exclude children completely from donating tissue or organs is too extreme a stance. The BMA, however, considers that it is not appropriate for live, non-autonomous donors to donate non-regenerative tissue or organs. However, there is no such clear legal prohibition in this country and some people argue that, in each individual case, the interests of the potential donor and the recipient must be balanced. An American example of the balancing of interests[97] concerned a minor with Down's syndrome who donated a kidney to his sister. The argument was made that his elderly parents would soon be incapable of caring for the donor, whereas a surviving sister could. The pressures on all the family members in such a case are hard to contemplate. Also despite apparent statistical evidence that it is safe, removal of a kidney is not innocuous and some donors do later become ill themselves or even, in exceptional cases, die.[98]

Bone-marrow donations by children to siblings are common.[99] It must be noted that bone-marrow donation poses relatively little risk or suffering and when another life can be saved with only minimal risk to a child donor, doctors feel there is an ethical imperative to try to save that life. The procedure must be explained to the potential donor and whose co-operation must be sought, unless the donor is a very young child who could not understand.

The subject of tissue donation by live minors is also discussed in chapter 1 (sections 1:7.1.2 and 1:7.1.3).

## 3:7 Research on children

Research which could equally well be carried out on competent adults with their consent, should not be carried out on any individuals whose capacity to understand, or freedom to refuse, is limited.

90

It is sometimes argued that it is unethical to include in any research projects individuals who cannot consent. Others argue that it may be unethical to exclude entire groups of people from research, since this is discriminatory and means there is a failure to seek measures which would improve their condition. In the BMA's view, research on people incapable of consenting is not unethical if it is governed by strict safeguards, including review by local research ethics committees (LRECs). The proposed research must not be contrary to the individual's interest, must pose only minimal risk, must be impossible to carry out using consenting subjects and must be designed to benefit others in the same category as the subject. The BMA's stance recognises that in some situations, knowledge to help children suffering from certain conditions can only be gained by research on children but in order to assess the arguments, it is first necessary to define "research".

### 3:7.1 *Defining research*

Chapter 8 discusses research issues in detail, drawing distinctions between therapeutic research where the aim is to benefit the individual, non-therapeutic research which involves procedures not of direct benefit to that person and innovative treatment which digresses from usual practice. In common with non-therapeutic research, innovative treatments may involve an unknown or increased risk for the patient but often the purpose is to benefit the individual. Any procedure whose primary focus is not the benefit of the person undergoing it must be subject to the strictest safeguards and ethical review: thus the highest and most rigorous standards must be applied to non-therapeutic research.

#### 3:7.1.1 *Therapeutic research*

Therapeutic research may involve research on the treatment of disease or its prevention, by vaccination for example, or research on diagnostic procedures. The aim is to benefit the individual. As with treatment, competent minors can consent to measures which are intended to produce benefit for them and parents or guardians can consent on behalf of immature children. Although the consent of a competent minor to therapeutic research is sufficient from an ethical viewpoint, doctors are advised to note the 1991 statements of the Medical Research Council[100] interpreting the legal position. The MRC advises that:

- When research projects involve young people between 16 and 18 years of age, particularly if there is some doubt as to the degree of understanding shown by the minor, it is good professional practice to seek the young person's permission to explain the research proposals to parents and, if the young person objects, to give these objections considerable weight.

- Where minors are under 16 but have sufficient understanding and intelligence, they can consent to medical treatment and age is of no importance. Researchers, however, should be reticent to proceed without the approval of a parent or guardian and should certainly not do so without the prior agreement of the LREC.

Legal advice issued by the Department of Health specifies that parental consent is required for participation in therapeutic research by a minor under 16.

### 3:7.1.2 Non-therapeutic research

Non-therapeutic research may or may not benefit the individual but its primary intention is to seek information. Both ethically and legally, non-therapeutic procedures involving minors are more difficult to justify than therapeutic research procedures.

Competent minors and non-therapeutic research: From both a legal and ethical viewpoint, the validity of minors' consent will depend on their understanding and intelligence, the information provided and the unpressured voluntariness of their agreement. As with any non-therapeutic procedure, the degree of understanding required must be commensurate with the seriousness and risks of the procedure. There is no clear legal requirement to consult the parents of a competent minor or obtain their consent. Nevertheless, it would be wise to do so unless the LREC rules this out. Competent minors may object to their parents being consulted and in such cases researchers should bear in mind the circumstances of the case, such as whether the minor is living independently away from the parental home and should seek guidance, if necessary from the LREC. Although the minor's age cannot be determinative, commonsense indicates that the younger the child, the more desirable it is to seek parental consent even though it must be noted that the legal validity of parental consent to non-therapeutic procedures is in some doubt. This is discussed below.

Immature minors and non-therapeutic research. Current attitudes reflected in the Children Act 1989 emphasise the responsibilities of parents, doctors and carers to act in the child's interest. Parents have duties rather than rights with regard to the child and are limited in the degree to which they can consent on the child's behalf to procedures which do not promote the child's welfare.

By definition, non-therapeutic research is not intended to favour the interests of the individual subject but it must not be contrary to the subject's interests. Research involving procedures contrary to the child's interests is unethical. There appears to be a broad consensus that participation by immature minors in non-therapeutic research is not necessarily unethical as long as:

92

- the research carries no more than minimal risk;

- it does not entail any suffering for the child;

- parental and LREC agreement is obtained;

- the child does not appear to object.

The law on children's participation in non-therapeutic research is less clear. However, researchers could look to the European Commission Guidelines on Good Clinical Practice for Trials on Medicinal Products, (published in 1990). The intention is that these guidelines will be incorporated into the national law of EC states. The guidelines require that research on subjects incapable of giving personal consent must be intended to promote the welfare and interest of the subject. Such research, the guidelines state, is ethically acceptable if the LREC, the researcher and the subject's legal representative agree that participation is likely to be in the subject's interests. The possibility of participation by immature minors or other people incapable of consenting is excluded by the requirement that research subjects must personally give written consent to being included in any non-therapeutic study.

As with treatments like organ donation, some argue that parents or guardians cannot legally consent to any treatment or procedures which are contrary to the child's interests. This is the opinion expressed by the Department of Health in 1991, which stated:

> "Those acting for the child can only legally give their consent provided that the intervention is for the benefit of the child. If they are responsible for allowing the child to be subjected to any risk (other than one so insignificant as to be negligible) which is not for the benefit of that child, it could be said that they were acting illegally."

### 3:7.2 Ethical responsibilities of researchers

Various bodies have debated the ethics of carrying out research or innovative treatments on minors and have expressed concern about the possibility of innovative therapies being repeated without being submitted as a formal research project, and about failed formal research projects being repeated. It is hoped that efforts such as those of the British Paediatric Association to keep a register of all paediatric research projects, and the requirement for all LRECs to publish annual reports, will reduce the risks of research on minors being duplicated unnecessarily. Researchers should make efforts to ensure that their project does not involve such duplication.

The relationship between the researcher and young subject has been given particular attention by the Institute of Medical Ethics[101] which recommends that:

- researchers recognise that the research enterprise should be a partnership with the child subjects and their parents or guardians rather than an activity undertaken on children;

- in assessing the risks of a research project to an individual child, researchers should take account not only of the risks of any proposed research procedures, but also of the cumulative medical, emotional and social risks to which the child is already exposed or may become exposed, whether or not as a consequence of the research interventions;

- researchers monitor whether the research procedures produce any emotional or behaviourial disturbance in the child and deal promptly with any such disturbance by referral, if appropriate. Moreover that the scientific evaluation of the research should take account of the emotional and behavioural outcomes for the subjects.

The BMA endorses these recommendations and adds one further recommendation of its own:

- that researchers be aware of the pressures which can lead some parents to volunteer their children for research and that, through discussion with parents, they attempt to minimise misconceptions and, if necessary, help them to identify the child's interests. Studies[102] show, for example, that parents who volunteer their children for medical research are likely to be significantly more socially disadvantaged and emotionally vulnerable.

## 3:8 Advice-lines and children and young people

The BMA has received enquiries from doctors associated with volunteers who provide advice by telephone to children and young people. It is not the Association's intention to encourage the growth of such services, which although helpful in some cases, raise complex issues. On the one hand it can be argued that recent scandals involving cases of alleged abuse in children's homes and other residential institutions highlight the need for responsible, independent people willing to listen to young people, since the statutory agencies appear to have failed in some cases. But if independent advice-lines similarly fail to deal adequately with the problems brought to them, they will not escape criticism even though they may have limited resources to solve hard cases.

The BMA is very much aware of the importance of listening to young people and respecting, whenever possible, their decisions about how problems might be handled. It is aware that GPs are involved in filling this role but recognises that teenagers do not necessarily feel confident about approaching their family doctor. The Association believes that informing young people about the confidentiality they can expect from GPs may be helpful.

The principal difficulties of independent people providing a service arise where there are questions of:

- liability for any harm arising as a result of the service being involved, either because erroneous advice was given or because the young person failed to take other necessary action believing, for example, that the advice line would solve the problem;

- confidentiality, including whether parents might ever be informed, in cases where the young person's identity is known.

Duties and liabilities accrue to people who hold themselves out as offering some form of care to others. Legally and ethically, once such a relationship of care is established, questions of liability and responsibility arise when a person who has accepted to give a form of care fails to prevent foreseeable harm befalling the person who is the object of that care. The GMC has expressed anxiety about the provision of telephone advice services to the general public by doctors, because of questions of liability if the wrong advice is given when the adviser has no direct contact with the enquirer. In such circumstances, doctors must ensure that enquirers consult their own doctors about the medical problems in question.

Although teenagers seeking advice are not the doctor's patients, by holding themselves out as people willing to consider teenagers' problems, doctors might be considered to have a relationship of care. If advice is given about how specific cases should be handled, the doctor would have ethical, and probably legal, responsibility for any foreseeable harm or error. Giving generalised advice rather than case-specific advice is less problematic. Liability and the likelihood of harm are reduced by encouraging callers to make contact with the respective professional agency.

Regarding confidentiality, the doctor should encourage the young people who call to confide in their parents, where this is appropriate. Following the Family Law Reform Act 1969, the Gillick judgement and the Children Act 1989, it is assumed that mature young people should be able to decide for themselves on issues which closely involve their welfare. The BMA feels that mature minors have a right to seek advice as they feel appropriate, and in confidence. The doctor should attempt to persuade young people to involve their parents, but confidentiality should generally be preserved if the young person refuses to do so.

In some cases, more harm might result from informing parents - who might deal very harshly with the young person - than from listening to and following the views of a mature minor. In exceptional circumstances, however, the situation may justify a breach of confidentiality, especially if there is a risk of harm to other people (see 3:5 above). The BMA recognises that some legal opinion disagrees with this view and considers that doctors owe a first duty to parents and should keep them informed of hazardous behaviour by the young person. This is not the view espoused by the BMA.

## 3:9 Summary

1　Children and young people should be kept as fully informed as possible about their care and treatment.

2　Definitions of who is a child differ considerably and there are no hard and fast rules. A person's status as baby, child or young person may vary and doctors should consider the context when making judgements.

3　For some treatments an individual may be considered a child and too immature to decide, for others the same individual may be considered to have sufficient capacity. When an individual does not have the capacity to make decisions about treatment, the doctor must do what is in that person's best interests.

4　The views and wishes of children and young people should always be sought and taken into account. The individual's overall welfare should be the paramount consideration and listening to young people's views is conducive to promoting their welfare in the widest sense.

5　There should be a presumption that young people have a right to make their own treatment decisions when they have sufficient "understanding and intelligence".

6　Although minors should be treated in such a way as to promote their personal responsibility, consistent with their needs, they should also be encouraged to take decisions in collaboration with other family members, especially parents, if this is feasible.

7　The informed consent of a minor to medical or psychiatric treatment depends not only on the minor's intelligence and understanding but also upon the quality of information given by the doctor. Patients need to understand the implications of their condition, the nature of the proposed treatment, its risks and side effects and the consequences of a failure to treat. These things should be explained at an age-appropriate level.

# 4 Reproduction and Genetic Technology

*In this chapter, the main focus is on ethical issues arising from the use of treatments to control fertility and from genetic technology. The chapter includes a discussion of contraception, with special emphasis on education about, and access to, contraceptive services by young people and the issues involved in post-coital contraception; abortion, the use of mifepristone and the doctor's rights of conscientious objection; sterilisation, including its use as an appropriate treatment for women with learning disabilities; products which have been used to control the libido of sex offenders. Also considered are infertility services, including the duties owed to various parties and possible problems concerning selective reduction of fetuses; and surrogacy, as a solution to childlessness. Ante-natal care and birth is briefly mentioned. Aspects of embryo research and the uses of genetic information and information obtained from pre-natal screening are considered .*

## 4:1 Introduction

### 4:1.1 *The issues*

The development of technology to exercise more control over the beginning and end of human life has been at the forefront of the scientific advances of the twentieth century. Such technology has often been seen in the past as the domain of clinicians, researchers and scientists but, as was noted in chapters 1 and 6, great importance is now given to the individual's ability to exercise control over his or her own body, including genetic material and other tissue. The issues discussed in this chapter concern not only individuals but, in some cases, their families and society at large. The technological developments affect the most intimate and profound aspects of human existence. They pose ethical, legal, social and psychological questions which have perturbed the whole of society. Many are too complex to be rehearsed adequately in such a brief guide and since our focus is on the practical questions which doctors raise, the philosophical debates which reproductive issues generate, are only briefly touched upon.

Control over one's body and genetic material, abortion, genetic manipulation, reproduction and parenthood are matters about which most people hold strong views. For many, such views are based on moral, religious or cultural convictions. Given the existence of such diversity of opinion, it is clear that some of these questions can never be resolved to the satisfaction of all sections of society but will be the subject of continuing ethical debate. While recognising that whatever is done "is going to be wrong from some point of view. It is not a black and white situation",[103] areas of broad moral concurrence can be sketched out. These areas are also regulated by legislation, including the Abortion Act 1967, the Human Fertilisation and Embryology Act 1990 and the Surrogacy Arrangements Act 1985, all of which are discussed in the BMA publication "Rights and Responsibilities of Doctors", 1992.

### 4:1.1.1 Conflicting claims to rights

Discussion of rights, or claims to rights, entails a variety of complex philosophical concepts, some of which are touched upon here. Reference is sometimes made to natural rights, to which each human being has automatic entitlement, but there is disagreement as to what such rights might entail or whether they indeed exist. It is often argued that a distinction should be made between negative rights, such as the right to be free of interference and positive or substantive rights, such as a right to demand appropriate health care. The fundamental distinction here is between a liberty and a right. Claims to positive rights are often seen as problematic in that they suppose that there is a corresponding obligation on other people to supply what the right-holder claims. A claim of a positive right to procreate, for example, implies that other individuals have a duty to co-operate to achieve the rights holder's aim and, that if required, the state has a duty to provide the necessary reproductive technology for every person who claims it, whereas negative rights simply require others to leave right-holders alone and not prevent them from procreating, for example, by non-consensual sterilisation.

Another way of looking at rights is to see them in a contractual sense, embodying the expectations we have as members of society. In return for paying taxes or health insurance, we have a right to health care and other services. By implicit agreement, the public expects that the state will provide access to a certain package of services and that each person has a right to share what the state makes available. Usually, however, there is no obligation for the state to provide every individual with every service but there is a (legally non-enforceable) expectation that it will provide a certain acceptable minimum (what that might entail is briefly discussed in chapter 12, see in particular section 12:4.2.1).

The so-called "right to life" raises many questions. Society considers it wrong, in most circumstances, to interfere in such a way as to deprive a human being of life. A right to self-defence is one of the few accepted justifications for killing a person. Arguments have been made comparing abortion to self-defence, if the pregnant woman's life is at risk, but flaws can be found in such arguments, some of which are mentioned in 4:3 below.

Not every person is necessarily thought to have the same rights as others. Some believe that only autonomous people have rights. According to this view, a senile person or a baby does not have the same rights as a competent child or adult, although a baby has the potential of achieving those rights and a senile person may have them intermittently.

Human beings who are completely non-autonomous are often said to lack "personhood", which is one of the criteria for possessing rights. The fetus and the embryo, for example, are seen by some as being very distant from the "personhood" which would confer rights. Others believe that from the moment of fertilisation embryos and fetuses should be recognised as having the same rights as children and adults to be free of any interference which is against their interests (see reference to sanctity of life in section 4:3.1.3 below). According to this view, other claims such as that of the pregnant woman to control her own body by seeking to abort the fetus or refusing a caesarean section, do not override the claim of the fetus to a right to life. People who hold this opinion see the rights of mother and fetus as equal, so that a decision would have to be based on a judgement of which rights-holder would suffer least damage. Thus the imperative to preserve a fetal life would be likely to outweigh any other consideration except the risk of death to the mother.

Many of the arguments touched upon above attempt to address the possibility of conflicting rights by drawing a line between those who have rights (or greater rights) and those who have none (or only potential rights). Even those who consider that non-autonomous people have no rights usually concede that society nevertheless has duties towards them. Society has a duty, for example, to ensure that the sterilisation of non-autonomous women is done in their interests rather than for the convenience of carers. A further point of common agreement is that all human beings command respect regardless of whether or not they are autonomous or have rights. Many people extend this respect to all that is potentially a human being. Fetuses, embryos, pre-embryos and, by logical extension, sperm and eggs have the potential to result in a unique person. Parliament can be seen as having drawn three dividing lines. It has defined what is permissible interference before and after the first 14 days after fertilisation (see discussion of embryo research in section 4:8 below.) Abortion in some circumstances is only permissible up to the 24th week of gestation and in other cases up to term (see discussion of abortion in section 4:3 below).

Thus the ethical dilemmas which arise in the discussion of fertility and reproduction include claims to certain rights or a clash of such claims. Society must find ways of accommodating the often conflicting desires of its members, whilst at the same time protecting the vulnerable and maintaining the respect due to human life.

99

### 4:1.2 *Background*

The techniques used in genetic and reproductive technologies are constantly evolving but the ethical questions they raise are often the familiar issues of consent, confidentiality and privacy, access to treatment and allocation of resources. In Britain, important recent debates on the issues include that of the Warnock Committee which reported[104] in July 1984 and laid the foundations for the enactment of the Human Fertilisation and Embryology Act in 1990 and the Clothier Committee which reported in 1992.[105]

### 4:1.2.1 *The Warnock Committee*

A committee of inquiry was appointed in 1982 under Dame Mary Warnock to consider "recent and potential developments in medicine and science related to human fertilisation and embryology; to consider what policies and safeguards should be applied, including consideration of the social, ethical and legal implications of these developments; and to make recommendations". Among its recommendations, the Warnock Committee saw a need for infertility services to be improved but, in fact, little has changed.[106]

In examining the various moral views put forward, the Warnock Committee also noted "an instinctive opposition" on the part of many people to "tampering with the creation of human life". As a consequence of this, the report was much criticised for implying that instinctive feelings have any relevance in the matter. Counter-opinion defended Warnock on the grounds that legislation must command wide support and that a popular instinct to react sensitively to the broad implications of issues such as embryo research and gene therapy is relevant to the continuation of the species. One significant point emerging from this debate is, perhaps, that society's views on these issues are not dictated by logic alone (although there need be nothing illogical about emotion or instinct).

### 4:1.2.2 *The Human Fertilisation and Embryology Authority*

The principal conclusion of the Warnock Report was that the human embryo could be used for research, subject to stringent controls. The Human Fertilisation and Embryology Act 1990 introduced statutory control, taking over from the previous Voluntary (subsequently Interim) Licensing Authority. Issuing licences for research and monitoring compliance with the provisions of the Act is undertaken by the Human Fertilisation and Embryology Authority (HFEA), which is discussed further in 4:8.3 below.

### 4:1.2.3 *The Clothier Committee*

In 1989 the Department of Health established the Committee on the Ethics of Gene Therapy, chaired by Sir Cecil Clothier, to "draw up ethical

100

guidance for the medical profession on treatment of genetic disorders ... by genetic modification". The Committee reported in early 1992, and among its recommendations was a proposal that an expert supervisory body be established to provide scientific, medical and ethical advice on matters relevant to the safety and efficacy of somatic cell gene modification, and its clinical use. In early 1993 the Committee gave approval for the first gene therapy trial in Britain.

## 4:2 Contraception

### 4:2.1 *Contraception and public policy*

The Chief Medical Officer's annual report for 1990 estimated that half of all conceptions in England were in some sense unwanted or unintended, indicating a clear need for better access for everyone to family planning information and services. Young people in particular need access to advice, as studies clearly link high rates of teenage pregnancy to restrictions on information about contraception and limited access to low-cost contraceptives.[107] Early teenage pregnancy and abortion rates in England and Wales fell in the 1980s.[108] Despite this improvement, in 1991, nine per cent of abortions in the UK were carried out on young women under the age of 16[109] and educational monitoring bodies identified a high degree of ignorance among adolescents about sexually transmitted diseases. In "The Health of the Nation",[110] the Government set targets for reducing by at least fifty per cent the rate of conceptions amongst the under-16s, and for improving sex education by the year 2000. This is an area where health professionals, especially GPs, have an important role, since many young people are likely to turn to their family doctor if they can have confidence that their requests for contraceptive advice or treatment will be kept confidential.[111]

The Government noted a need for greater co-operation between various agencies, including health and education services, the voluntary sector and users of services. The NHS Management Executive issued guidelines in 1992 to all regional health authorities, highlighting service accessibility and the importance of providing information; the guidelines drew particular attention to the needs of young people. GPs and practice nurses are taking an increasing role in primary-care family planning. Some doctors, however, have a conscientious objection to providing contraceptive advice or treatment and may choose not to provide such services. Nevertheless, in the BMA's view, doctors with a conscientious objection to providing contraceptive advice or treatment have an ethical duty to refer the patient promptly to another practitioner or family planning service (see also 4:3.2 below). Patients are often unaware that they can register with another GP for contraceptive services only (see chapter 3, section 3:3.1.2).

## 4:2.2  Contraception and the under-16s

Controversy about the issue of "under-age" contraception is a recurring phenomenon. The BMA has a clear policy, based on the Gillick[112] judgement, that the patient's maturity and understanding of the nature of the consultation and of the treatment proposed should be the guiding factors. It is sometimes argued that very young patients may not understand either the concept of confidentiality or the implications of the treatment they request. They may have an erroneous impression of the purpose of contraceptives. An example would be that of a 9-year-old seeking contraceptives because she knows older friends have them. Kennedy[113] raises this hypothetical case but such cases are likely to be exceptional. Minors who seek contraception are usually either sexually active or intending to be so. In such cases where the patient understands the treatment, her autonomy and confidentiality should be respected. The BMA emphasises the importance of the doctor trying to persuade the patient to agree to parental involvement but if the patient refuses, the Association considers there is a duty to maintain the confidentiality of the consultation. Even if the doctor is unwilling to supply contraception on the grounds of the patient's immaturity the BMA still maintains a general duty of confidentiality unless there are very exceptional reasons for disclosing information without consent. Such reasons might occur when, for example, the request for contraception arises in the context of sexual exploitation, incest or other sexual abuse. In such very exceptional cases the doctor has a duty to protect the patient and this may eventually involve a breach of confidentiality, although with counselling and support the patient may feel able to agree to disclosure. Nevertheless, it is important that doctors avoid making completely unconditional promises about secrecy to individual young people, while at the same time making it clear that confidentiality as a general principle extends to all consultations. (Confidentiality issues are discussed further in chapter 2; the autonomy and best interests of minors are discussed in chapter 3, see in particular section 3:3.1.2).

## 4:2.3  Post-coital contraception

The development of drugs which prevent the establishment of pregnancy after intercourse has blurred the boundary somewhat between contraception and abortion. For those who believe that human life begins at fertilisation, post-coital birth control is a form of abortion. Therefore some doctors who do not object to providing contraceptive treatment in advance of intercourse may feel a conscientious objection to post-coital treatment. Others argue that techniques which prevent implantation are not the same as abortion and define conception as a process which includes both fertilisation and implantation. This is the view taken, for example, by the British Council of Churches[114] which has stated that "a woman cannot abort until the fertilised egg has nidated and thus become attached to her body".

Any GP who has an objection to providing post-coital contraception should refer the patient without delay to another doctor.

## 4:3 Abortion

### 4:3.1 *BMA policy and background to the abortion debate*

The BMA represents doctors who hold a wide diversity of moral views about abortion. The Association itself makes no policy statement about the morality of abortion. Nevertheless, this implies that there are circumstances in which the BMA considers that abortion is acceptable, unlike euthanasia, which the BMA unreservedly rejects. In the 1970s and 80s, the Association approved policy statements supporting the 1967 Abortion Act as "a practical and humane piece of legislation"[115] and urging that the same legislation be extended to Northern Ireland.[116] The BMA also supports the rights of doctors to abstain from participating in abortions on grounds of conscience. In emergencies, doctors with such a conscientious objection are ethically required to take action to try and save the mother's life and in other cases there is a duty to ensure that the pregnant woman receives non-directional counselling about abortion.

In order to understand the very contentious background to the abortion debate, it may be helpful to mention briefly the main strands of the argument. People generally give one of three common types of response to abortion. They thus fall into three groups ranging from a pro-abortion to an anti-abortion stance:

- Those who support the wide availability of abortion and consider that abortion is not wrong in itself and need not involve undesirable consequences.

- Those who consider that abortion is permissible in some circumstances but that unlimited free choice for abortion may result in undesirable social consequences.

- Those who feel that abortion is wrong and can never, or only rarely, be permissible because it violates the fetal right to life or the sanctity of life in general.

There are also a number of common arguments which can be divided very roughly into these classifications.

### 4:3.1.1 *Arguments in support of abortion being made widely available*

The arguments in support of abortion being made widely available tend not to recognise fetal rights or to acknowledge the fetus to be a person. According to some, abortion is a matter of a woman's right to exercise control over her own body. The "self-defence" argument has been made[117] that a woman is entitled to expel an entity which threatens her autonomy

103

(although many people would find unconvincing the analogy of a fetus and an intruder breaking into a house). Philosophers who judge actions by their consequences alone could argue that abortion is equivalent to a deliberate failure to conceive a child and since contraception is widely available, abortion should be too. Some think that even if the fetus is a person, its rights are very limited and do not weigh significantly against the interests of people who have already been born, such as parents or existing children of the family. The interests of society at large might outweigh any right accorded to the fetus in some circumstances, such as if, for example, overpopulation or famine threatened that society. In such cases, abortion might be seen by some people as moving from a neutral act to one which should be encouraged. (Some societies have apparently encouraged infanticide for just such reasons, as being for the greater good.[118])

Similarly, utilitarians who see a duty to promote the greatest happiness and maximise the number of worthwhile lives, could argue that there should be as few as possible unwanted children in the world. Utilitarians also consider that it is sometimes wrong for a woman to refuse to have an abortion.[119] For example, when the fetus is so abnormal that its quality of life will be drastically impaired, Glover considers "it will normally be wrong of the mother to reject abortion". For many people, however, this borders dangerously on arguments for eugenics (see 4:10 below) and, in practical terms, it presupposes the infallibility of pre-natal diagnosis.

### 4:3.1.2 The middle position

Adherents of the middle position argue that abortion may be justified in a greater number of circumstances than those conceded by anti-abortionists but that it would be undesirable to allow abortion automatically and without restriction in every case. To do so might incur undesirable effects, such as encouraging irresponsible attitudes to contraception. It could also lead to a devaluation of the lives of viable fetuses and trivialise the possible psychological effects of abortion on women and on health professionals. Some people feel uneasy about the possibility of abortion being viewed as an automatic or routine solution. They may point out that children who are initially unwanted are often greatly loved once they are born or, if not, they could be adopted by people who would love them.

Some believe that the embryo starts off without rights but acquires them at some point during its development, unless it is seriously malformed to the degree that it is unlikely ever to achieve autonomy or personhood. The notion of developing fetal rights and practical factors, such as the possible distress to the pregnant woman, nurses, doctors or other children in the family, gives rise to the view that early abortion is more acceptable than late abortion. Some people support the middle position on pragmatic grounds, believing that abortions will always be sought by women who are desperate and that it is better for society to provide abortion services which are safe and which can be monitored and regulated, rather than to allow "back-street" practices.

### 4:3.1.3 Arguments against abortion

Some people consider abortion wrong in any circumstances because it fails to recognise the rights of the fetus or because it challenges the notion of the sanctity of all human life. Some argue that permitting abortion diminishes the respect society feels for other vulnerable humans, possibly leading to their involuntary euthanasia. Those who consider that an embryo is a human being with full moral status from the moment of conception see abortion as killing in the same sense as the murder of any other person. Similarly, they see contraceptives such as the IUD, or other products which make the womb inhospitable to implantation, as forms of murder. Those who view abortion as a form of homicide cannot accept that women should be allowed to obtain it without legal repercussions, however difficult the lives of those women are made as a result. Comparisons are made with what would be said about women proposing to kill their elderly parents or children, if caring for such dependents became very burdensome.[120]

Such views may be based on religious or moral convictions that each human life has infinite value, which is not diminished by any impairment or suffering that may be involved for the individual living that life. It is also often said that only God can give life or take life away. Another argument is that abortion, like embryo research, uses humans merely as a means to an end in that abortion can be seen as a discarding of a fetus in which the pregnant woman no longer has any interest.[121] Many worry that the availability of abortion on grounds of fetal abnormality encourages prejudice towards any person with a handicap and insidiously creates the impression that the only valuable people are those who conform to some ill-defined stereotype of "normality".

Some people who oppose abortion in general, concede that it may be justifiable in very exceptional cases[122] such as where it is the result of rape or the consequence of exploitation of a young girl or a mentally incompetent woman. Risk to the mother's life may be another justifiable exception, although the "self-defence" argument is criticised by those who maintain that, in defending oneself, it is only justifiable to use the minimum force necessary to preserve one's own life. Thus it could not be justifiable to abort a fetus if the life of both fetus and mother could be saved by any other solution, such as arranging the premature delivery of the fetus in conditions in which it would be likely to survive. This may sometimes overlap with the doctrine of double effect, which permits a doctor to carry out a good action, the foreseeable side-effect of which is bad. According to this argument, a pregnant woman with cancer of the womb can be saved by hysterectomy even though the inevitable but unintended consequence is the death of the fetus. By this reasoning, however, it would be impermissible intentionally to kill the fetus in order to save the mother.

### 4:3.1.4 The legal position

The law[123] can be said to take a middle course as described above. Abortion remains illegal but no offence is committed if the pregnancy is terminated by a registered doctor in compliance with certain conditions. Two registered doctors must believe that the pregnancy has not exceeded 24 weeks and that its continuation would involve greater risk than its termination to the physical or mental health of the pregnant woman or other children of the family. After 24 weeks' gestation, a pregnancy can be lawfully terminated only if it is necessary to do so to prevent grave permanent injury to the physical or mental health of the woman, or to reduce a risk to her life, or if there is a risk that the fetus would suffer from such physical or mental abnormalities as to be seriously handicapped after birth. To avoid an offence, abortion must also be carried out in an NHS hospital or a place approved for the purpose by the Secretary of State.

### 4:3.1.5 Public attitudes

There is no unanimity in society on the question of abortion but there seems to be general agreement that public attitudes towards abortion have changed significantly in the last two decades. From 1983 to 1987, public support for lawful abortion in all circumstances increased significantly,[124] partly because it is increasingly portrayed as an issue of women's rights. Support grew even among religious groups, such as Catholics, traditionally seen as opposed to abortion.[125] The Government Statistical Service, noting the shift in attitudes, concluded that the apparent rise in abortions in the early years after the 1967 Abortion Act was mainly due to women, who might previously have sought illegal abortions, now seeking an abortion which complied with legal requirements. According to the Government's statistical experts, the increase in terminations in more recent years cannot be attributed solely to changing fertility and contraception patterns but must also be due to changing attitudes towards abortion. Nevertheless, some people fear that the development of products which terminate pregnancy without surgical intervention will lead to irresponsible attitudes to abortion.

### 4:3.1.6 Medical abortion

The use of mifepristone, in particular, has been extensively debated. It is licensed in the UK in combination with a prostaglandin to achieve medical abortion at up to 9 weeks' gestation, and is effective alone when administered within 72 hours of intercourse. Multicentre clinical trials of mifepristone have shown the drug to be a safe, effective alternative to surgical abortion and acceptable to women seeking terminations. Under the terms of the Abortion Act 1967 two doctors must support the woman's request and the termination must begin and be monitored through an NHS unit or licensed premises. The ethical issue raised by its use is apparently that mifepristone makes abortion too "easy"; the implication being that women may undertake the procedure too lightly. Some have predicted that the availability of such early abortion may result in a diminished sense of moral responsibility to avoid unwanted pregnancy, leading couples to neglect to take contraceptive measures. Informed commentators,[126] however, have argued that the decision to terminate an unplanned pregnancy is unlikely to be trivialised in this way and have criticised the attitude that appears to claim that abortion requires punitive aspects for the woman in order to be taken seriously.

The Royal College of Obstetricians and Gynaecologists has concluded that the continuing "need for abortion should be seen, not as evidence of widespread sexual irresponsibility, but rather as evidence of an intention only to have wanted children and as an expression of widespread difficulty in the management of the sexual part of life".[127]

### 4:3.2 *Conscientious objection*

Some doctors object to abortion on moral grounds. The Abortion Act 1967 carries a conscientious objection clause which permits doctors to refuse to participate in terminations but which obliges them to provide necessary treatment in an emergency when the woman's life may be jeopardised. The BMA is frequently asked to give an opinion on the scope of the conscience clause and has been helped in this task by a Parliamentary answer on the matter.[128] This made clear that conscientious objection was only intended to be applied to participation in treatment, although hospital managers had been asked, according to the Parliamentary answer, to apply the principle, at their discretion, to those ancillary staff who are involved in the handling of fetuses and fetal tissue. This is also the view that emerged from the House of Lords' discussion in the Janaway case.[129]

#### 4:3.2.1 *Legal views of doctors' obligations*

The Lords were asked to interpret the regulations concerning the conscience clause when a doctor's secretary (Janaway) refused to type the referral letter for an abortion and claimed the protection of the clause. Lord Keith summed up the case, saying:

> "The issue turns on the true construction of the words 'participate in any treatment authorised by the Act'. For the applicant it is maintained that the words cover taking part in any arrangements preliminary to and intended to bring about medical or surgery measures aimed at terminating a pregnancy, including the typing of letters referring a patient to a consultant. The health authority argues that the meaning of the words is limited to taking part in the actual

procedures undertaken at the hospital or other approved place with a view to the termination of the pregnancy."

He went on to say: "The regulations do not appear to contemplate that the signing of the certificate would form part of the treatment for the termination of pregnancy". Therefore it would seem that GPs cannot claim exemption from giving advice or performing the preparatory steps to arrange an abortion if the request for abortion meets the legal requirements. Such steps include referral to another doctor as appropriate. The BMA's Legal Department has considered the matter and takes the view that failure to make such a referral could give rise to a claim for damages if, because of the failure, there is a delay in eventual referral and an inability to obtain a termination.

### 4:3.2.2 BMA advice

In the context of GP practice, the BMA's policy on conscientious objection can be summarised in the following points:

a)  There is a distinction between legal and ethical obligations. Doctors should be aware of both.

b)  The legal implications of the Janaway case can be interpreted to support the view that GPs have an obligation in law to carry out the preliminary paperwork for terminations by signing the statutory form when the request for termination complies with the legal requirements. It is also arguable that general practitioners are entitled to decline to complete the form on grounds of conscience alone but that standards of good practice might require them to take some other action in the patient's interest. In such a case, good practice might assume legal importance if a case went to court. However, the full legal position is not entirely clear, since it requires interpretation of case law, GP terms of service, good practice and the NHS Act 1977.

c)  Having noted the legal view, the BMA does not consider that there is a comparable ethical obligation for a doctor personally to complete the statutory form. Completion of the form is a legal requirement for abortion and therefore arguably an integral part of the abortion procedure. The BMA considers that this falls morally within the scope of the conscience clause. Other preliminary procedures, such as clerking in the patient or assessing the patient's fitness for anaesthetic, are incidental to the termination and are considered outwith the scope of the conscience clause.

d)  Patients should receive objective medical advice regardless of their doctor's personal views for or against abortion. BMA policy[130] is that a patient seeking termination of pregnancy has a right to receive balanced medical counselling from her chosen doctor and a second opinion if she wishes. As is discussed in chapter 1 (section 1:2.4), doctors have a general duty to ensure that patients are provided with as much information as the patients need to make a decision. In any circumstance where an individual doctor is unable to do this, the patient should be referred to a colleague who can.

### 4:3.3 *Delay in referral*

Much concern has been expressed about avoidable delays in referral. It is unethical to delay referral to another practitioner. Unreasonable delay with the intention, or the result, of compromising the possibility of a termination being carried out is unethical and may possibly leave the practitioner open to litigation. Referral need not be a formal procedure. In some cases, it may simply consist of arranging for the patient to see a partner in the practice. In other cases, it will involve arranging a specific appointment with a colleague in another practice. It is not sufficient simply to tell the patient to seek a view elsewhere since other doctors may not agree to see her without an appropriate referral.

## 4:4 Sterilisation

Male or female sterilisation is usually expected to produce permanent sterility (although this is not necessarily the outcome). Some people have conscientious objections to sterilisation for contraceptive purposes. In some religious teaching, for example, only therapeutic sterilisation is acceptable. Within society as a whole, however, sterilisation appears to be viewed as an acceptable form of family planning as long as the individual is adequately informed of the implications of the procedure and no pressure is exerted upon the patient.

Non-consensual sterilisation, however, has been the subject of intense debate for several reasons. The harm against which it seeks to protect may not be sufficient to justify the invasion. Also it may expose the patient more easily to sexual abuse. And it can be seen as contravening a fundamental freedom to reproduce.

### 4:4.1 *Consent*

As is discussed in chapter 1 (section 1:2.1) on consent, the patient's agreement to treatment is valid only when adequate information about the procedure and its implications has been provided. The degree of patient understanding should be commensurate with the gravity of the treatment: in other words, where the procedure is irreversible, the need for patient understanding is at its greatest.

Any treatment affecting an individual's reproductive capacity also has potential implications for that person's spouse or partner. In the past, consent to treatments such as sterilisation was sought routinely from the patient's spouse. This is now acknowledged to be unacceptable unless the patient gives specific consent for the partner to be consulted. It is good practice, however, to encourage patients to discuss such procedures with their partners.

### 4:4.2 Sterilisation of people with learning disability

Individuals with learning disabilities have varying degrees of difficulty in making decisions which influence the course of their lives. Like all patients, they should be encouraged to make for themselves all those decisions the implications of which they broadly understand and with which they feel comfortable. The rights of people with learning disabilities to enjoy sexual relationships in privacy has been an issue of historical debate. Contraceptive services for people with learning difficulties should not impede the exercise of autonomy more drastically than is essential to protect against an unwanted pregnancy or the transmission of disease. In the past hysterectomies, or other forms of sterilisation, may have been carried out prematurely, on young women who might have coped successfully with other forms of contraception and who might have been capable of making their own decisions about motherhood at a much later stage. This point was implicit in a 1976 case[131] where the judge refused to authorise the sterilisation of an 11-year- old, pointing to the frustration and resentment the patient would be likely to experience in later life, arising from her inability to have children. To perform a sterilisation on a woman for non-therapeutic reasons and without her consent, the judge said, would be a violation of the individual's basic human rights to have the opportunity to reproduce. The debate about rights was taken forward but not resolved in the legal cases of "B" and "F".

### 4:4.2.1 Re B and the right to reproduce

In the case of B,[132] the House of Lords decided that a young woman of 17, with learning disability, could be sterilised without her consent. The Lords held that it was in her best interests and the case was rushed through, on the grounds that while the patient remained under the age of 18 consent could be given on her behalf by virtue of the court's wardship jurisdiction. The decision was widely criticised. Many found the pace of the judgement inappropriate.[133] Some argued that in relation to the patient's immediate need for contraceptive treatment sterilisation was not the best available option,[134] since she was not sexually active and might have had potential to exercise control over her own life. The case addressed the "right to reproduce" as a fundamental human right and this issue, in particular, was subsequently debated by many commentators.

Analysing the judgement, many experts[135] agreed that there could be no absolute right to reproduce since, among other things, this would i) infringe the rights of others by requiring another person to co-operate in conception, and ii) entail access by right to all means of assisted reproduction (see also 4:5.1. below). A right to exercise autonomy in choosing whether or not to reproduce is recognised but this hinges upon the ability of an individual to make rational choices. (It also implies that the individual is, or could be, physically able to procreate.) A right to reproduce would also carry implications for the child so produced, whose parents might not be capable of caring for it. Clearly cases must be decided on an individual basis, bearing in mind the potential of individuals with learning disabilities to marry and care for children at a later stage of their lives.

Of continuing concern, however, are allegations of sexual abuse of mentally disabled adults and the possibility that contraception, rather than other procedures, such as measures to protect the individual from unwanted interference from other patients or family members, might be seen as part of the solution. In the B case, it was suggested by the media[136] in support of the sterilisation decision, that the overriding consideration should be to protect B from sexual exploitation. Yet it is perplexing to understand how sterilisation can be thought to achieve this and it is inappropriate for such measures to be seen as a substitute for care.

### 4:4.2.2 Re F and the definition of "best interests"

Re F[137] is important, not only for issues of reproduction but for any question concerning the medical treatment of adults who are unable to consent for themselves. In this case the House of Lords set out for the first time the law in relation to such treatment. It specified that in all cases involving the treatment of an incapable adult, the treatment must be "in the patient's best interests", which was defined as:

- necessary to save life or prevent a deterioration or ensure an improvement in the patient's physical or mental health;

- in accordance with a practice accepted at the time by a responsible body of medical opinion skilled in the particular form of treatment in question.

It was further indicated that doctors may have a common law duty to provide necessary treatment for adults who cannot consent but that some procedures should not be carried out without the court's approval. Sterilisation (unless for therapeutic reasons) is such a procedure because of its intended irreversible nature which deprives the individual of what is, according to one judge, "widely and rightly regarded as one of the fundamental rights of a woman, the right to bear a child".[138] Only one judge in this case went as far as to say that all such sterilisation cases must

111

go to court, and in practice there has been a marked reluctance among doctors to regard this as an operation which requires court authorisation, with the result that many people remain concerned that individuals with disabilities continue to be sterilised unnecessarily, without recourse to the courts. The BMA emphasises that only on unambiguous therapeutic grounds should such treatments be carried out without judicial review. The Official Solicitor has issued a practice note which provides legal guidance on this matter.[139]

### 4:4.3 *Other measures*

In 1989, the BMA discussed the ethical implications of using Zoladex/Goserelin to control the libido of sexual offenders. The Association expressed concern about the lack of research on the long-term effects and the potential genetic effects on eventual offspring. The issue also raises important questions about unpressured valid consent and whether doctors can feel confident that such treatment is in the patient's best interests. If the patient is incapable of giving valid consent, doctors should seek a further medical opinion before providing this treatment. Competent detained people can give valid consent but their opportunity to give free consent may be limited. When detained people seek such medication in anticipation of early release, doctors must ensure that they provide such patients with information and counselling about the implications of treatment. (See also the discussion of surgical implantation of hormones to reduce male sexual drive in chapter 1, section 1:8.1).

## 4:5 Assisted reproduction

Assisted reproduction raises moral and social issues of profound importance. When donated gametes are used, artificial reproduction challenges our basic concepts of family relationships, personal identity and the definitions of "mother" and "father".[140] The material used in these techniques represents, in a very real sense, the "immortality" of the donor and although little study has been made of the subject, it seems that some donors later come to regret giving away their genetic material. As new techniques evolve, not only can offspring be created from the frozen gametes of people who are now dead but, by using fetal ovarian tissue, it is possible to create a child whose genetic mother was never born.

Assisted reproduction is needed because the inability to procreate is a common and distressing problem. Although statistics in this area can only be an approximate guide, one in ten couples are said to be infertile[141] and one in seven experience some difficulty in conceiving. In many societies, infertility has been stigmatised. There has been much debate, however, about whether involuntary childlessness is a medical issue. The Warnock Committee concluded that infertility is a condition deserving a medical remedy. Others think that infertility in itself cannot be classified as an illness since many infertile people lead normal, healthy lives. Treatment of infertility is often seen as a medical matter while childlessness is seen as a social problem, the remedy for which should not use up NHS resources. This argument is sometimes put forward to justify the relative scarcity of NHS funded treatment centres, which in turn may lead to greater selectivity in the consideration of people who should have priority to receive treatment. Another important point in choosing which infertile people to treat concerns the interests of the potential child.

### 4:5.1 *Access to treatment*

The question of access to fertility treatment raises some of the same issues as the sterilisation debate, particularly whether a "right" to bear children exists and whether it is encumbent upon the state or doctors to ensure that such a right is met. We have already seen that the use of the language of rights in this context is of dubious value and problematic, given that "meeting the rights" of some people will undoubtedly have serious consequences for others - not least the child.

#### 4:5.1.1 *Fitness for parenting*

Assisted reproduction exists to satisfy the desires of infertile people for children. Yet only the desires of some will be met, as only a proportion of those desiring treatment will be accepted, (and for only a proportion of them will there be a baby). This implies that clinics establish criteria of "fitness for parenting", which applicants must meet before they are accepted for treatment. While some would see this as discriminatory against the infertile since society does not generally attempt to prevent unsuitable parents from conceiving naturally,[142] others consider that by intervening with treatment to help people have children, doctors have special responsibilities to ensure that the child will not be greatly disadvantaged. Clearly doctors must ensure that potential patients are medically suitable for treatment. It would be unethical to undertake treatment without first medically assessing the likelihood of that treatment proving successful for that patient and so informing the patient.

#### 4:5.1.2 *The need for a father*

The Warnock Report warned that "this question of eligibility for treatment is a very difficult one"[143] demanding social judgements which go beyond the purely medical and require multi-disciplinary assessment. Current assessment procedures for infertility treatments appear to vary widely. Many clinics appear to operate on the premise that such treatments should only be made available to applicants who are married or in stable heterosexual relationships. Attempts to enshrine this in law during the passage of the Human Fertilisation and Embryology Bill through

113

Parliament met with failure. This left unregulated the question of eligibility for treatment, apart from the requirement that clinics must take into account the welfare of the potential child, including its need for a father. This not only has implications for single women but also for couples in which the male partner has a poor long-term prognosis. In France,[144] for example, between 1984 and 1990, 61 young couples sought donor insemination because the male partner had been diagnosed as HIV-positive. Of these eight were treated, resulting in five live births but three of these children were fatherless at birth or soon after. This gave rise to debate about the ethics of selecting applicants for treatment, not least because the fact that the mother tested HIV-negative prior to insemination, could not guarantee the absence of HIV infection for her and her child.

Discussion about the need for a father is one very important element of pre-treatment counselling when patients seek assisted reproduction. In this country, there has been little open debate about the selection criteria which are actually used and little published research[145] is available about how eligibility is assessed in practice. Factors such as age of the couple, duration of their relationship, history of illness in either partner and area of residence may all affect applicants' acceptability. Fertility treatments have been denied to people whose lifestyle doctors consider unsuitable[146] and the court did not find this unreasonable, except if there was a blanket policy of refusal to treat members of particular religious or ethnic groups, for example.

While it may be easy to identify clearly such extreme forms of discrimination as unacceptable, the correct procedure in individual cases, which can involve a variety of complex factors, may be much harder to define objectively. For example, how should doctors assess widows whose ability to experience the reality of their bereavement and recover from it, is linked to a desire to bear their dead husband's genetic child by use of his frozen sperm? The HFEA takes the view at present that clinics which provide infertility treatment services alone and do not conduct research do not need to maintain an ethics committee.[147] Unfortunately, this means that such centres have no independent, non-clinical source of advice and support in cases of extreme difficulty or sensitivity. The BMA would welcome all clinics having access to such independent scrutiny of difficult cases although Douglas implicitly questions whether this would bring about any real change since her study appears to indicate that the final decision on whether to offer treatment in a particular case rests generally with a medical person rather than a multi-disciplinary team or an ethics committee, where these exist.

The BMA has rejected the notion of establishing hard and fast rules on eligibility, as part of a general refusal to classify individual patients into groups. It insists that legally accepted medical procedures are the subject of clinical judgement applied in each individual case.

In 1978, in correspondence with Sir George Young MP, the Association stated the need:

"for a full investigation of any couple seeking artificial insemination by donor (AID) and in this respect we would expect the doctor to consider most carefully the overall family situation, the needs of his patient and most importantly the welfare of any child who might be born into the family as a result of AID. This would apply whether the couple seeking AID was of a heterosexual or homosexual (lesbian) nature. Although one might be tempted to generalise about any given situation, the provision of medical advice and treatment for each individual patient must be a matter for decision by the medical practitioner concerned".[148]

As stated above, our view is that doctors would benefit from the views of ethics committees in difficult cases.

### 4:5.2 Consent to treatment of infertility

When a woman consents to fertility treatments, not only does she agree to undergo potentially hazardous medical procedures, she also makes uniquely difficult decisions about her future and that of many of her embryos. Pre-treatment counselling must include explanation of the risks of the procedures and their chances of success. The HFEA is also addressing the need for centres to make public their success rate. In the past, the BMA has occasionally received worrying reports from GPs that women, who for medical reasons had no realistic chance of conceiving, had been accepted for private fertility treatment. While the rights of patients are recognised, the BMA stresses the need for doctors and the health care team to provide the frank information necessary if an informed choice is to be made.

### 4:5.3 Duties to the different parties

In many circumstances, doctors' duties are primarily focused on the patient before them. In assisted reproduction or surrogacy arrangements, there is another party to be considered, that is the child born as a result of medical intervention. Disputes about the ethical obligations, if any, owed to the unborn child continue unabated. The BMA's general view is that the fetus deserves respect but as a non-autonomous being does not have absolute claims which can override those of an autonomous person, usually the mother.[149] In the case of any form of assisted reproduction, however, the ethical claims of the child and the doctor's responsibilities to it assume greater weight, since doctors who intervene to generate a pregnancy have particular duties to ensure that the resulting child is not foreseeably disadvantaged. It is on these grounds that doctors must make an assessment of potential parents seeking treatment. The child is the most vulnerable party and doctors' obligations are held to be significantly

115

greater than in any case where the doctor assumes management of an already existing pregnancy. The BMA has expressed dismay that the HFEA does not accord the claims of the potential child pre-eminence in such contexts but instead sees the child's interest as deserving of equal consideration as those of other parties.

If the child's claims are considered to be paramount, it may be unethical, for example, for doctors to assist in generating a pregnancy with the purpose of providing a child to donate material for transplantation to a sibling. The best interests of the potential child, however, are difficult to assesss when the alternative is non-existence. Such cases raise many complex moral issues about using particularly vulnerable individuals as a means to an end and generating pregnancies which may be terminated if the desired features (such as the correct tissue match for transplantation) are absent. The BMA considers that there should be serious public debate about the principles involved.

In all cases of assisted reproduction the doctor's duty involves ensuring that adequate assessment and counselling has been provided for the woman or couple receiving treatment. The doctor must be satisfied that all concerned have considered the implications, including the possibility of some genetic or other defect in donated genetic material and the resultant handicap in the child.

### 4:5.4 *Multiple pregnancies*

One of the results of the development of assisted reproduction is the increase in high order births. Pregnancies involving several fetuses carry increased risks of premature birth, handicap such as cerebral palsy and perinatal mortality. It has been estimated[150] that the incidence of prematurity increases from 10 per cent in single births to more than 75 per cent in triplet pregnancies; and perinatal mortality rises from 17 per cent in triplets to over 40 per cent in sextuplets. Although high order births carry increased risk, on occasion the actual number of fetuses in the pregnancy only becomes clear at birth,[151] which means it is impossible to counsel the parent(s) properly about the medical risks and social consequences. Until comparatively recently, there has been little information about the problems encountered by neonatal units in dealing with high order births, and about the long-term difficulties of parents. At the end of the 1980s, the Department of Health supported the world's first national study of triplets and higher order births.[152] This threw light on the social and physical problems in this group. It also contributed to an ongoing debate about the ethics of using resources to treat very low birthweight babies, some of whom will require repeated hospital admissions or special educative facilities throughout life.[153]

High rates of multiple pregnancies after ovarian stimulation, transfer of several eggs or embryos after in vitro fertilisation (IVF), or gamete intrafallopian transfer (GIFT) have led to the practice of fetal reduction to ensure the survival of some.

### 4:5.5 *Selective reduction of fetuses*

Selective reduction is the killing in the womb of one or more fetuses in a multiple pregnancy. A particular fetus may be selected because it shows signs of abnormality or weakness, or a random choice may be made, simply to increase the survival chances of other fetuses. While the practice raises some of the same issues as abortion regarding the respect due to human life and the moral arguments about sacrificing a non-autonomous fetus in order to minimise risk to the mother (and, in this case, to other fetuses) it also involves additional issues, since the fetuses who are killed have usually been created by reproductive technology. Like gender selection, (see 4:5.6 below), selective reduction is a procedure which has arisen from medical necessity but which could arguably be offered as a consumer choice to parents who have not undergone assisted reproduction and who are not prepared to accept a natural multiple pregnancy. The ethical issues as to whether it is acceptable selectively to reduce for reasons of parental preference for a single child or twins remain to be debated.

In law, the selective reduction of fetuses in multiple pregnancies is regulated by the Human Fertilisation and Embryology Act 1990. Some still see the procedure as posing medical, ethical and psycho-social problems, not least because of the paucity of information about how women and their partners cope with the experience and its after-effects. It is said,[154] for example, that women are insufficiently informed about selective reduction, including the subsequent sense of loss and grief that many parents experience.

Selective reduction cannot be performed earlier than six weeks after conception and most are carried out between eight and fourteen weeks' gestation. A lethal injection of potassium chloride is usually made into the heart of one or more of the fetuses. The procedure itself is not without hazard and the risk of obstetric complications is far from negligible. Delayed spontaneous abortion of all embryos is one risk, which varies according to the technique used. Other risks include maternal infection and some possible risk of fetal malformation.[155] All agree on the need for discussing these problems with patients and abiding by their decisions, but some people feel there is also a need for the involvement of ethics committees and for a re-examination of current practice, in order that greater efforts be made to minimise multiple pregnancies. According to some commentators,[156] this is where one of the dilemmas lies, since the transfer of three embryos or eggs in IVF or GIFT has come to be accepted practice internationally, although some centres have shown evidence that equally high pregnancy rates can be achieved by transferring only two eggs or embryos.[157] There is no regulation of ovulation induction practices.

### 4:5.6 *Gender selection*

Several techniques exist for selecting the gender of children. Primary selection may be achieved through sperm-sorting (although expert opinion suggests that this is not an effective technique) or through timing of insemination. Secondary selection takes place after fertilisation, by pre-implantation diagnosis or after the embryo has implanted in the womb, when prenatal diagnosis may lead to an abortion if the fetus is not of the desired sex. The law, however, does not permit termination of pregnancy on grounds of fetal sex alone, although it allows abortion in instances where the mother's mental or physical health would be impaired by continuation of pregnancy. In some cases, the pressures brought to bear on a woman to produce a child of the desired gender may so affect her health.

Gender selection is often sought in order to eliminate the risk of passing on gender-linked diseases such as Duchenne muscular dystrophy. It may also be sought for social or cultural reasons. When sperm-sorting was initially advertised to the public, the procedure had not been validated scientifically and doubts continue to be raised about it. The BMA considered that couples might be exploited financially by an unproven procedure and that, if the procedure failed, this might give rise to them seeking abortion of a fetus of the "wrong" sex. It was also concerned that gender selection might reveal discriminatory attitudes against females.

In early 1993, the HFEA issued a public consultation document on the issues, the results of which will be available later in 1993. The BMA also organised an open debate to hear the views of a wide range of professionals and interest groups. The results of this are available from the BMA's Ethics Division.

The main arguments which have been advanced are:

- Freedom of choice should be encouraged if this is not likely to produce foreseeable harm. If it is particularly important to some families, should they not be entitled to choose their child's sex? In some religions, for example, certain rituals can only be performed by sons; but

- if freedom of consumer choice is the standard criterion, arguably it may also be applicable to other decisions, resulting in "designer children".

- The balance of the sexes would be upset since many people value males more than females; but

- while this argument is undoubtedly true in some cultures, there is no evidence collected in this country to substantiate this claim. Some people are of the opinion that most of those who want to make a choice would opt for a balance of males and females. This might suggest that freedom of choice in this area might not lead to overall population imbalance, although it might in some sections in the community.

118

- Some are concerned that most people would choose to have a male child first and that this would have an adverse psychological effect on younger daughters. It would also serve to perpetuate society's existing sexual stereotypes and prejudices about the status of women; but

- some would argue that the solution is not to ban gender selection but to tackle the root of the problem and break down effectively society's prejudices. Alternatively gender selection for social reasons could be restricted to parents who already have some children.

- Some believe that gender selection should be approved on utilitarian grounds since it would make more families happy. If people prefer sons, they will treat them better than daughters. Thus allowing couples to choose would increase the number of happy children and diminish the abuse or neglect of unwanted children.

- The ability to plan the sex composition of one's family may give rise to trivial or misleading attitudes.

- Some argue that gender selection is preferable to people seeking abortion at a later stage and that to allow choice would reduce the number of abortions. Although abortion on the grounds of fetal gender is not legally permitted, some have speculated that it is practised by unscrupulous doctors theoretically on grounds other than gender choice.

- People might have fewer children as some parents continue having children until they have one of the desired sex. When overpopulation is a concern choice may help limit population size.

Early in 1993, the BMA concluded that sex selection for social and/or medical reasons is ethically acceptable. If, however, sex selection is offered in the UK, it should be properly regulated and licensed by the HFEA. This will safeguard patients from unsafe practices and will ensure that they receive the same professional assessment and counselling that people seeking infertility treatments currently receive.

### 4:5.7 *Rights to know one's genetic background*

Individuals' needs to know their genetic background is a matter of continuing debate. Doctors sometimes ask whether it is justifiable to modify a child's health record at parental request in order to conceal the child's genetic origin or the fact of adoption. The BMA does not consider that a child's medical record should be automatically marked to indicate that the patient is not the genetic offspring of the supposed parents. In some rare cases, for instance if there is a history of hereditary disease within the family, it is important to be able to identify the patient's true genetic background. In most situations, however, it is not clear that children produced by assisted reproduction who are unaware of their genetic background, are disadvantaged when compared with a child who has been conceived naturally: in the latter case, the presumed father may not be the genetic father. Susceptibility to many diseases is usually determined by testing the individual (who may or may not want to know the outcome) rather than other (supposed or real) genetic relatives.

The BMA and the HFEA encourage parents to be frank with children about their origins. The Association has also expressed concern about the possible effect upon children and young people of stumbling upon the truth inadvertently, which might occur through minors exercising a right of access to their medical records. It advises GPs to discuss these issues with parents in the hope that young people will be properly prepared.

The HFEA holds a register of donors of sperm, eggs and embryos and, in exceptional circumstances, could divulge that information. The absence of a clear right to know one's genetic origins has concerned some people. In 1991 the Secretary of State for Health was asked in the House of Commons what action was going to be taken, in respect of information about their donor parents, for children born as a result of infertility treatment. She drew attention to the Human Fertilisation and Embryology Act 1990 which can require the Authority to give specified information at the age of 18 (or earlier if the minor is intending to get married) to an applicant born following treatment services involving the use of donated gametes. She went on to say that this raised profound issues which required wide-ranging consultation and that therefore there was no intention to introduce regulation in the near future.

## 4:6 Childlessness and surrogacy

As has been mentioned previously, there is much debate about whether medicine has a role in alleviating childlessness, which some see as a social rather than medical matter. Surrogacy represents a controversial solution to childlessness, raising many concerns about the exploitation of women and the under-valuing of children who can be commissioned and "bought". Surrogacy arrangements are often compared to adoption procedures although some[158] argue that they should be regarded very seriously as a distinct way of establishing a family, and be set clearly apart from adoption. A principal difference between adoption and surrogacy is that surrogacy satisfies the desires of intending parents by creating children who would not otherwise have existed, whereas adoption seeks to meet the needs of existing children for a family. Doctors need not necessarily be involved in establishing conception in surrogacy arrangements but where they are involved, doctors are held to have special responsibilities to the child (see 4:6.1 below).

The Surrogacy Arrangements Act 1985 prohibits commercial surrogacy arrangements but permits non-commercial activities and does not ban payment of expenses to a surrogate mother. The BMA has issued two reports on surrogate motherhood. The most recent[159] was published in 1990 after a working party chaired by Sir Malcolm Macnaughton had debated the issues for two years. In this report the Association supported the view that surrogacy should be an option of last resort, in which the interests of the potential child must be paramount. The BMA advised doctors to be extremely cautious about agreeing to help with such an arrangement but considered that it would be undesirable to prevent all medical involvement in surrogacy arrangements.

### 4:6.1 *The doctor's duties in the surrogacy arrangement*

The 1990 BMA report contains brief guidelines for doctors. These guidelines apply to cases where a doctor's help is sought in order to initiate a surrogate pregnancy. Once such a pregnancy has begun - with or without medical intervention - the doctor's ethical obligations to the surrogate mother and the child are no different from those owed to any mother and child who are the doctor's patients. In particular, it must be emphasised that a woman who has become pregnant as the result of a surrogacy arrangement is entitled to precisely the same maternity care as any other pregnant woman.

The Association considers that it would be unethical for doctors to be associated with the initiation of a surrogate pregnancy if they have not first satisfied themselves that the level of all the foreseeable risks is acceptable to all the parties involved. In the case of the child to be conceived, the combined total of all the foreseeable hazards should not be greater, taking account of all the circumstances including the surrogacy, than that which doctors could properly and responsibly impose on any other child whose conception lay within their professional powers.

Surrogacy presents many difficult problems. The BMA recognises that the procedure is unacceptable to some doctors, either for reasons of conscience or because the risks are so great they would not wish to have anything to do with any form of surrogate pregnancy. If doctors take that view, the BMA considers that it would not be unethical for them to refuse to undertake the necessary procedures but their ethical obligation in that case is to refer the patient(s) to someone else. Once a doctor has decided to take part in a surrogate arrangement, it is important that overall care of all participants and adherence to the BMA guidelines, should be ensured by one doctor.

If doctors are willing to consider taking part in the initiation of a surrogate pregnancy, they should, together with appropriate counsellors, first ensure that both they and all the parties are fully aware of the kind and degree of all the risks associated with such an arrangement. These risks are of two kinds: those generally associated with pregnancy, and those which are peculiar to surrogacy.

### 4:6.2 *Problems with surrogacy*

A number of risks particularly related to surrogate arrangements are discussed in the BMA report. They include the risk of a handicapped child which might be rejected by both the surrogate and the commissioning parents; the danger that the surrogate will lead an unhealthy life which might have implications for the unborn child, risks of psychological damage to the surrogate, or to her existing children who see a sibling given to another family, psychological harm to the child itself, and the risk that the surrogate may seek to keep the child.

The BMA emphasises that a doctor who is considering being involved in the initiation of a surrogate pregnancy must first establish the probability of each of these risks, and must make all the enquiries necessary to establish those probabilities. This must involve the fullest discussion with all the parties concerned in the surrogacy arrangement.

### 4:6.3 *BMA conclusions and recommendations*

The main conclusions and recommendations of the BMA 1990 report are that:

a) The welfare of the potential child should be the first consideration.

b) Surrogacy should only be a last resort where the commissioning couple suffers from infertility due to a medically recognised disorder, and where all other appropriate means for enabling them to have a child have been tried, and have failed. It would be unethical for a doctor to take part in the initiation of a surrogate pregnancy merely to suit the convenience of a commissioning mother who is in fact capable of conceiving, and bringing the pregnancy to term without undue risk.

c) The parties likely to be affected by a surrogacy arrangement are all the members of the respective households and families, and all their existing or future children - including, as the most important, the child or children who would not be conceived but for the doctor's intervention. The practitioner owes ethical obligations to all these parties.

d) Only women who have partners and who have already had one child or more should be considered as potential surrogates, since the surrogate should be aware of what is involved in pregnancy and labour and should ideally have the support of a partner.

e) It is inadvisable for the commissioning couple and the surrogate mother to be aware of each other's identity.

The relationship between the surrogate and the commissioning parents, is often raised in debates about surrogacy. Glover,[160] for example, notes the surrogate's longing for a close friendship with the commissioning couple as a key element in many English, French and American surrogacy arrangements. The commissioning couple, he says, normally do not want a continuing relationship with the surrogate. In countries where payments to surrogates are permitted, payment of the fee is often intended to terminate the relationship and wipe out any debt which the commissioning couple might feel towards the surrogate. In producing its own report, the BMA was aware of the potential for psychological damage to any of the parties to the surrogacy arrangement and cautioned those considering such arrangements to reflect on its many possible risks and drawbacks.

## 4:7 Ante-natal care and birth

Some questions of patient choice in ante-natal care and birth are briefly mentioned in chapter 11 (section 11:2.2.3) where the problem of patients choosing an option, such as home delivery, in circumstances which present increased risk for the unborn child, is discussed.

As a general point, the BMA emphasises the importance of liaison between GP, midwife and consultant in domino arrangements. As is discussed in chapter 11 (section 11:2.2.3), it stresses that where GPs do not agree to be involved in a home confinement which they consider dangerous, the patient should not feel abandoned by the doctor and nor should the GP be excluded, since he or she will have continuing care of the family. GPs should ensure that the patient is aware of their views and that the GP retains the obligation to respond in any emergency which might arise. In such cases, the midwife may be willing to supervise the confinement. In others, the midwife may believe the choice to be inappropriate but nevertheless be obliged to attend if the patient is unwilling to accept the joint advice of doctor and midwife.

### 4:7.1 *The autonomy of pregnant women*

The limitations which society is prepared to place on a woman's freedom of choice regarding the management of her pregnancy and labour are unclear. Unlike the United States, where there has been much debate about court orders detaining pregnant women in hospital or authorising caesarians, in Britain there has not been much discussion until relatively recently about compulsorily treating pregnant women against their will. For some time, a number of American obstetricians[161] have been pointing to the problems associated with court-ordered interventions, which often rest on dubious legal arguments and can adversely affect maternal and infant health by, for example, encouraging pregnant women to go into hiding.

In this country, attempts to override refusal of treatment by competent pregnant women have usually been rebuffed in the courts.[162] Department of Health statistics on maternal deaths 1985-87, indicate some cases where women have died after declining various treatments without steps having been taken to involve the courts to override a competent patient's refusal. Such cases are deeply tragic for the individuals concerned and the health professionals who offer treatment but these rare cases have been seen as a risk which society must allow in order to protect the integrity and autonomy of all competent patients.[163] Some fear that usurping the decision making rights of a competent pregnant woman demeans women in general and sets a precedent for invading the bodies of some patients in order to benefit other patients. The idea that a woman should be forced to undergo surgery for another's benefit has been widely rejected. Where the woman's own life is also jeopardised, the right of competent patients to decline life-prolonging treatment has been invoked.

In 1992, however, in the case of Re S,[164] the High Court authorised a caesarian on a competent patient who refused the operation on religious grounds. The procedure failed to save the baby and the judgement evoked much criticism[165] regarding both its unclear legal basis and its procedural deficiencies (the pregnant woman was not given an opportunity to be heard).

### 4:7.2 Balancing maternal-fetal moral claims

As is briefly mentioned in 4:1.1.1 above, many people who do not consider that non-autonomous beings have rights, nevertheless concede that we have duties towards them. The BMA's general view is that some duties are owed to the fetus even though its claims may not supersede the mother's claim to autonomy over her body. The relative development of the fetus is an important consideration when conflicting claims must be balanced. The more developed the fetus is, the greater may be its moral claims and the mother's freedom of choice may be thought subject to greater moral constraints. In this context, for example, the BMA has recognised that all patients have a right to make an advance directive refusing life-prolonging treatment but that doctors must also weigh up their moral obligations to the unborn child if such a directive is invoked to withdraw treatment from a pregnant (and now incompetent) woman.

Useful guidance has been given on how a pregnant woman's claims to freedom of action may be weighed against the risks her actions entail for the fetus.[166] This involves identifying the morally relevant factors in each individual case, such as the degree of harm to the fetus, the importance the woman attaches to her choices and the degree of autonomy she has (as opposed to being dependent on drugs, for example, or to having been misinformed). According to this system, the following facts are among those to be considered:

124

- The more serious the risk of harm to the fetus, the more compelling may be the mother's duty and the greater the need on the part of the mother to show compelling reasons for not complying with it.

- Another factor is the risk to the mother herself from a proposed surgical intervention. The more serious the risk associated with the proposed intervention or other stipulated regime, the less strong may be the claim of the fetus.

- The reasons for the mother's choice or conduct. It may range from mere convenience to religious conviction, concern for her own health or concern for the fetus' or future child's health. That is to say, it may range from the trivial to the serious. The more trivial it is, the less justified the mother may be in seeking to rely on it.

- The degree of uncertainty about prenatal diagnosis must also be considered. (In some American cases of court-ordered caesarians, the women delivered healthy babies by natural means before the court order could be enforced). The greater the degree of uncertainty, the less it would justify limiting the woman's freedom of choice.

Kennedy emphasises that this mechanism is not intended as a checklist for answering difficult cases. Nevertheless it provides a framework by means of which moral arguments can be applied. In contrast, one of the enduring concerns arising from the S case has been the court's failure to give adequate explanation of its moral reasoning or proper justification for the decision.

## 4:8 Embryo research

The issue of embryo research is often portrayed as the clash of diametrically opposed viewpoints, with scientists anxious to push forward to understand and control the creation of life while "at least half the human race needs, and frequently prefers, a mystery".[167] The issues raised by embryo research require continuing debate even though legislation currently governs what is permitted (see also chapter 8, section 8:8.1.5). The Human Fertilisation and Embryology Act 1990 permits research on the embryo up to 14 days after fertilisation, at which time the primitive streak appears. Until the 14th day after fertilisation, cells are pluripotential and can develop into one embryo or twins or degenerate entirely.

### 4:8.1 *Status of the embryo*

Many of the arguments raised about embryo research turn on how we classify the embryo, since its perceived rights depend upon its status. The Warnock Report considered the ethical and moral principles which should be considered in determining the status of the embryo but declined to address whether or not the embryo is a person or a chattel. It concluded that human embryos should have special status and many agree that, being neither, they should occupy a separate category from both autonomous beings and things. The contention that the embryo is fully human does not command wide support but its human origin and potential must be recognised and respected. Those who assign full human status to the embryo oppose research upon it since this causes its destruction, while those who believe the embryo has no moral status see no objection to embryo research. Following the latter line of thinking, it can be argued that "if the moral reasons which justify abortion are sound then we should permit embryo research and experimentation on the same terms and set a limit to such research at the same point as the upper limit for abortion".[168] Others, however, draw a distinction between the very early embryo (pre-embryo) prior to the development of the primitive streak and the embryo proper, acknowledging only the latter to be a potential human being, which therefore requires to be protected from research.

### 4:8.1.1 "Spare" embryos

Embryos used in research come from two sources. They may have been created with a specific intention of providing research material or they may have been created as part of an IVF procedure, to which they are now surplus and would otherwise be allowed to perish if the gamete donors do not wish them to be used by other infertile people. Some of the people who believe that embryos have, or should have, moral status, believe that research on them can never be ethical. Others consider it is only ethical when the embryos are "spare". Adherents of this view assume that the creation of more embryos than is strictly necessary for IVF is unavoidable for medical reasons and argue that to use them for research is not worse than destroying them and may bring about good. Opponents may agree that the creation of surplus embryos is unavoidable but may still object to profiting from what they see as a necessary evil. There has been much debate about whether it is ethical to produce embryos exclusively to provide research material.

In the mid-1980s[169] there was extensive discussion within the BMA about the ethics of researching on "spare" embryos and the creation of embryos specifically for research. Opinions within the Association were sharply divided on the question of whether human life could be created for the purposes of research although there was wide acceptance of the need for such research relevant to clinical problems such as contraception, diagnosis and treatment of infertility and inherited diseases. There was little objection to research on "spare" embryos but some people who supported research worried that this would not provide sufficient embryonic material.

One line of argument laid importance on the doctor's intention in creating embryos. If the intention was to promote the interests of the embryo (by establishing a hopefully successful pregnancy) this was distinct from creating embryos with the sole intention of ultimately destroying them.

The moral issues were rehearsed at meetings of the BMA Council and the Annual Representative Meeting. Those who argued that doctors must have the intention of creating a child (although they might thus create "spare" embryos as a side effect) were over-ruled. The BMA confirmed its belief in the need for research involving embryos and refused to rule out the possibility that embryos might be created for this purpose, although it also stressed that "the prime objectives" of in-vitro fertilisation concerned the production of normal children. This echoed the majority view of the Warnock Committee, which had also been divided on this issue. Attempts in the House of Lords to limit research to "spare" embryos were also defeated by 214 votes to 80.[170] (Creation of embryos for research is legally regulated by the terms of the Human Fertilisation and Embryology Act 1990).

Parliament can be seen as generally endorsing the philosophical view that "if it is right to use embryos for research then it is right to produce them for research. And if it is not right to use them for research, then they should not be so used even if they are not deliberately created for the purpose".[171]

### 4:8.2 *Moral arguments*

Various interwoven strands of thought can be identified concerning the moral status of embryos:

- The embryo has the potential to develop full human capacities. The counter argument to this is that so do the contents of a petri dish containing sperm and egg but we do not assign special moral status to those contents.

- Some argue that embryos are human beings. The use of humans for research which is not in their interests and will result in their destruction is morally wrong. Some who see a value in the results of embryo research nevertheless oppose such research, since the benefits are bought at a price which they consider to be unacceptable. The counter-argument is that respect and moral status can only be related to human personhood and the embryo is simply a collection of cells. Personhood is seen by many as the key element which distinguishes human from other life-forms. Lacking personhood, embryos are as equally valid as subjects for research as plants and animals. Some supporters of this line of reasoning see embryos as entitled to more respect than other life-forms but not deserving of or endowed with the absolute respect which would prevent useful research to help those who have achieved personhood.

127

- Another view is that from fertilisation, the embryo is a unique individual with the same rights as any other person, by virtue of its potential for development. This is again countered by those who see personhood as the important criterion and the possession of rights as being dependent upon the ability to exercise autonomy. Some see the development within the embryo of brain tissue, at about 10 weeks' gestation, as the beginning of individuality and rights. Others consider that personhood resides in the individual's sense of self-awareness, which does not develop until well after birth and is lost in dementia or unconsciousness. In this view, the possible harm which might be done to potential human beings through embryo research is balanced against the suffering of actual humans which could be prevented by embryo research.

Some have criticised the lack of logic in the way in which the arguments about the embryo's potential for development are used by the Warnock Committee and others. They argue that if the potentiality argument is good, it is good against all non-actualisation of human potential and it rules out research on human eggs, sperm and embryos at any stage, as well as favouring unlimited procreation.

Many people distinguish between research which destroys the embryo and research intended for its benefit, encouraging strictly therapeutic interventions designed to rectify chromosomal defects. This brings in the strongest argument favouring embryo research, in that the preventive approach to genetic disease is preferable to attempting to alleviate the effects of major, crippling disease.

### 4:8.3 *The Human Fertilisation and Embryology Authority (HFEA)*

The HFEA governs embryo research. Each research protocol must relate broadly to one of the stated categories of research aims. These are:

a)   promoting advances in the treatment of infertility;

b)   increasing knowledge about the causes of congenital disease;

c)   increasing knowledge about the causes of miscarriage;

d)   developing more effective techniques of contraception;

e)   developing methods for detecting the presence of gene or chromosome abnormalities in embryos before implantation;

f)   endeavouring to increase knowledge about the creation and development of embryos and enabling such knowledge to be applied.

128

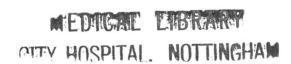

## 4:9 Gene therapy and research

In 1992 the BMA published its report, "Our Genetic Future", on the science and ethics of genetic technology. Its main conclusions in relation to the impact of genetic technology on the health and wellbeing of people are summarised below.

### 4:9.1 *Gene therapy*

Human genetic modification should be restricted to the treatment or prevention of serious disease. Somatic cell gene therapy, the correction of defective genes in particular tissues of the body, affects only the individual concerned and therefore is no different in principle from other routine and widely accepted therapies such as organ transplantation. As such, somatic cell gene therapy raises no new ethical issues but as with all innovative therapies it should be subject to rigorous ethical appraisal and used only when there is no alternative available or when it offers genuine advantages, such as safety or efficacy, over other types of treatment. With these reservations, the Association considers that somatic cell gene therapy has considerable potential.

Germ-line gene therapy, on the other hand, involves modifying genes in the reproductive cells which would cause changes not only to the genetic make-up of individuals but also to their descendants. At present the risks associated with germ-line gene therapy, such as genetic damage during the modification process or the loss of a gene with hidden advantages from the gene pool, are impossible to evaluate and there is a general consensus, shared by the BMA, that germ-line gene therapy should not yet be attempted. In the UK it is currently prohibited under the Human Fertilisation and Embryology Act 1990.

### 4:9.2 *Genetic screening*

Genetic screening may take a number of forms: for example, screening for carrier status of recessive genetic diseases such as cystic fibrosis or sickle cell disease; presymptomatic predictive screening for dominant disorders such as Huntington's disease; or pre-natal screening of fetuses for a range of genetic conditions. Each form of screening raises specific ethical issues but there are also some issues which are common to all genetic screening. Screening should always be accompanied by appropriate counselling so that individuals and couples may make informed choices. Participation in screening should be on a voluntary basis and if someone were to refuse screening, for whatever reason, it should not jeopardise either that person's rights, or his or her children's rights, to subsequent care or state benefits. Information about an individual's genetic make-up, like all medical data, should, in principle, be treated as confidential. However, it is recognised that particular difficulties may arise

129

in this area of medicine as genetic information about one person may have profound significance for other family members. The Association nevertheless considers that genetic information should not be made freely available within the family and that any breach of confidentiality without a patient's consent would have to be justified on the basis of the severity of the disorder in question and its implications for other family members.

### 4:9.2.1 Pre-natal screening

In many families where there is a previous history of genetic disease, it is now possible to screen fetuses for the particular disorder and offer couples the option of termination of pregnancy if the fetus is found to be affected. For couples who will not countenance a termination other options may be available, depending on the disorder, such as egg or sperm donation, pre-implantation diagnosis or adoption. Of course, some couples may choose none of the options and decide simply to "wait and see".

Many factors may influence a couple's decision to accept pre-natal testing, such as the severity of the disease, the probability that a child will be born with the disorder and the availability of treatments for the condition. In addition, social, moral, religious and cultural factors, and family considerations may play an important role in the couples' choices. The Association, in "Our Genetic Future", did not wish, therefore, to be drawn into making decisions about which diseases would or would not justify pre-natal screening services. The BMA argued, however, that pre-natal testing should not be allowed for morally frivolous reasons such as detection of traits which have no disease association, but which may not be considered "desirable".

## 4:10 Eugenics

"Eugenics" is the term used to describe the science of producing healthy or fine offspring. In itself, the term need carry no pejorative overtones. However, because of its associations with Nazi experiments it is today generally used pejoratively.

All parents hope for healthy children and most are prepared to take steps to avoid the transmission of disabling traits (although views of what constitutes "disablement" may differ). The legislation permitting abortion up to term on grounds of fetal abnormality is partly based on the premise that for a person to be born with very severe abnormality is undesirable, possibly even for the person so affected, for whom the alternative is no existence at all. Some argue that the concept of eugenics, like the idea of abortion on the grounds of fetal handicap, discriminates against people who have handicaps. Others maintain that to try and avoid handicap is no more unacceptable than to try and eliminate it by curing whatever disease causes it.

130

The fear which underlies the pejorative use of the term "eugenics" is that if practised, eugenics might become the basis for the imposition of compulsory measures on some people either not to procreate or only to produce offspring who fit within some pre-defined scale of what is acceptable. This is the fear that might be raised by Glover's comment (see 4:3.1.1) about the moral duty to seek an abortion in some cases. Such a "moral duty" might be seen as underpinning an assumption that "those who are genetically weak should be discouraged from reproducing or are less morally important than other persons and that compulsory measures to prevent them from reproducing might be defensible".[172] Harris, however, argues that it is not the genetically weak who should be discouraged from reproducing but rather that, when there is a choice to be made, everyone should be discouraged from producing children who will be harmed by their genetic constitution. Perhaps the acceptability of such a premise depends on how "discouragement" is defined and whether society would be prepared to bring pressure on individuals who have differing views, such as that it is not for parents or doctors to decide such matters.

## 4:11 Summary

The issues which are raised by the discussion of different aspects of reproduction and genetic technology are too wide-ranging to be helpfully summarised into a list of points, although common concerns about respect for humanity and freedom of choice run through many of them.

As has been mentioned throughout this chapter, reproductive issues touch upon deeply held convictions and perceptions about what constitutes a human being or a person, about identity, about the family and about the sense of one's own characteristics living on in some form after one's death. The way society draws lines for some procedures - allowing abortion on viable fetuses in some circumstances but prohibiting embryo research outside a very restricted framework - may well seem inconsistent and arbitrary. It must be emphasised that particularly in the area of reproduction and gene therapy there must be constant re-evaluation of the issues involved. Without such continuing re-evaluation there is a risk that decisions will be based merely on past accepted practice or on an intuitive distaste for certain proposals. As we argue in chapter 13, intuition has its place but must be congruent with ethical reasoning.

# 5 Caring for the Dying

*This chapter and the one which follows it deal with aspects of medical treatment at the end of life. This chapter concentrates on the relationship between patient and health team as the patient's condition is recognised as terminal. It looks at "medical friendship", the skills and virtues expected of health professionals which might be particularly important in this context and the influences exerted by the hospice movement. Patient rights are discussed and emphasis given to the importance of frankness and communication between the health team and the patient. Family support for the dying person is briefly mentioned, as is the need for carers and health professionals to receive support to help them deal with stress and bereavement.*

## 5:1 Introduction

Our original intention was to discuss all ethical issues concerning the end of life in one chapter. It was felt, however, that discussion of good quality terminal care should be separated from issues such as euthanasia and non-resuscitation, which are discussed in chapter 6. A common element in both chapters is the emphasis on listening to the views of the patient whether these views be expressed at the time or through an advance directive.

Doctors should be aware that the relationship between patient and doctor may subtly change when there can no longer be any expectation of restoring the patient to health. As the patient moves into a terminal stage, the focus will shift to support, ensuring the best quality of life and coming to terms with the situation. However, this shift should occur within the context of continuity. The general practitioner's role is often a continuing one, involving the whole family. The hospital health team may have treated the patient through previous stages of the disease or the patient may already have received care at home or in day-centres from hospice staff. When death becomes inevitable, the aim of treatment alters but this does not affect adherence to fundamental principles. Treatment is always patient-centred. The primacy of patient consent and confidentiality is undiminished, even though at the end of life people close to the patient may be drawn into decision-making.

Some people argue that medical ethics is excessively dominated by these issues of consent and confidentiality and the individual's competency to exercise them, to the virtual exclusion of other values such as care and commitment. At the end of life in particular, respect for each of these values should blend together in order to treat the whole patient by seeking to alleviate both physical and mental anguish. In many respects, this chapter simply draws attention to accepted practice. Nevertheless, since many patients fear that their rights may be compromised at the end of life, we believe it to be a valid and worthwhile exercise to rehearse the basic ethical principles in this particular context.

Death is an intrinsic part of life but a part which, generally, we all find hard to contemplate with equanimity. It is the event, more than any other in our existence, which emphasises the fundamental aloneness of the individual. Often, however, it is not death itself that people dread, but the manner, time and even place of death. Fears about "the threat of unacknowledged pain, denial of opportunity to talk about dying, impersonal institutions and technologised death" have been reflected in the literature from a wide variety of sources.[173] Many still harbour these fears. As is discussed in chapter 6, the upsurge in interest in measures such as advance directives, testifies to a broadly felt need for individuals to exercise some control over their dying process.

Various commentators have analysed society's attitudes to the dying. Some see a common perception of disease as being a deviation from the norm. Illness is perceived as excluding people from ordinary society, resulting in isolation, secrecy and loss of autonomy - all of which have characterised the experience of being sick. Most dying is done by the elderly, who have tended to live in relative obscurity on the periphery of society, so that terminal illness and death have often been hidden.[174] Society, however, now comprises a large elderly population whose rights and needs, while still not adequately met, are increasingly articulated. The development of HIV infection among young people may also radically affect the perception of death as being largely confined to the elderly. The pejorative social implications which presently surround the disease, however, have tended to increase secrecy and discrimination.

Some have seen community involvement in hospice provision over the last quarter of a century as a manifestation of a general change in attitudes to death. The hospice movement has shown that the period leading to the end of life can be one of personal development and strengthened relationships. Similarly, the isolation of sick people in general is being broken down by specialised medical and nursing groups as well as by voluntary organisations and self-help groups which support sufferers of particular diseases and their families.

## 5:2 The medical role

Patient expectations about the scope of the medical role have increased. Doctors and the health team are expected to fulfil multiple roles, providing medical skills, psychological support, and scientific and philosophical insight. Although this approach might be thought to conform with the spirit of Hippocrates who took the view that every physician should be a philosopher, it raises the question of the type of training, with which doctors need to be provided if they are to meet these demands. The issue of such training very much concerns the Association.

### 5:2.1 *Training*

For many medical students the first encounter with the human body occurs in the dissection-room, with no sense of the deceased as a person. Death has traditionally been represented as a failure of medical effort. Medical training, reflecting wider attitudes in society, has tended to the view that attempts to extend life should be made almost regardless of the circumstances. Such views are undergoing reappraisal as health professionals respond to patients' claims to choose among the treatments on offer. Nevertheless, many patients still fear that a full battery of medical technology will be gratuitously employed to prolong their dying. Training must include the importance of listening to patients.

The BMA is encouraged by the growing recognition that training in a range of skills, including communication and providing emotional support, needs to be given to health professionals who care for dying patients. It is clear that regardless of how well intentioned doctors may be, their relationships with their terminally ill patients can be severely and irrevocably damaged by inadequate communication skills. Particularly in relation to treatment at the end of life, it is imperative that all doctors receive training in recognising patients' needs for comfort, counselling, more or less detail, or simply a breathing space prior to receiving more information. It is our belief that such training must fully recognise the importance of the doctor's role in dealing with the patient's psychological pain as well as his or her physical symptoms. Senior clinicians who have developed the appropriate skills are invaluable role-models. They have an ethical duty to share this expertise, just as much as their other clinical skills, with less experienced colleagues. In this context, doctors may also profit from the high levels of expertise acquired by other professionals, including specialised nurses and other colleagues.

### 5:2.2 *The GP's role*

Although it calls upon the same skills and judgement, the experience of death in general practice is somewhat different from the experience of death in hospital. The GP has usually known the dying patient for some time and is not faced with the task of beginning a relationship with a patient who may already be in a state of crisis. Ideally, doctor and patient will already have established a dialogue and the GP is likely to be familiar with the patient's values, relationships and general circumstances. These may have been discussed in detail if the patient has chosen to draft an advance directive. The doctor will often be aware not only of patients' attitudes to the provision of information and their ability to deal with it over a short or longer time-span, but also of the patient's views about treatment or non-treatment. The GP may also have insight into whether the patient's consent or refusal is compromised by pressure from relatives. In many areas, local guidelines have been produced on the handling of cases where such pressure may also amount to exploitation or financial abuse of an elderly or confused patient.

For GPs, the patient's death is often not the end of a process, since they may have a role in caring for the bereaved if these people also happen to be the doctor's patients. Having obligations to other people close to the patient may present particular dilemmas for the GP. Sometimes the relatives let it be known that, in the event of a life-threatening disease being diagnosed, they do not wish the patient to be fully informed of it. The GP may need to explore with them the fears which lie behind such a request in the hope that these fears can be overcome and improve communication between all concerned. Patients also may not wish those close to them to be aware of the prognosis. In such circumstances, the doctor should counsel the patient about the desirability of preparing those close to him or her. Vital last opportunities for communication or reconciliation may otherwise be lost. Part of the general perception of a "good death" involves patients and those close to them sharing the experience as fully as possible and supporting each other. The GP is often best placed to help the patient in preparing others to come to terms with the situation. (See also 5:3.4.1 below.)

The potentially extended responsibility of the GP to others in the family may give rise to particular difficulties, especially if anticipatory grief makes the relatives critical of the doctor. This is again an area where well developed communication skills help to minimise difficulties which have no complete solution.

## 5:3 Approaches to care

Care of the dying must be founded on the same ethical principles as the treatment of all other patients. Health professionals caring for the dying are aware of the continuing importance of respect for patient autonomy, provision of information for decision-making and the safeguarding of patient confidentiality. Patients, however, may need reassurance that these fundamental concepts will not be glossed over. Although doctors often may find it easier to talk to those close to the patient rather than to the actual patient, this is a breach of confidentiality, and quite apart from that, giving information to relatives first can cause difficulties with patient insight later in the illness. While the patient remains competent, extension

135

of the doctor-patient dialogue to include relatives and others should not take place without the patient's acquiesence. (See also chapter 2, section 2:4.2.1 for possible exceptions.)

### 5:3.1 *The hospice/palliative care movement*

The modern hospice movement was established in the 1950s and, although providing actual care for a very small minority of terminally ill patients, has exerted a tremendously positive influence and has raised the standards of terminal care. It has shown how effective symptom relief, good communication and psychologically supportive care can permit patients to live out their remaining lifespan to the fullest possible extent. Organisational audit of palliative care services supports work on general standards for the care of the dying but also promotes the principle that this philosophy of care is equally applicable throughout the course of a life-threatening disease, from diagnosis onwards and in any health care setting. Home-care schemes, run by hospice staff, which began in the late 1960s, have given rise to a wide range of programmes throughout the NHS for supporting patients and families at home.

In 1992, a National Council for Hospice and Palliative Care Services was established to link the work of regional organisations, in the same way as was the Scottish Partnership Agency for Palliative and Cancer Care co-ordinates services in Scotland. It liaises with bodies involved in palliative care and seeks to promote the highest standard of clinical care, professional education, audit and research. The BMA welcomes the growth of such advisory bodies, seeing a particular need for non-palliative specialists to have access, on an individual basis if necessary, to the pain control expertise developed in the hospice setting. The dilemma for non-specialists in confronting apparently intractable pain in seriously ill patients was brought home in 1992, when a doctor was convicted of the attempted murder of a patient whose pain he was unable to assuage.[175] The continuing dilemmas of coping with such situations are discussed in chapter 6 (section 6:2.2.3) but it is to be hoped that they will be significantly reduced by increasing access to palliative specialists.

It is essential that doctors master techniques to control pain and distressing symptoms. In addition to the technical skills required, the doctor needs to be able to develop a relationship with the patient. Dying patients may show a wide range of emotions and the doctor must be able to respond appropriately. In this sphere, the educative influence of experienced hospice staff cannot be over-valued.

It is clear, however, that not all patients wish to receive hospice care and ideally patient autonomy should dictate where care is provided. It is equally clear that the total annual figure of cancer deaths alone outnumbers the availability of hospice beds (there are thought to be about 150,000 cancer deaths annually but only about 2,500 hospice beds in

England and Wales.[176] Currently some 15 per cent of cancer patients are treated in hospices during their terminal period although many more are treated at home by hospice staff). Nevertheless, the movement has focused attention on the importance of tailoring expertise in palliative and counselling skills to individual requirements.

### 5:3.2 *Keeping a distance*

Traditionally doctors have been taught to concentrate on the mechanisms of treatment. They have found it easier and safer for their emotional survival to distance themselves from the emotional issues surrounding death and mental deterioration. Thus doctors have sometimes found it particularly difficult to discuss prospective death where general degenerative processes and mental deterioration are involved (where questions of quality of life often arise) and easier when death is a clear probability in relation to a definable disease.[177] There is now greater public awareness of conditions such as dementia and greater willingness to discuss their implications. Because patients have a particular need to know in advance about potential degeneration of mental faculties in order to decide whether an advance directive is an appropriate measure for them, it is important that information about this be given sensitively in good time. Advance directives are discussed fully in chapter 6 (section 6:3.3).

Dying patients have often complained that they are avoided and "written off" by doctors who may feel threatened by their inability to offer a cure. While distancing oneself may be helpful for the doctor, it is not helpful for the patient or relatives. In our view, there must be a middle ground upon which a mutually respecting relationship can be built. Dying patients want reassurance that their doctor is interested in them as individuals right up to death.

### 5:3.3 *"Medical friendship"*

The concept of partnership between doctor and patient appears throughout our discussions in this book. That partnership might also be described as "medical friendship", a view of which is given below. Granted, it digresses somewhat from currently popular moral approaches to patient care, nevertheless the notion of friendship serves to illustrate a valid approach, which is not inconsistent with the fundamentally rights-and-duty-based theories which might seem to predominate. Although emphasis is rightly given to the patient's right of personal autonomy and the doctor's duty to provide adequate information, a further important consideration is the establishment of trust between doctor and patient.

Hippocratic tradition gives pre-eminence to the doctor's responsibility to benefit and not harm the patient. This responsibility was developed in the classical-mediaeval concept of the role of virtue in medicine. "Medical

137

friendship" describes the relationship between the virtuous physician and the patient and arises from the observance of the virtue of beneficence.

Modern medical training may give the impression that the scope of the doctor's role is limited to what applied medical knowledge can do for an individual patient. Accordingly, doctors are seen as acting for the good of the patient when they apply objectivity, scientific integrity and conscientiousness to the exercise of professional expertise. When Thomas Percival was drawing up one of the first English codes of medical ethics in 1803,[178] character traits such as tenderness and steadiness were emphasised as essential for doctors. Nowadays, doctors are sometimes criticised for concentrating only on acquiring a high level of technical skills and failing to give enough attention to listening to and establishing rapport with the patient or demonstrating characteristics such as sympathy. This falls short of the essential requirements of "medical friendship" which requires compassion, empathy, advocacy, beneficence and perhaps most of all, a willingness to be involved.

The concept of "medical friendship" would seem to be particularly relevant and potentially therapeutic in the treatment of the dying. This is not a denial of rights-based or duty-based ethics, but a recognition that the provision of medical treatment is considerably more complicated than providing patients with information and a list of options. The vulnerability and dependence of the sick person at the end of life makes it all the more important that there is trust and confidence as well as the observation of rights and duties. Doctors should, and generally do, approach the dying with a deepened sense of how crucial it is to respond with sensitivity and feeling to patient need. Virtues of character such as veracity, honesty, integrity and courage are seen as important, in addition to the requisite diagnostic and technical skills, in order to practise medicine optimally. To avoid paternalism, such a relationship must reflect patients' rights to make choices and doctors' duties to empower patients.

Doctors are expected to act in the patient's interests and to place those interests above their own. In practical terms, this means that a doctor cannot, for example, refuse to treat a patient on the grounds that the patient's condition might pose a threat to the health of the doctor.[179] Patients' interests may be separated into diverse components such as their personal values and perception of their own best personal and medical interests. There may be conflicting components within a particular case or conflicts may arise between patients and other people: according to the circumstances different weights will be accorded to different interests. For example, the patient may prefer a course of treatment which does not necessarily give the best clinical outcome but is most compatible with the patient's lifestyle and values. Patients' personal interests may take precedence over their medical interests. In other cases, however, if the patient is unconscious or otherwise unable to express an opinion, there may be disagreement between the people involved in clinical decisions as to what course of action is in the patient's interests. People close to the patient may be able to say what would have been the patient's view of his or her own best interests and thus a hierarchical order can be established among the conflicting values.

### 5:3.4 *The changing relationship*

Various studies have attempted to define a point at which the attitudes of health professionals change as the patient enters what Kubler-Ross[180] terms the "pre-death" stage. The patient recognises that death is approaching and medical and nursing staff, acknowledging that the patient is indeed dying, move towards managing the death by concentrating on palliative care. A patient's acknowledgement of the approach of death is often a time for important communication.

"Palliative medicine" is the term used to describe the care of patients with active, progressive and far advanced disease, a limited prognosis and for whom the focus of care becomes quality of life. It is important that this change in focus is clearly recognised by patient, relatives and staff. Such recognition allows discussion of the management of death and bereavement. Some patients put the phase of struggling behind them, and come to a different perspective. Part of the staff recognition that death is approaching may involve symbolic acts such as removing all the previously prescribed medication and concentrating on pain control and communication.

### 5:3.4.1 *Facing reality*

In contrast with the changing awareness of the pre-death stage, all are familiar with the atmosphere of collusive disregard of reality, which has too often characterised the final months of life for many people as the patient and relatives try to protect each other from the truth. Even when doctors are willing to assist the patient and the family to face up to the inevitability of death, they often encounter strong social pressures to preserve an overly optimistic, rather than an honest, approach. Pressure to prevaricate should be resisted, but at the same time it should be recognised that individuals require varying degrees of time and support to assimilate what they are told.

The role of the health team in this situation includes attempting to help the patient and those close to the patient to face the reality in a compassionate way. Unwittingly, different members of the health care team sometimes contribute to the confusion because they hold different goals and objectives and are therefore giving different advice and information to the patient and relatives. Good communication between members of the health care team is essential and minimises the risks of conflicting messages being given.

139

# 5:4 Doctors' duties

The focus of this chapter is the individual needs of the dying patient. Having stated previously that we believe it to be worthwhile to explore other values rather than to concentrate solely on the themes of rights and duties, nevertheless we recognise the necessity of considering how both doctor and patient interpret these concepts. Thus, some aspects of the doctor's perceived duties to the dying patient are explored before proceeding to the claims the patient may lay upon the doctor.

## 5:4.1 *The doctor's duty to respect patient autonomy*

The principle of patient autonomy requires the empowering of patients through the provision of information. It is often in connection with the choices patients wish to make about controlling the end of their lives that doctors find patient autonomy most problematic. (See also 5:5 below on patient rights and chapter 6, section 6:3.2 on patients' rights to refuse life-prolonging treatment.)

As patients usually have ambivalent attitudes towards receiving information about a terminal prognosis doctors may have difficulty in carrying out their general duties to observe the patients' rights because of the way an individual patient chooses to exercise those rights.

### 5:4.1.1 *Provision of information*

Respect for patient autonomy involves sensitivity to the amount of detail required by individual patients and to the pace at which they may be prepared to receive it. This may be illustrated by an anecdote concerning an elderly patient, in whom a life-threatening condition was suspected. The patient underwent the necessary diagnostic tests but her comments left it unclear to the clinician whether or not she wished to know the full implications of the results. In further discussion, the patient eventually made clear that she did want to know this information but at a later stage, so that she and her family could enjoy Christmas first. Autonomy was enhanced rather than compromised by the clinician's withholding of information until the agreed time. The important point is that the cue came from the patient, not the doctor.

In our view, the dialogue between doctor and patient should include informing patients when there is medical uncertainty. There may be a number of reasons for uncertainty. Perhaps there is no "best treatment" for the patient's condition, or it is not clear how much the disease process has advanced. As stated previously, it must be recognised that both doctors and patients sometimes feel ambivalent about total frankness. Doctors may feel that by acknowledging uncertainty they are undermining the patient's confidence in the profession at a time when the patient most needs reassurance. Doctors may think that by presenting an appearance of certainty, which the circumstances do not justify, they are able to give a sense of hope and optimism, which may in itself be therapeutic. The difficulty for each doctor is how to evaluate the implicit messages from the individual patient in the face of a perhaps more generalised pressure from relatives to paint an optimistic picture.

### 5:4.1.2 Truth-telling

Honesty between doctor and patient is a key element in the partnership. The BMA stresses frankness and also the need to explore gently issues with the patient rather than brutally confront an unprepared patient with the truth. There is a school of thought, however, which places values such as beneficence above truth-telling, particularly in relation to news of terminal illness. Patients or their relatives occasionally complain to the BMA that information, especially about degenerative illness, has been given prematurely, before the onset of acute symptoms, and has thus deprived the patient of a period of "blissful ignorance". A major problem with such an approach is that it assumes an ability on the part of the doctor to know what is best for the patient. The view taken throughout this book is that individuals must make that assessment for themselves and need information in order to make it. In some cases patients need to know in order to take appropriate health measures to delay the progress of the disease. Information at an early stage may allow the patient time to accomplish plans which would be impossible later. Therefore the BMA strongly recommends that the primary objective must be frankness throughout the doctor-patient relationship, although individual circumstances may sometimes modify this ideal.

Amongst any group of people, however, there will be some who do not wish to know the full implications of their prognosis but we believe this can be reconciled with patient autonomy. When a doctor decides to convey to the patient something less than the full implications of the illness, such a decision must be based on the perception that such withholding is the patient's clear desire rather than the doctor's interpretation of what is best for the patient. The aim must be to prepare the patient to receive the information. This advice could easily be over-simplified and used as an argument for depriving patients of choice. We believe, however, that doctors are very much alive to these difficulties.

## 5:5 Patient rights

Various attempts have been made to construct a bill or table of rights for patients and since those nearing the end of life are envisaged as being particularly vulnerable, such statements sometimes make specific reference to dying patients. The language of rights presupposes that others have corresponding duties to see that rights are respected. However, few rights can be absolute, since rights may impinge upon, or conflict with, the equally important rights of others. These issues are discussed further in general terms in chapter 12 which deals with the allocation of resources, and more specifically below with relation to the so-called "right to a good death" (see 5:5.4).

Earlier in this chapter we put forward the view that the treatment of dying patients must be based on the same ethical principles as that of other patients, observing the same rights of autonomy and confidentiality. It is sometimes asked whether the dying acquire additional rights which they do not have as ordinary patients. The usual response to this is that while the dying may have a greater claim on our attention and compassion, they may not override the rights of others. The dying may acquire great power over those around them and make unjust or unreasonable demands on their families or on health professionals. Doctors must, however, constantly examine what appear to be unreasonable demands and question the criteria by which they appear unreasonable. Such demands often arise from an unexplored need that should be addressed. Nevertheless, there may be situations where doctors have a responsibility to tell patients that their rights and authority are limited. Thus, one of the major challenges to doctors caring for terminally ill patients is how to handle those patient demands which are founded on claims of autonomy and choice, but which cannot be satisfied.

### 5:5.1 *Rights of autonomy and choice*

In many contexts the patient's right of autonomy is seen to be somehow in conflict with the trust which ideally should exist between doctors and patients: the latter feeling a need to demand something as of right because they do not trust that the doctor is doing what is best for them. In our view, however, the concepts of autonomy and trust are not mutually exclusive. Trust and autonomy are both supported and enhanced by dialogue and sensitive communication.

Problems frequently arise because trust has faltered. A typical example concerns a treatment which a patient desires but which, in the view of the doctor, is not in the patient's best interest. Treatment which was previously helpful may no longer be effective. The clinician may propose another, which implicitly recognises that the patient is entering the final phases of illness. For symbolic and emotional reasons, as well as a possible conviction that the old treatment could still be beneficial, the patient invokes the rights of autonomy and choice. It is not a question of the patient being deprived of the information which would support the doctor's advice but rather that the patient is not ready to acknowledge the validity of the information and may seek further medical opinions to prove the doctor wrong.

Doctors are not obliged to provide a treatment which they consider not to be in the patient's interest, but sometimes a compromise can restore trust. Such a compromise might involve either another medical opinion or postponing for a limited period the proposed change of treatment. When neither of these options is possible, and trust appears irrevocably lacking, it may well be in the patient's best interests to be referred to a colleague. It is tragic for the doctor-patient relationship if, as a result of some misunderstanding or lack of rapport, a doctor feels unfairly criticised, or a patient is beset by doubt, about the management of the illness.

Dilemmas often arise when patients have exhausted all the treatment possibilities of conventional medicine and places their last hopes in an unproven therapy. This is not a problem if the clinician is willing to take responsibility for supervising such therapy, either because it alleviates symptoms or because it provides a psychological benefit to the patient and does no harm. It is immensely more difficult when the clinician believes that the therapy in question can achieve nothing or could even be harmful if its implementation causes a delay in more useful treatment being given. After advising patients of the reasons why they cannot support the proposed therapy, it is our advice that clinicians should not appear to abandon those patients but should continue with all those aspects of care which lie within the clinicians' control.

### 5:5.2 *The right to information*

As is discussed more fully in chapter 1 (section 1:2.4) and chapter 8 (section 8:6.2), the BMA's advice is that doctors should seek to be as frank as possible with patients. In the past, information was withheld on the grounds that it would distress the patient and in some exceptional cases as indicated in 5:4.1.2 above, this argument may still be relevant when based on a clear cue from the patient. Sometimes information is held back because further confirmation of the diagnosis is required. Depending upon the patient's receptivity and desire for information, we believe honesty to be the best policy from an early stage.

### 5:5.3 *The right to privacy*

Privacy in the sense of confidentiality is discussed fully in chapter 2 but there are also other aspects of privacy, such as the freedom from interference by others. This involves a right to a freedom from medical intervention when their patients have declined treatment (see chapter 6, section 6:3.2) or patients' right to be heard and to have their beliefs respected. Doctors and other health professionals should seek to explore whether the patient has a need for spiritual care and if this is being met by pastoral counselling. The dying person may wish to discuss personal, moral or spiritual problems, knowing that health professionals will not only safeguard the confidence of discussions but will also refrain from imposing their own moral or religious advice. Perhaps most difficult of all for the health professional is the aspect of privacy which is embodied in the patient's right to reject not only treatment, but all the other offers of help or advice.

### 5:5.4 *The right to a good death*

In our view, patients clearly have a right to be looked after by caring, sensitive and experienced professionals who will attempt to understand the patient's needs and support patients facing the process of their own death. What is sought, however, by some who espouse this right, is not simply a right of access to the best available terminal care, but also the acknowledgement that the patient has a right to choose to die by electing "voluntary euthanasia". This is an area where we believe that the wishes of the individual may conflict with the rights of others. This is discussed fully in chapter 6 (section 6:8).

For many people, one facet of a peaceful death is the knowledge that their religious or cultural beliefs concerning appropriate treatment of their bodies after death will be respected. It is important that health professionals discuss with the patient, if appropriate, or with those close to the patient, how the body will be handled after death to conform with the individual's cultural or religious customs while it remains on hospital or hospice premises.

### 5:5.5 *The right to support*

Dying should not be an event suffered in isolation. When the patient's symptoms have been adequately controlled and communication is a possibility, the crisis of dying, like the other crises of life, can become an opportunity for reconciliation and growth. Ideally, support for the patient should come from family members and other people close to the patient.

## 5:6 Caring for the carers

### 5:6.1 *Those close to the patient*

Care of the dying usually involves provision of comfort to those close to the patient. Good communication and team care at an earlier stage can help to ease the pain of bereavement. Much preparatory work falls to specialised nursing staff or to GPs. After the patient has died, it is usual and comforting to see death as a release for the patient, but a sense of guilt and fear of criticism often prevent people from also admitting beforehand that the death of the patient may represent a relief for them.

### 5:6.2 *Support for the medical team*

It is increasingly recognised that caring for dying and bereaved people also takes its toll on health professionals specialising in terminal care.

Forming necessarily impermanent, although rewarding, relationships with patients is draining and being constantly exposed to suffering, helplessness, uncertainty, anger and loss is demoralising for health staff. Fortunately awareness of the importance of stress-management skills and the prevention of "burnout" is growing.

Colleagues, senior staff and managers need to provide support and to ensure that all health professionals have opportunities for discussion of particular and general problems. Such support must ensure a fair distribution of difficult burdens, since problems may arise when willing individuals fail to recognise their own needs. Continuing education and regular appraisal are vital elements in coming to terms with this work - or with the fact that one is unsuited to it. The setting aside of regular time to learn about research and ways of working with the dying is essential and helps health workers to keep their work in perspective within the whole spectrum of care. Regrettably because admitting one's difficulties in coping may have professional and career implications, we feel it is important that those who care for the dying should consider seeking counselling and support in a confidential and non-hierarchical setting outside the place of work.

## 5:7 Summary

1   Trust, confidence and dialogue are vital aspects of the doctor-patient relationship at all stages. At the end of life, the importance of, and need for, a good relationship is obvious.
2   Medical training should include the particular skills necessary for caring for the dying such as symptom relief techniques, effective communication, counselling and stress management.
3   Respect for the patient's autonomy and confidentiality must be no less at the end of the patient's life than at other times.
4   Patients have the right to exercise their autonomy and control to the fullest possible extent at the end of their lives. Doctors provide patients with information to enable them to do this but, particularly at the end of life, the doctor-patient relationship demands more than the simple provision by the doctor of a list of options.
5   Good communication between all members of the health care team is essential.
6   Dying patients must be seen and treated as whole individuals. There is a need to respect all aspects of their life and personality and address the patient's mental as well as physical pain.
7   Patients have a right to be looked after by caring, sensitive and experienced professionals who will attempt to understand patient needs and help patients to face death.

8   Dying should not be an event suffered in isolation but should ideally involve those close to the patient.
9   The quality of life for the dying patient may be as important as the length. Patients have the right to be allowed to die with dignity when they do not desire further treatment.

# 6 Cessation of Treatment, Non-Resuscitation, Aiding Suicide and Euthanasia

*Introduction and background to the debate. An attempt to set a framework of guidance including reference to fundamental principles of autonomy, justice, beneficence and non-maleficence and an examination of how values may conflict. The lessons which might be drawn from practice in the Netherlands and the difficulties in interpreting the evidence. Professional standards, the law, personal morality and conscientious objection. Non-treatment decisions including patient consent and refusal, broaching difficult issues with patients, advance directives and proxy decision-makers. Standards of assessment including quality of life and best interests. Resolving disputes between decision-makers. Withdrawing treatment, withdrawing nutrition. Non-resuscitation decisions and guidelines including the importance of communication between members of the health team. Aiding suicide. Euthanasia. Summary.*

## 6:1 Introduction

In the previous chapter on "care of the dying", we attempted to draw the attention of the public and profession to where we believe the true focus of the debate about the end of life should lie: the provision of a high standard of palliative care and support, the aim of which is to sustain and prepare the patient and the family for the inevitable approach of death.

In chapter 5, we have tried to show that death is not a medical failure and that the doctor's ability to relieve the suffering associated with dying is a positive achievement. Health care extends over all phases of a patient's life and into his or her death. Health care professionals are required to provide good quality service at all times. A good death is therefore a proper part of good health care. The health team is urged to support, and not to appear to abandon, the dying patient. The importance of such attitudes is well recognised with regard to palliative care and in this context we also discussed the necessity for effective pain and symptom control. We do not consider a doctor should seek to achieve a "good death" for a patient if this means aiming to bring about a premature death.

147

### 6:1.1 *Aim of this chapter*

In this chapter we aim to establish a broad framework, within which doctors can scrutinise and resolve individual cases. We examine three broad themes: ceasing treatment, aiding suicide and euthanasia. Such issues, concerning as they do, the end of life, are central to philosophy, religion and medical ethics. This chapter cannot hope to reflect the full range of thinking on these matters: what it does attempt is to give plain and practical guidance for doctors. Unavoidably, complex themes are evoked, some of which are debated more fully in other parts of this book. Among them are important questions of individual freedom, for both patients and doctors, who have a right to abstain from participation in treatment they consider unacceptable. Questions are also raised about the nature of consent, including consent given in advance or on behalf of other adults. Furthermore, in contexts where patients cannot express their own views, doctors are accustomed to being asked to assess what constitutes that person's "best interests" or to outline the possible benefits of continued treatment. This requires some examination of the criteria for such assessment, including whether death can ever be in a patient's "interest" and whether treatment given to a permanently comatose person, for example, can be considered to "benefit" that person. A common thread is sought through widely differing situations.

The focus of the chapter is on treatment options for the individual. Therefore some issues traditionally associated with death but not linked to treatment of the dying individuals are discussed elsewhere. Principal among these is organ donation, which involves the dead in producing benefits for the living. This issue is discussed in chapter 1 on consent (section 1:7.1.4 and 1:7.1.5). It may seem self-evident to state that the duty of confidentiality remains the same for all patients but nevertheless it bears repetition. This duty is not, for example, modified by a patient's suicide attempt, request for euthanasia or approaching death. General principles concerning confidentiality are outlined in chapter 2.

## 6:2 General purposes of the debate

### 6:2.1 *The categories of medical action*

Four categories of medical action can be considered relevant to this debate.

a)   The alleviation of distress by use of opioids and sedatives in such dosages that the patient's life will, or may, be shortened. The use of such drugs does not inevitably lead to the shortening of life. In some cases sedating with anxiolytic drugs may be the only way to alleviate patient distress. Such drugs should not be withheld. Effective pain and symptom relief at the end of life must be a first priority. The

Association believes that fewer patients would seek to end their lives prematurely if they felt assured of a pain-free end, and this should be attainable for the vast majority of patients. The BMA regards control of physical pain and distress where the treatment required, for example, anxiolytic drugs, is acceptable to the patient, as an essential facet of ethical medical practice. Under no circumstances should such medication be rationed. Some patients will choose to endure a degree of pain in preference to any loss of alertness. Such a choice is consistent with patient autonomy and the accepted concept of continually adjusted care. Thus patient refusal of pain control, as refusal of any treatment proposal, must be respected and does not affect the right of the patient to receive supportive care or comforting, or to change his or her mind at any time regarding refusal.

b)  The term "non-treatment" is used of medical decisions not to give a specific treatment even though the application of that treatment would probably prolong the patient's life. As chapter 1 (section 1:6.1) recognises, competent patients have a right to refuse any treatment, including life-prolonging treatment. Such a right is undisputed. Decisions by doctors not to provide or to withdraw treatment, without patient authorisation, raise a separate issue, which is part of the subject matter of this chapter. Doctors have a responsibility to use their considered judgement with regard to appropriate treatment, and a duty not to provide or continue treatment which they feel is not in the patient's best interests.

c)  Aiding suicide is not an activity which concerns doctors alone, since any person can do this. It is usually understood to consist in providing the means or advice to commit suicide. To be an accessory, it is apparently sufficient that the individual (i) knew that the particular deed was contemplated and (ii) that he or she approved of or assented to it and (iii) that his or her attitude in respect of it in fact encouraged the principal offender to perform the deed. The prescription or supplying of drugs with the intention of enabling patients to end their lives falls within this category, as may the provision of advice or literature on the subject.

d)  An active medical intervention to end life is commonly termed "euthanasia". The literal meaning of "euthanasia" a gentle and easy death, has no untoward ethical implications. The term has come to be associated with the "mercy killing" of people suffering from painful and incurable disease. It can, however, be used to refer to all forms of, and motivations for, bringing about death by medical means or by medically qualified people. The qualifiers "active" and "passive" are often applied to "euthanasia" but do not lead to

149

precision in argument. We have tried to avoid imprecision in this discussion, by referring to medical interventions to end life when this is what we mean.

Among these options, (a) and (b) can be distinguished from (c) and (d) by the intention behind them. Society recognises that there is a range of clinical decisions whose effect may be to bring forward or delay death. When the side effect of a treatment hastens death, doctors lack an intention to kill. In such cases, it is not the doctor who causes death but the patient's illness or injury. Such acts or omissions by a doctor have "an incidental effect of determining the exact moment of death" but are not considered "the cause of death in any sensible use of the term".[181] On the other hand, the law makes clear that "no doctor, nor any man, no more in the case of the dying than the healthy, has the right deliberately to cut the thread of life."[182]

To some people, however, decisions not to resuscitate, not to treat a treatable condition, to prescribe sedatives, to help patients to obtain lethal drugs or intentionally to administer a fatal dose may simply seem progressive steps on a continuum of possible medical options. Clearly, all may result in the death of the patient and this will have been foreseen at the time of making the decision. In the view of the law and the majority of the medical profession, such a range of options cannot be subsumed under the rubric of clinical decision-making. The last options are distinguishable from the others on several grounds, not least of which is their clear illegality. Even more fundamentally, they change irrevocably the ethical relationship between doctor and patient.

The BMA firmly maintains that, if doctors are authorised to kill or help kill, however carefully circumscribed the situation, they acquire an additional role which is alien to the traditional one of healer. In some circumstances it may be that neither patient nor carers, and perhaps not even the doctors themselves, can be quite certain which role has been adopted. The available evidence[183] suggests that some doctors placed in this position adopt psychological defence mechanisms which enable them to avoid the pain of trying to reconcile two distinct and conflicting roles. Moreover doctors would be acting in a way which many see as radically inconsistent with recognising the dignity which belongs to every human being.

### 6:2.2 Conflicting imperatives

Decisions about the provision or withdrawal of treatment always have importance for the individuals involved. When, however, those decisions have life or death implications, interests far wider than those of the individual case are called into play. The way in which the professional and society resolve the dilemmas posed by life or death cases reflect our most deeply held moral beliefs about the value of life and the qualities which make it valuable; the scope and limits of individual autonomy and the balancing of benefit for one patient with the possibility of causing harm to other patients. Nowhere are the conflicts between ethical imperatives more acute than in the debate about treatment at the end of life. If society is prepared, as it seems to be, to overrule the desires of some individuals in pursuit of a perceived wider public good, the grounds for such a view must be carefully analysed and open for public debate. (See also chapter 12 on rationing and allocation of health care resources, since rationing decisions may involve similar concepts of a balance between satisfying in full the needs of one individual or meeting the lesser needs of a much larger number).

In chapter 13, we have discussed some of the moral values to be considered in arriving at ethically justifiable decisions. There, we have also pointed out the difficulties inherent in any effort to rank these moral values in order of priority. The potential for conflict between them is particularly illustrated when they are applied to life or death decisions.

*6:2.2.1 Autonomy and justice*

We have consistently emphasised the importance of patient autonomy and rights, reflecting the weight society assigns to individual freedom of choice. Supporters of a right to die often present this issue as one of personal liberty, maintaining that therefore individuals should be entitled to assistance to end their lives at the time and in the manner they choose. The BMA, however, maintains that autonomy has limits. The rights of one group cannot be permitted to undermine the rights of others. Recognising a legal right to die would have implications for the whole of society and, perhaps, most particularly for its vulnerable members.

Thus many doctors fear that even a limited change in the legislation would bring about a profound change in society's attitude to euthanasia. By removing legal barriers to the previously "unthinkable" and permitting people to be killed, society would open up new possibilities of action and thus engender a frame of mind whereby some individuals might well feel bound to explore fully the extent of those new options. Once a previously prohibited action becomes allowed, the argument goes, it may also come to be seen as desirable - if not by oneself, then as something which might be recommended for others. The specific fear being that those "others" will typically be the elderly: a particular worry at a time when an increasingly ageing population is raising the question of imbalance between financial providers and financial dependents in many developed countries. The choice of exercising a right to die at a chosen and convenient time could become an issue all individuals would have to take into account, even though they might otherwise not have entertained the notion.

In Germany in the 1930s voluntary euthanasia led to an extension of the practice of euthanasia beyond those who sought it. This raises the

151

common "slippery slope" argument that permitting voluntary euthanasia may result in non-voluntary euthanasia since the safeguards against the latter would have been weakened or because the reasoning underpinning claims for a right of voluntary euthanasia could easily be extended to those incapable of making any claim for themselves.

Similarly in the United Kingdom, a social environment which recognised the right to die, we argue, would bring about a fundamental shift in social attitudes to death, illness, old age and disablement. It would encourage the labelling of people by group and result in some groups who presented problems being seen as more expendable. It would also change the public view of the role of the profession in an irrevocable way and undermine the trust that patients have in doctors. At present, the Netherlands is the only model, the only place where we can look for guidance as to whether or not an acceptance of euthanasia does bring about wide-ranging changes in society's attitudes to euthanasia. Euthanasia in the Netherlands remains a punishable offence, but its practice has a degree of legal sanction in that doctors who follow medical guidelines, approved by Parliament, are guaranteed immunity from prosecution. Many find the Dutch evidence difficult to assess. Although batteries of statistics resulting from the Remmelink[184] report have been issued, the interpretations drawn from the statistics appear variable and somewhat difficult to compare, partly due to different definitions adopted by commentators as to what constitutes "euthanasia". We therefore make only brief reference here to the Dutch situation.

Despite the difficulties of obtaining an unambiguous overview, one indication of the views of Dutch society might be seen in the admission[185] in 1987 of one leading paediatric oncologist that he supplies young patients with poison which would enable them to commit suicide, some with parental consent and others without. A subsequent opinion poll[186] indicated that almost 70 per cent of the Dutch public supported this course of action. Furthermore, while the Royal Dutch Society of Medicine has declared support for the non-voluntary euthanasia of neonates, minors, mentally retarded people and elderly people suffering from dementia in those "cases in which one can suppose that were the patients able to express their will, they would opt for euthanasia", the BMA opposes such views, not least on the grounds that such comments appear to classify whole groups of people as particularly eligible for premature death. BMA members are generally very far from seeing such measures as a solution. British doctors' anxiety typically appears to centre on whether more could be done to solve the problems which make patients' lives intolerable, rather than focusing on allowing such lives to end. The difference in attitudes is apparent. What is difficult to know, however, is whether such Dutch attitudes are genuinely reflected in the published material and if so, whether they have been affected by changes in practice in the Netherlands or pre-date them.

Interestingly, it has been claimed that the medical decisions and patterns of treatment prior to patient deaths in the Netherlands are similar in many cases to those generally considered acceptable in this country. One extrapolation[187] from the Remmelink report indicated, for example, that 38 per cent of all deaths in Holland involve a medical decision relevant to the end of life but that most of these would have been considered acceptable practice in other countries.[188]

Other views of the same material express a differing opinion, suggesting that almost one third of all euthanasia deaths in the Netherlands do not meet strict criteria and that the practice of euthanasia is being informally extended.[189] Some 1,000[190] (0.8% of all deaths) Dutch cases a year apparently involve the active termination of the patient's life without the patient requesting it. Such medical interventions do not meet the Dutch criteria for euthanasia and theoretically could be a cause for prosecution.

Various interpretations of the Remmelink report abound but all seem to agree that the so-called rules of careful conduct (official guidelines for euthanasia) are sometimes disregarded. Breaches of rules range from the practice of involuntary euthanasia to failure to consult another practitioner before carrying out euthanasia and to certifying the cause of death as natural. Some would see this as lending credence to the view that even careful circumscription of the practice cannot guarantee observance of the rules. The existence of rules permitting euthanasia in some circumstances might well have the effect of making instances of non-voluntary euthanasia, or even medical error, harder to detect.

The BMA fears that, were the law in this country to be relaxed, euthanasia would become an option for anybody facing death. That does not mean that everyone would seek euthanasia but some people might realistically fear that others would choose it for them. This too is exhibited to some degree in the Netherlands where studies appear to indicate that some elderly people fear their lives will be ended without their consent[191] and that, in fact, families request euthanasia more often than the patient.[192] This may be because, as has been shown in many studies, relatives perceive the patient as enduring worse suffering than patients themselves report.

The aim of this chapter, however, is not to analyse the Dutch situation but rather to look at how changes in practice may alter attitudes. If the option of active medical intervention to end life were on the British agenda, the BMA believes that the climate of opinion in which care at the end of life is considered would be radically altered.

All members of society must be guaranteed equal protection from pressure. It is frequently argued that if a patient's desire to be killed by a doctor were recognised as a legitimate right, elderly or disabled people might see their lives as burdensome to others and feel pressured to choose to end them. It is possible that the rights of some to choose how they die would undermine the rights of others to live and the demands of justice would be ignored.

### 6:2.2.2 Beneficence and non-maleficence

Similar arguments could be constructed to show that on the question of a right to die, (ie to be killed) individual autonomy can also come into conflict with the medical duties to do no harm and to benefit others. To some extent, however, such arguments are dependent upon the definitions of "harm" and "benefit". For people who would prefer to control and end their lives, "harm" is seen in the contradiction of their wishes, or the physical pain or indignity that might accompany death. "Benefit" lies in the removal of such concerns. Such a viewpoint is based on the predicate that some people who would prefer to be dead, would indeed be better off dead. What doctors find difficult with this argument is its logical consequence. If death is a benefit that competent people can choose, then incompetent people in comparable situations should not be deprived of it. The concept of voluntariness can quickly be lost. Also, some people might request euthanasia because of feeling they are a burden to others. Beneficence would require that they be assured of their worth and that efforts be made to avoid the impression that their lives lacked value.

Doctors are trained to recognise that they have a duty to benefit others and to avoid risk of harm unless this is outweighed by potential benefit to the patient. In the traditionally accepted medical view, life implies "benefit" and death implies "harm". So, to ask doctors to benefit patients by causing their death or harm them by not doing so, appears to many doctors a contradiction in terms.

In the BMA's opinion, "beneficence" is reflected in the profession's efforts to achieve total pain control for patients nearing the end of their lives. It considers that accepting patients have a right to die might well interfere with efforts to achieve such high standards of pain control since it would sometimes prove an easier option to kill the patient than investigate the proper management of relief.

Hospices have now demonstrated that in the majority of cases pain can be controlled by an appropriate analgesic in appropriate doses at regular intervals. The World Health Organisation's guidelines involve the use of an "analgesic ladder", including non-opioids, mild and strong opioids. The WHO publication "Cancer Pain Relief" states that "complete pain relief was reported by 87 per cent of patients, while acceptable relief was achieved in a further 9 per cent and partial relief in the remaining 4 per cent.[193] Methods of pain control are continuously being improved.

In contrast, a fairly recent Dutch study,[194] based on patients admitted to the Netherlands Cancer Institute, indicated that for 54 per cent of patients (42 cases out of the final 79 studied) cancer pain was inadequately managed, but with relatively better management being offered in hospital than at home.

Some might be tempted to draw the conclusion from this that less attention may be being given to effective training in controlling pain when the option of actively ending the patient's life is available. To draw such a conclusion may be to place too much significance on one example but the BMA remains concerned that eliminating the patient rather than striving to eliminate the pain may seem an easier solution.

Despite the availability of effective pain management measures, misconceptions among health professionals in the past led to the under-treatment of some patients.[195] There has previously been hesitation among doctors and nurses about providing the necessary degree of pain relief because of concern about drug tolerance, addiction or fear of shortening the patient's life. Yet numerous studies[196] indicate that psychological dependence occurs rarely in cancer patients receiving narcotics for pain and, in any case, the possibility of such dependence should not be a major obstacle to narcotic use, especially in terminal-stage patients. It is now emphasised that relief of physical and mental distress must be the first aim of treatment at the end of life.

### 6:2.2.3 A continuing dilemma

The BMA recognises, however, that for a very small minority of patients it may not be possible to control completely pre-terminal pain and distress by conventional means. Even hospices, which can confidently claim to control suffering in most cases, recognise that in a small number[197] of cases modern palliative care may be insufficient. The additional expertise provided by experienced anaesthetists, surgeons or others may, however, provide solutions for individual cases.

The task of assessing where the patient's "benefit" lies in such cases poses immense problems for doctors, on a scale rarely broached by other professionals. Clearly, the profession must hope soon to arrive at the situation where all pain and distress can be controlled by skilled management. Until that time, however, there will be exceptional cases where death is inevitable but slow and sedation may be the only solution. Some argue that in some such cases, and when the dying patient and the doctor "stand in a special relationship", a caring doctor may take exceptional action and also be exempted from the legal rules and moral principles to which all other doctors and members of society are subject.[198] The BMA however would not wish to see any change in the law. Its view is based on the principle that any moral stance founded on the permissibility of active termination of life in some circumstances may lead to a climate of opinion where it becomes not merely permissible but desirable, as discussed above. The BMA considers that doctors must always be answerable before the law and the General Medical Council for the decisions they make. Doctors who have patients with apparently intractable pain should ensure that they seek expert advice from specialists in symptom control regarding the management of pain including the use of anaesthesia and nerve blocks. In our view, the primary focus must be an effective training in control of pain and distress.

It is increasingly found that some patients will choose to tolerate a little pain if the quality of life is otherwise good: experience suggests that pain, even when modestly present, is often the least of the issues affecting quality of life. In our experience, many requests for euthanasia are not based on the presence of pain, but on the patient's increasing sense of worthlessness and dependence on others. Only by provision of skilled and compassionate palliative care, including "medical friendship", can the patient have a restored sense of worthwhile identity. Willingness by society to supply or condone euthanasia will merely confirm the patient's sense of worthlessness, resulting in a society where individuals are not deemed valuable unless demonstrably useful.

### 6:2.2.4 The imperative to use technology to the full

Some claim that contemporary medical practice is conducted in a climate of tension between the emphasis on respecting patient autonomy on the one hand, and an increasingly complex array of medical technology on the other. In other words, conflicting with patient autonomy and the individual's claim to control the end of life, are technological measures which can prolong that life and of which doctors feel bound to make full use, irrespective of patients' wishes. The BMA, however, feels such a view to be outdated and does not believe that doctors feel compelled to use technology "because it is there". Many of the practices that were controversial in the care of the dying patient a few years ago are now widely accepted. Do-not-resuscitate orders, for example, non-existent a few years ago, are now commonplace. Also the profession is increasingly persuaded of the value of measures such as advance directives. (The importance of discussion between doctor and patient in regard to both advance directives and do-not-resuscitate orders is discussed in 6:3.3 and 6:6 respectively.)

### 6:2.3 The law

Throughout this handbook emphasis is placed on what are perceived as ethical obligations, which may not necessarily be identical to legal duties. On the question of euthanasia, however, there is perceived to be a commonality between law and ethics. Despite an apparently increasing level of public interest in many countries in the possibility of doctors intervening to end life, there is little indication that law-makers would welcome change. Their resistance may be based on much the same reasons as those of doctors in many countries, who fear that a change in the law would divorce medical practice from its ethical roots. This reflects the profession's view that liberalising the law on euthanasia would herald a serious and incalculable change in the ethos of medicine. Although there is evidence that some doctors admit privately that they have taken active steps to hasten death,[199] it is generally held within the profession that individual doctors must be accountable for such decisions. Since the mid-19th century the BMA has considered that doctors cannot be held to a single and invariable ethical rule that applies to all patients in all circumstances. Equally, the exceptional case in no way invalidates the general rule.

Effective management of pain and distress which has the side-effect of curtailing life, is an acceptable and indeed necessary option of ethical practice. Dosage which is augmented in order to cause death is not. The law too lays great weight on the intention behind the action. The deliberate taking of life is categorised as murder and the courts have ruled that doctors are not entitled to special consideration.[200] Thus, a doctor acting with the intention of causing the patient's death can claim no special privilege and must be prepared to face the closest scrutiny of the law.

Doctors cannot rely entirely on the law for clarification of their duties, since the application of legal maxims to specific cases is often subject to complex and variable interpretation. In recent years, some widely differing legal cases concerned with the provision of life-sustaining treatment have laid emphasis on a general presumption in favour of life but only if the treatment confers some benefit and is not burdensome for the patient. (This is discussed further in 6:3.6.1 below.) The law recognises the right of refusal of life-sustaining treatments by a competent patient, but assessment of competency is left vague. Furthermore, many issues concerning patient autonomy, as expressed through health care proxies, are not covered by current English law.[201]

### 6:2.4 *Professional standards*

Professional standards provide guidance for doctors and may also carry weight in law. The General Medical Council states that doctors must obey the law and have proper regard for the welfare of patients. In 1992 the General Medical Council reiterated that treatment whose only purpose was to shorten the patient's life was wholly outside the doctor's professional duty to a patient and fell short of the high standards which the medical profession must uphold.[202] In the past, patterns of treatment affecting the survival of whole groups of patients, such as handicapped neonates, have been developed and then changed with little consultation with either families or other health professionals. While some consider it appropriate to make such treatment decisions only with the involvement of those directly concerned, it is clearly a matter of public policy that such important procedures are subject to review. Such review measures, in addition to the role of the GMC, are also discussed in 6:4.2 below.

157

### 6:2.5 *BMA policy*

A wide spectrum of opinion will be found within the medical profession but the BMA believes that the majority of doctors in the United Kingdom do not support euthanasia. BMA policy opposing euthanasia was established in 1969, when the Association's annual meeting affirmed the fundamental objects of the medical profession as the relief of suffering and the preservation of life. The issues were further addressed in a BMA publication in 1988, the conclusions of which are discussed in 6:8 below.

### 6:2.6 *Personal morality*

The protection of life is fundamental to the practice of medicine. Some, however, envisage this goal of sustaining life as an absolute imperative. People who hold such a view, consider it an ethical or religious duty to protect human life in all forms and all circumstances. Considerations as to the views of the patient or the patient's quality of life are considered secondary. Life in the quantitative sense must be maintained and prolonged because it represents a value in itself. As is discussed in other sections of the book (for example, chapter 4, section 4:3.1.3, on abortion) this perspective poses complex difficulties for doctors who espouse it. The intention never to kill an innocent human being does not, however, imply a positive requirement always to prolong life. Historically the two positions are quite distinct although they are frequently confused. The Association advises its members to consider their own views and to inform patients at the outset of any absolute objection they have to the principle of limiting treatment. Competent patients then have the opportunity to consider consulting another doctor or re-considering their own stance regarding a wish to refuse treatment in some circumstances.

## 6:3 Cessation of treatment/non-treatment decisions

There are a number of reasons why a treatment which might prolong life is not given. It may be that the patient refuses the treatment. If the patient is incompetent, doctors may believe that the side-effects and burdens of the treatment outweigh any benefits an extension of life would bring. Doctors might consider the treatment futile, in the sense that it would not achieve the desired effect for that particular patient. Scarcity of resources should never be a factor in deciding whether treatment is desirable, but the absence of resources may make a desired treatment impossible. Finally, doctors may think that even if the life-prolonging treatment is provided, its consequences either in terms of pain, psychological stress, loss of liberty, or restrictions of life style are so clearly unacceptable to the patient that the treatment may reasonably be withheld. Surveys[203] have indicated, however, that doctors are particularly reluctant to adopt this last way of thinking and will, in many cases, provide treatment for their patients in situations where they would have declined it for themselves if in their patient's place.

In these circumstances, when we talk about not prolonging life, it should be understood that active intervention to end life is not in question and nor is the withdrawal of care. In this sense, "treatment" and "care" are distinguishable insofar as treatments change according to clinical decisions but care must always continue until the very end of the patient's life.

### 6:3.1 *Patient consent to treatment*

The need for dialogue between doctors and patients as a background to the patient's continuing consent to treatment is discussed in chapter 1 (section 1:2.4) but assumes particular importance when the matter at the centre of discussion is the patient's death. Some consider the emphasis on patient autonomy to be misplaced, seeing this as a concept which fails to recognise the practical limitations on patients' options and the undoubted fact that doctors do influence patients, even inadvertently, by the way in which they present information. In the BMA's view, the stress on patient autonomy represents a genuine striving for partnership in decision-making between doctor and patient. This can only be done on the basis of shared information and guidance about diagnosis, prognosis, realistic treatment options and the patient's view of these. Great emphasis is given, therefore, to providing patients with sufficient information to allow them to exercise their autonomy in choosing treatments.

### 6:3.1.1 *Discussion of non-treatment*

All things being equal, the person best placed to assess what is being gained from life is the person living that life. Individuals facing deterioration of mental or physical health will require advice to assess the potential quality of their own lives and decide whether certain treatments should be accepted or declined. They will need to know, for example, whether a proposed treatment is likely to affect cognition or longevity, improve quality of survival over a limited time or impose burdensome side-effects. Patients' informed assessment of such factors may lead them to decline certain life-prolonging treatments.

The principle that doctors should discuss with patients in advance the circumstances in which the patient might choose non-treatment is difficult to implement. In the past, it was often said that patients, if asked in advance, would find it too distressing to contemplate non-treatment or non-resuscitation in their own case. In some instances, this is likely to be true and certainly it cannot be considered ethical to force reluctant patients to exercise all of their acknowledged rights of self determination whether they like it or not. However, an indication must be sought regarding the patient's attitude to such a discussion. Ian Kennedy in his 1980, Reith lecture remarked:

"The doctors realised that some patients may indeed have wished to know the truth but, since without asking they could not know which patients, they managed the problem by not telling anyone. This may have proved the ideal coping mechanism for the doctors. But it meant that only the patient who insisted on the truth and was confident enough to be persistent, got his way".[204]

Current practice recognises that it cannot be assumed that patients prefer to be protected from potentially upsetting decisions. Patients who retain rational faculties often indicate directly and indirectly the pace, scale and manner in which they wish to be involved. Those close to incompetent patients are usually consulted regarding non-treatment and non-resuscitation decisions and have the opportunity to reflect what patients themselves might have chosen.

It would be facile to underplay the anxieties or anger experienced by many patients when faced with a choice between harsh options. Supportive measures such as counselling or exploring different treatment strategies, including complementary practices, are explored in chapter 5 (section 5:5.1).

When individuals are unable to assess their life potential either because the necessary information was not given at the right time or because of incapacity, they are vulnerable to others making such decisions on their behalf. The BMA sees the possibility of danger and arrogance in the assumption that doctors can properly assess the quality of others' lives. This is not to say, however, that doctors can avoid making such assessments and this is discussed further below.

### 6:3.2 *Patient refusal of treatment*

No treatment can be given contrary to the wish of competent patients even if necessary to save life.[205] The BMA receives many enquiries on this matter and it is clear that doctors and nurses experience great anxiety when patients refuse life-saving treatment. Unfortunately, the situation may then become confrontational and this may have the effect of reinforcing the patient's refusal without the reasons for it being fully explored. The health care team should seek to explore the patient's reasons and correct any misunderstandings. Alternative measures which might be acceptable to the patient should also be discussed. Independent pastoral counselling could be made available, if this is acceptable to the patient. The patient should be fully informed in a non-directional manner of the potential effects of non-treatment but should also be assured that supportive care and treatment for pain will be available at all times.

In the real world, circumstances are seldom entirely clear-cut and measures are sometimes taken which doctors suspect the patient would decline if conscious and given sufficient opportunity. Attempted suicide

160

cases are often treated on the assumption that the person's judgement was temporarily impaired: legal opinion[206] has confirmed that where there is genuine doubt about the competence or voluntariness of a refusal of treatment, doctors should give treatment as if in an emergency. It is not simply a case of doctors assuming paternalistic attitudes but of reflecting society's desire to see life preserved if there is doubt about the rationality of the patient choosing suicide or non-treatment. Clearly, when an individual has decided that he or she wishes to die, doctors should not conclude that that person's competence is impaired. Nevertheless, in cases where any doubt exists, it is vital and proper to take steps to verify that patients are competent when they choose options which appear to be clearly contrary to their interests and survival. An emergency psychiatric assessment may be valuable in these circumstances.

It is traditional to cite the example of Jehovah's Witnesses to demonstrate a premeditated and widely shared group commitment against certain treatments. Although it is sometimes assumed that such examples occur more frequently in text books than in reality, the enquiries which the Association receives from members indicate that appropriate treatment of Jehovah's Witnesses is not merely a matter of academic concern, but rather of deep soul searching. It frequently requires doctors to act in a way they find profoundly disturbing. Nevertheless, the BMA reiterates the familiar advice that the decisions of a competent patient regarding non-treatment must be respected. Furthermore, patients whose competence is judged to be temporarily impaired can only be treated until they have regained the rational ability to decide.

The BMA recognises that patients who fear loss of competence are able to make valid decisions in advance about treatment or procedures. Thus the Association confirms its commitment to the fundamental right of patients to accept or reject, through advance directives, treatment options offered to them.

### 6:3.3 *Advance directives*

Advance directives[207] are one means of expressing in advance the patient's consent to, or refusal of, treatment. They are documents which patients draw up while mentally competent, to indicate their views of certain treatments at a later stage.

The most obvious disadvantage of drafting an advance directive is that patients may fail to foresee the particular circumstances of their own case and this may give rise to confusion about their wishes. The likelihood of this eventuality is diminished when patients have gained particular insight into the phases of their disease and the likely treatment options. For this reason, the BMA has very strongly recommended that any patients who wish to draft advance directives should ensure that they are well informed and do so with the benefit of medical advice. It has also recommended that this initiative should become part of a continuing dialogue between doctor and patient so that both are fully apprised of the other's opinion. As part of this exercise, it is advised that doctors should notify patients of the risks as well as the advantages of such a document.

The possibility of patients inadvertently misdirecting their doctors by an inadequate appreciation of the circumstances or of the evolution of new treatments led the Association to recommend strongly that advance directives should not be legally binding upon doctors, but legal cases in 1992 and 1993[208] indicated that an anticipatory decision which is clearly established and applicable to the circumstances would be as legally binding as any current decision made by a competent patient. The BMA believes that mutual respect and a common accord is better achieved without legislation. Furthermore, not only does the mechanism of an advance directive permit the patient to refuse the treatment offered but it may be used by patients who wish to request every possible life-prolonging treatment, including those which are clinically inappropriate or which might distort resource allocation. Some patients may request illegal procedures such as active euthanasia or may have informally indicated a change of view to that recorded in the directive. Although the Association has concluded that it would be impractical for advance directives to have obligatory status in all cases, it stresses that, all matters being equal, they should be regarded as a valid expression or refusal of patient consent to particular procedures.

### 6:3.3.1 Responsibilities of patients

The BMA recognises that there are risks involved in taking advance directives seriously and patients should be aware of the need for very careful thought in drafting. Patients will require assistance to make choices appropriate for them. Ideally, such discussion should not be a single event but a continuing process between patient and doctor. It is important that patients who make advance directives take steps to ensure such dialogue.

The onus for ensuring that the advance directive is appropriately drafted and available for those to whom it is addressed lies with the patient. The BMA suggests that patients who have drafted an advance directive carry a card indicating that fact as well as lodging a copy with their doctor.

While any coherent statement drafted by a competent person is worthy of consideration, patients must be aware that a poorly drafted document may complicate rather than clarify the situation and is more likely to be regarded as irrelevant. In cases where treatment options cannot be predicted, a simple statement of the patient's views may be more helpful than a complicated document which tries to cover all possibilities.

The BMA recommends that any person making an advance directive updates it at regular intervals. Five years is suggested as an appropriate interval for patients to review their decisions. The possible nomination of a health care proxy (6:3.5 below) may represent a safeguard for patients in the event of an advance directive being made many years prior to illness and unchanged despite changing circumstances. Such cases of unrevised directives will exist but are unlikely to present a profound dilemma for doctors, since instructions written so previously can clearly only give the most general of indications, if that, of the patient's ultimate views.

### 6:3.3.2 Responsibilities of doctors

As is mentioned above (6:2.6) any doctor who objects to the principle of an advance directive should inform the patient accordingly. Some patients may want to reconsider their own views in the light of this and re-assess the value they assign to having an advance directive: others may consider changing their doctor. It is not acceptable for doctors to give patients a tacit impression that an advance directive would be respected when the doctor, for reasons of conscience, has no intention of doing so.

### 6:3.3.3 Late discovery of an advance directive

Questions often arise about the ethical status of discontinuing a course of treatment which has been initiated prior to the doctor's awareness of the advance directive, and which is contrary to the patient's wishes. The BMA considers that late discovery of an advance directive after life-prolonging treatment has been initiated is not grounds for ignoring its provisions. If practicable, treatment should be discontinued in accordance with the directive once it is known. If the patient has nominated a proxy decision-maker, that person's opinions should also be sought to confirm the patient's likely view.

### 6:3.3.4 Application to non-terminally ill patients

Most people are unlikely to wish to deprive themselves of the possibility of any treatments when they have a chance of recovery. Thus, it is usual for the advance directive to be considered as valid only from the point at which doctors advise that there is no realistic anticipation of the patient's recovery. Although a usual provision of the advance directive is that it assumes importance only when the patient is terminally ill, this is not a necessary requirement. "Terminal" itself requires interpretation and, in some cases, individuals may wish to specify a refusal of treatment, if incompetent, even though death is not imminent. An example of such circumstances arises with regard to the persistent vegetative state.

Patients in persistent vegetative state (PVS) may survive for decades in insentience and therefore may not be regarded as terminally ill in the usual sense of the term. Thus, when such patients have drawn up a directive questions may be raised about whether it should be observed, given that the advance directive usually comes into play when the patient is nearing the end of life. If, however, an advance directive has been drafted, the

163

BMA believes it should be accorded the same weight as any other valid expression of a competent patient's opinion. Ethically, if specified in the advance directive, all medical treatments can be withdrawn from the PVS patient when sufficient time has elapsed for the PVS diagnosis to be independently confirmed and there is no reasonable prospect of further recovery (12 months is currently recommended). This view was held to reflect the legal position by Lord Keith in the 1993 House of Lords' decision in the Bland case.[209] (See also 6:5 below).

### 6:3.4 *Procedures for patients who have never been competent*

Advance directives cannot help patients who have never been competent or who were unprepared for a deterioration in competency. Other methods of decision-making must be evolved for such individuals. The principal motive for establishing such procedures is to enable treatment rather than authorise its withdrawal but in some instance the latter case may arise. In 1991 the English Law Commission embarked on an examination of all the alternatives for reform of the law, including expansion of guardianship measures and the role of the Court of Protection. This process will take some time. The BMA has put forward its own proposals for a decision-making procedure based on a three-tier approach.[210]

In addition to considering mechanisms for patients who have never been able to express an opinion, the Law Commission is also looking at other options for patients for whom an advance directive is not convenient or appropriate. Among these are proposals for extending enduring powers of attorney to health care decisions and the appointment of proxy decision-makers.

### 6:3.5 *Health care proxies*

Competent individuals can appoint, in advance, another person to act as a proxy decision-maker for them, should particular circumstances arise. For example, patients with a condition which they know may lead to dementia, may wish to appoint in advance, a proxy to convey their views about various treatment options when they, themselves, can no longer do so. The precise role, powers and title of a proxy decision-maker are not defined by either custom or law (even in Scotland where tutors dative may exercise this role). Pending clarification in law, the BMA believes that in cases where such a person has been nominated by the patient, the criterion to be followed in decision-making would be that of "substituted judgement", with the agent acting as a sympathetic interpreter of the patient's own values, rather than attempting to judge the patient's best interests.

The proposed system of health care proxies has the advantages of meeting the circumstances which arise rather than being tied to the particular words of the advance directive and reflecting the patient's true wish, so respecting patient autonomy. It should also be possible to challenge, and if necessary displace, a substitute decision-maker whose actions are mischievous.

The health care proxy and the advance directive are quite separate measures. Patients can choose either measure or combine the two. In some cases where patients have opted to express their views through an advance directive, this may need to be interpreted in the light of the circumstances. Clearly, there is greater likelihood of the individual patient's views and values being reflected by the patient's own nominated health-care proxy, who is familiar with the patient's opinions.

### 6:3.6 *Quality of life*

The patient's opinions about prolongation of life may have been formulated on the basis of an appreciation of the quality of life that might be expected to follow treatment. Similar assessments of quality of life are likely to be used by doctors making treatment and non-treatment decisions on behalf of others who are incompetent. In the BMA's view, life should be cherished despite disabilities and handicaps. Nevertheless, life is not to be indefinitely sustained in all circumstances, for example, where its prolongation by artificial means would be regarded as inhumane and the treatment itself burdensome. The BMA does not, therefore, espouse a strict vitalist "sanctity of life" approach, although it recognises that some of its members do.

The judiciary has made clear that a doctor cannot "be under an absolute obligation to prolong the patient's life by any means availalbe to him, regardless of the quality of the patient's life. Common humanity requires otherwise, as do medical ethics and good medical practice accepted in this country and overseas".[211]

Most people would agree, that a noticeable shift has occurred towards more decision-making being based on "quality of life" assessments, particularly perhaps in the United States of America, where medical decision-making appears to be dominated by the issue of autonomy and the quality of life which the particular individual patient, now incapacitated, would have found acceptable or unacceptable, according to the opinions of those close to him or her.

### 6:3.6.1 *An intolerable burden*

Efforts to prolong life might be regarded as intrusive in circumstances where the patient's capacity to experience life and to relate to others is very severely impaired or non-existent. Although this must be a matter of careful individual consideration, the courts gave some guidance in the 1990 case of Baby J, who was severely brain-damaged at birth. J's life expectancy was uncertain and although he was expected to die before late adolescence, he was not terminally ill. The court held that "where a ward

165

of court suffered from physical disabilities so grave that his life would from his point of view be so intolerable if he were to continue living that he would choose to die if he were in a position to make a sound judgement, the court could direct that treatment without which death would ensue from natural causes need not be given to the ward to prolong his life, even though he was neither on the point of death nor dying".[212] This judgement therefore recognises limits to the doctor's duty to treat. It can usefully guide, but not determine, the ethical and moral responsibilities in other, apparently similar, cases.

It was also made clear, however, that the court would never sanction positive steps to terminate life. The medical profession generally supported the court's decision. In such cases, the withholding of certain treatments which sustain life is ethical, provided that caring attention to the patient's comfort is sustained.

### 6:3.7 *Non-treatment in the patient's best interests*

The doctor's role is to maintain quality of life through the relief of suffering. When cure is not achievable, treatment options may be more concerned, for instance, with either prolonging a limited life-span, or attempting to provide the best quality of survival. Surgical resection to relieve symptoms might be considered, for example, because while it may not offer greater longevity, it will give better quality survival for the time the patient has left. In other cases, the side-effects of treatment may be painful or burdensome and thus the justification for treatment is questionable.

Usually, the preferences of the patient should prevail but if the patient is incompetent, the doctor, together with those close to the patient, must act in his or her best interests. The consent of people close to the patient is not legally valid but often relatives are able to reflect what the patient would have wanted. As is stressed elsewhere in this book, the term "incompetence" covers a wide range of varying or fluctuating abilities and does not simply mean that the patient has no preference or no voice in the choices made. Rather it implies that the importance accorded to those preferences must be individually decided. In the case of total incompetence, such as when the patient is unconscious, a non-treatment decision is often supported by the people close to the patient, reflecting what they believe to be the patient's view.

In deciding whether the administration of potentially life-prolonging medical treatment is in the best interests of the patient who is incompetent, the health team must consider three main factors:

- the possibility of extending life under humane and comfortable conditions;

- the patient's values about life and the way it should be lived;

– the patient's likely reaction to sickness, suffering and medical interventions.

Some have argued that where there is real doubt as to whether a proposed treatment is in the patient's interests, treatment should be withheld. The grounds for such a position are that the common bias of doctors towards treatment, whether resting on a technological imperative or a vitalist viewpoint, are unjustified. The BMA believes that although doctors should not give treatment simply because it is available, in cases of doubt about the best interests of the patient, the presumption should be in favour of prolonging life. This is particularly so if most people would consider that life to be of acceptable quality.

### 6:3.7.1 Doctors' responsibilities to incompetent patients

In cases of doubt the BMA suggests the key points can be briefly summarised as follows:[213]

a) The doctor must discern as far as possible the patient's current medical situation, the likely course of the disease in the absence of interventions, the full range of potentially useful interventions and the likely course with each of these.

b) The doctor should try to ascertain the patient's own values and preferences, which should be given importance in choosing between options.

c) Information about all alternatives which might be beneficial should be discussed with those close to the patient, who may be able to reflect the patient's values and preferences.

d) If it is not clear which of the options would most accord with the patient's values, the doctor and those close to the patient should identify the plan of care that would generally be considered to most likely advance the patient's interests.

### 6:3.7.2 The persistent vegetative state

As is discussed above, when treatment or non-treatment decisions are based on arguments about the patient's best interests, doctors need an objective mechanism for assessing these interests. Much recent debate has concerned the application of best interests criteria to patients in the persistent vegetative state (PVS).[214]

PVS patients have lost the function of the cognitive past of the brain - the cerebral cortex. Definitive diagnosis of the condition cannot be made in the early months and the BMA has been greatly concerned by the possibility of a premature labelling of patients as being in PVS and therefore potentially deprived of treatments which might benefit them.

167

The BMA recommends that possible diagnoses be reviewed after the patient has been insentient for one year. If PVS is confirmed in accordance with BMA guidelines, doctors have the difficult task of assessing the patient's best interests. Guidance on this matter has been provided by the House of Lords where it was stated that when:

"a patient is brought into hospital in such a condition that, without the benefit of a life support system, he will not continue to live, the decision has to be made whether or not to give him that benefit, if available. That decision can only be made in the best interests of the patient. No doubt, his best interests will ordinarily require that he should be placed on a life support system as soon as necessary, if only to make an accurate assessment of his condition and a prognosis for the future. But if he neither recovers sufficiently to be taken off it nor dies, the question will ultimately arise whether he should be kept on it indefinitely. That question can only be answered by reference to the best interests of the patient himself, having regard to established medical practice. Indeed, if the justification for treating a patient who lacks the capacity to consent lies in the fact that the treatment is provided in his best interests, it must follow that the treatment may, and indeed ultimately should, be discontinued where it is no longer in his best interests to provide it.

The correct formulation of the question is of particular importance in a case where the patient is totally unconscious and where there is no hope whatsoever of any amelioration of his condition. In circumstances such as these, it may be difficult to say that it is in his best interests that the treatment should be ended. But if the question is asked, as in my opinion it should be, whether it is in his best interests that treatment which has the effect of artificially prolonging his life should be continued, that question can sensibly be answered to the effect that it is not in his best interests to do so.

Even so, a distinction may be drawn between (i) cases in which, having regard to all the circumstances (including, for example, the intrusive nature of the treatment, the hazards involved in it, and the very poor quality of the life which may be prolonged for the patient if the treatment if successful), it may be judged not to be in the best interests of the patient to initiate or continue life-prolonging treatment, and (ii) cases in which, so far as the living patient is concerned, the treatment is of no benefit to him because he is totally unconscious and there is no prospect of any improvement in his condition. In both classes of case, the decision whether or not to withhold treatment must be made in the best interests of the patients".[215]

(See also 6:4.2.1 and 6:5 below).

*6:3.7.3 Conflict between decision-makers*

Where a medical procedure can offer an enhanced quality of life without imposing suffering on the incompetent person, there will be no dilemma. Problems only arise when present suffering must be weighed against a limited or dubious benefit or there is disagreement between decision-makers as to where the patient's best interests lie. An example of just such a case was provided in 1992. It concerned a young child with advanced cancer; the doctors were pressing for continuing treatment, despite opposition from the child's mother. The latter wished to spare her son further suffering in view of doubts about the efficacy of the treatment, the prospect of resulting handicap and the uncertainty as to the child's long-term survival. Non-treatment decisions in similar cases are made every day and this particular case was only important because the disagreement about what constituted the child's best interests attracted media attention.

The case, however, exemplifies a number of dilemmas. The child, although young, had sufficient experience of painful treatments to be made miserable by the prospect of more and he expressed his own opposition. (In chapter 3, the dilemmas of weighing the child's viewpoint with other considerations are discussed at length. See particularly section 3:2.) If the treatment proved successful in ensuring survival there was nevertheless a strong chance of brain damage, which the family found almost as difficult to contemplate as the child's death. Although ethics place the interests of the patient as pre-eminent above the problems of the family, it must be recognised that in reality it is sometimes difficult to disentangle the two. Yet, there was a small but significant chance that the child would survive with manageable handicaps to a reasonable age. Some doctors felt convinced it was a chance worth taking or possibly even worth taking the case to court to ensure treatment.

When conflict arises between the responsible doctor and those close to the patient, it is regrettable and additionally traumatic to all if the case needs to be resolved at law. Counselling, discussion and further medical opinions may help bring about agreement. It is not suggested that health professionals align to impose their views on lay people but rather that they recognise that it is difficult and sometimes impossible for relatives to sustain a position in which they believe in the face of expert medical opinion. Time and effort should therefore be given to resolving the conflict or, if possible, the decision should be postponed so that further thought can be given to it. As is discussed above in the section on proxy decision-makers, measures must be taken in the rare cases involving a mischievous proxy or a proxy who stands to benefit indirectly from one course of treatment in preference to another.

It is sometimes suggested that if the person who opposes the recommendations of the health team is emotionally distant from the patient and others close to the patient support the proposed course of action, the latter should prevail. In some countries this is codified, with the views of a spouse, for example, taking precedence over those of a cousin. In the United Kingdom, there is no such clearly established hierarchy of decision-makers and since no person can legally consent or refuse treatment on behalf of another (except in Scotland where a tutor dative may be empowered to do so), the views of those close to the patient are principally important as an indication of the latter's own wishes.

## 6:4 Withdrawing treatment

### 6:4.1 *Ethical importance*

Sometimes, where there is uncertainty as to its benefits, there is a reluctance to initiate a course of treatment because the doctor believes that once begun that treatment must be sustained. Also, some cultures still prefer to withhold treatment initially, rather than withdraw it after it is in place. This is not the BMA's view: we can see no ethical difference between initial non-treatment and withdrawal of a treatment which is shown to be unsuccessful in achieving the desired effect. The BMA believes that where there is doubt, treatment should be given, although this may eventually be modified or even withdrawn as clinical prognosis becomes clearer.

Very often queries about withdrawing or withholding treatment concern elderly confused patients, or incompetent patients with chronic conditions, who have been resuscitated and subsequently ventilated; the usual objections are that treatment is futile given the low quality of life which remains. Similar cases could arise, however, if treatment had been initiated before a doctor knew about the existence of an advance directive since doctors are often very reluctant to discontinue a procedure once started.

Despite the practical difficulties of withdrawing treatment at any stage, it is difficult to justify continuing any treatment when it becomes evident that the patient does not benefit from it. The definition of "benefit" is itself complex and can be variously defined. Some would see a benefit to the patient in the carrying out of that individual's wishes even if this meant the withdrawal of life-prolonging treatment and the patient's death. Others question, for example, whether incompetent patients who cannot understand the potential benefits of painful or distressing treatments such as chemotherapy can be said to benefit from them. Unlike competent patients, they cannot weigh the drawbacks and side-effects against an expected, or at least potential, gain. It is also questioned whether the continuation of purely vegetative reflexes, as in the case of patients in persistent vegetative state (PVS), constitutes any benefit for such patients. Benefit must be judged in terms of the individual patient. Judgements should not be based on the prospect of benefit to others. The ability to make complex judgements about benefit requires compassion, experience and an appreciation of the patient's view point. Doctors who may have to make such decisions should call upon the expertise of other health professionals and for certain decisions they will require guidance from the courts.

### 6:4.2 Review measures

Life and death decisions concerning treatment and non-treatment are of such importance to society that some people believe they should not be left solely to the individuals concerned but should be subject to some form of review. Various forms of review are possible.

#### 6:4.2.1 Legal review

In recent years, it has been the custom in Scotland for doctors and those close to patients diagnosed as being in a persistent vegetative state to make decisions about withdrawal of hydration and nutrition. In each case, the doctor reports the full circumstances to the Crown Office, which may initiate further enquiry if it feels this is necessary. In England, the 1993 House of Lords' decision in the Bland case established a procedure, whereby each case of PVS in which withdrawal of treatment was being considered should be subject to legal review.

#### 6:4.2.2 Peer review

Peer review means the profession monitors and maintains its own standards. It should include not only team discussions of unusual or problem cases, but also regular reviews of routine work and keeping up to date with procedures and treatment decisions by reading the relevant medical journals, which draw the profession's attention to possible developments.

#### 6:4.2.3 Review by ethics committees

In the United States, institutional ethics committees provide a multidisciplinary forum for the audit of difficult cases. A network of such committees has also been established in the Netherlands. In Britain many specialised units, such as neonatal intensive care units, have assembled multidisciplinary teams to provide health care. These teams also discuss difficult cases before a decision is made in a manner comparable to the institutional ethics committees. Furthermore, the BMA's proposed mechanism[216] for decision-making on behalf of mentally incapacitated adults provides for a committee to review all controversial treatment decisions.

## 6:5 Withholding nutrition

Doctors have questioned whether artificial nutrition should be classified as a treatment, and therefore be subject to clinical discretion, or whether it is in a separate category from medical treatments. The BMA's view that artificial feeding or hydration are medical treatments was confirmed by the House of Lords' decision in February 1993. The question may arise in two contexts: either because the patient refuses nutrition or because the patient is incompetent and usually unconscious and thus has a very low quality of life.

### 6:5.1 *Patient refusal of nutrition*

In the United Kingdom, competent patients cannot legally be forcibly fed although the courts have authorised such treatment for a competent person under 18 years of age.[217] From an ethical viewpoint, adults can refuse any form of medical treatment either at the time it is offered or in advance.

Lawyers believe that there are strong legal grounds for complying with instructions to withhold nutrition or hydration if this has been indicated by the patient in an advance directive.

### 6:5.2 *Withdrawing nutrition from an insentient patient*

The BMA welcomed the judicial ruling in the Bland case in 1993 which confirmed that medical treatment, including artificial nutrition and hydration, can be lawfully discontinued in some cases, where no recovery is expected. The House of Lords specified that there can be no blanket ruling and each case, in which discontinuation of artificial feeding from an insentient patient is proposed, should be referred to the courts. The Association believes that this decision accords with good medical practice with regard to patients in the persistent vegetative state and has issued a guidance note on PVS.[218]

## 6:6 Do-not-resuscitate orders

The issue of the resuscitation of patients who suffer cardiac or respiratory arrest is one which will have a bearing both on advance directives and on other mechanisms for making non-treatment decisions. Cardiopulmonary resuscitation (CPR) can be attempted on any individual in whom cardiac or respiratory function ceases. Such events are inevitable as part of dying and thus CPR can theoretically be used on every individual prior to death. It is therefore essential to identify patients for whom cardiopulmonary arrest represents a terminal event in their illness and for whom CPR is inappropriate.

### 6:6.1 *Discussion with the patient*

Although many health professionals may have reservations about raising the issue with patients, experience indicates that if it is discussed in a sensitive and realistic manner by an appropriately trained person and at an appropriate time, patients are not made unnecessarily anxious by the topic. It would be unethical to make a do-not-resuscitate order on any patient who is capable of expressing an opinion, without consulting his or her views.

### 6:6.2 *Communication between carers*

"Do-not-resuscitate" (DNR) orders may be a potent source of misunderstanding and dissent amongst doctors, nurses and others involved in the care of patients. Many of the problems in this difficult area would be avoided if communication and explanation of these decisions could be improved. Communication with the patient is particularly important although this may clearly be impossible in an emergency. The Chief Medical Officer has made it clear[219] that the responsibility for resuscitation policy lies with the consultant concerned and that each consultant should ensure that this policy is understood by all staff who may be involved, and in particular by junior medical staff. Unfortunately, in many cases discussion and consultation about the resuscitation of a patient is carried out by staff who are the least experienced or, the least well-equipped to undertake such sensitive tasks. The UK Central Council for Nursing, Midwifery and Health Visiting (UKCC) considers that the decision should first be recorded by the doctor before it can be reflected in the nursing treatment notes.

### 6:6.3 *Guidelines*

In a survey it conducted, the Royal College of Nursing (RCN) found that most health authorities and health boards had taken steps to ensure that appropriate health-workers were proficient in CPR. However, the problem of who should - and who should not - be resuscitated had not been addressed and several authorities said they would welcome guidance. Such guidance has accordingly been drawn up and agreed upon by the BMA, the RCN and the Resuscitation Council (UK). The factors surrounding a decision whether or not to initiate CPR involve complex clinical considerations and emotional issues. The decision arrived at in the care of one patient may be inappropriate in a superficially similar case. These agreed guidelines, therefore, should be viewed as a framework, providing basic principles within which decisions regarding local policies on CPR can be formulated. The full guidelines are available from any of the signatory bodies, including the BMA, but some of the principal points are noted here.

a)  It is agreed that CPR should be routinely undertaken in all patients who suffer cardiac or respiratory arrest except:

- Where the patient's condition indicates that effective CPR is unlikely to be successful.

173

- Where this is not in accord with the recorded, sustained wishes of the patient when mentally competent.

- Where successful CPR is likely to be followed by a length and quality of life which would not be acceptable to the patient.

b) The overall responsibility for DNR decisions rests with the consultant in charge of the patient's care. This decision should be made after appropriate consultation and consideration of all aspects of the patient's condition. The perspectives of other members of the medical and nursing team, the patient and with due regard to patient confidentiality, the patient's relatives or close friends, may all be valuable in helping the consultant to reach a decision.

c) Sensitive exploration of the patient's wishes should be undertaken. This should ideally be carried out by the consultant concerned, in some circumstances, for example, when a patient is at risk of cardiac or respiratory failure or has a terminal illness. Such discussions should be documented in the patient's record.

## 6:7 Aiding suicide

Suicide differs from euthanasia in that the act of causing death is performed by the patient, not the doctor. Reported cases concern the prescribing of sleeping pills with the knowledge of their intended use, and/or discussing the required dosage with the patient. In its 1992 Statement of Marbella, the World Medical Association[220] confirmed that assisted suicide, like euthanasia, is unethical and must be condemned by the medical profession. Where a doctor intentionally and deliberately enables an individual to end his life, the doctor acts unethically.

Attempting to commit suicide is not a criminal offence but it remains illegal to assist someone to commit suicide. The latter is punishable by up to 14 years' imprisonment, although for a number of years there have been calls for the de-criminalisation of aiding the terminally ill to commit suicide. The Canadian Law Commission, in particular, considered this matter in 1982[221] and concluded that the reluctance of the legislature in many countries to make an exception for assistance given to terminally ill people to commit suicide was based on the fear of the excesses or the abuses to which it might lead.

The Commission put forward examples of cases where incitement to suicide could not be considered morally blameless, for instance, when, for their own financial advantage, someone encouraged a depressed relative to commit suicide. It considered that the law might legitimately fear the difficulties involved in determining the true motivation of the person committing the act of assisting suicide, but pointed out that cases involving truly altruistic assistance to a terminally ill person who wishes to die are rarely prosecuted.

Doctors are not likely to be accused of aiding suicide for financial benefit, but as with questions of euthanasia, some might fear that less attention would be given to solving patients' pain control problems or finding a civilised way to relate to consistently perverse or disruptive patients, if they could be assisted to kill themselves. Furthermore, for some patients, with the advance of disease comes a reduction in the decision-making capacity because of the effects of drugs or of the disease. Assisting such patients to commit suicide can hardly be differentiated from an action by the doctor to end their lives. It is believed[222] that doctors who play a role in suicide keep the fact secret and therefore do not consult colleagues or ethics committees for confirmation that the patient has made a rational decision.

Ethicists argue that there is no moral difference between knowing terminally ill people will take a fatal dose they have obtained and watching them do so after having provided them with the drugs. The distinction is difficult to justify on grounds of logic and some would argue, as with euthanasia, that when someone is determined to end their life, the act is better done with supervision and comforting support rather than bungled or prolonged by lack of expertise. Our response, however, must be similar to that made to calls for the legalising of euthanasia. To legalise a doctor's participation in a patient's suicide would undermine a fundamental principle in support of the value of life. In neither case would it prove possible to restrict the deliberate ending of life to cases of terminally ill people, and once established the practice could be extended widely and be open to abuse. People who might be seen as a burden or who fear that others see them so might feel encouraged to commit suicide.

Thus, the BMA considers that doctors should not assist, either directly or indirectly, their patients to commit suicide.

## 6:8 Euthanasia

Doctors have a duty to try to provide patients with a peaceful and dignified death with minimal suffering but, as is indicated throughout this chapter, the BMA considers it contrary to the doctor's role deliberately to kill patients, even at their request. Such requests from young and severely handicapped patients present one of the hardest problems of day to day care, perhaps only surpassed in difficulty by the exceptional cases of great physical and emotional suffering discussed in 6:2.2.3. Clearly, doctors have a very profound sympathy for such patients who find living intolerable for varied reasons.

Nevertheless, despite the compassion felt for the individual, there is a widespread misgiving within the profession about compromising principles to suit particular circumstances. In the early 1970s, Hare reflected something of the pragmatic approach usually attributed to doctors:

"Doctors would do well, having adopted some fairly simple set of principles which copes adequately with the cases they are likely to meet, to dismiss from their minds (at least when they are doctoring) the possibility of there being further exceptions to their principles. For doctors, like all of us, are human, and if once they start thinking, when engaged on a case, that this case might be one of the limitless and indeterminate set of exceptions to their principles, they will find such exceptions everywhere. There may be - in fact there certainly are - cases in which soldiers ought to run away in battle. But if soldiers were all the time asking themselves whether the particular battle in which they were fighting might be such a case, they would run away every time. The temptation to special pleading is too great. A doctor once said to me in connection with the proposal to allow euthanasia: 'We shall start by putting patients away because they are in intolerable pain and have not long to live anyway; and we shall end up putting them away because it's Friday night and we want to get away for the weekend' ".[223]

In chapter 5, we discussed communication and palliative measures. While neither will entirely eliminate requests for euthanasia, if practised they might, it is to be hoped, lessen the anxieties which sometimes give rise to such requests. It is clearly recognised, however, that for some people, choosing when and how they want to die is a fundamental matter which they wish to have recognised as a civil right and that they are not going to change their minds about this. How the profession responds is a delicate matter.

That there are patients who hold these views deeply and sincerely makes it all the more important that doctors take a positive, active approach to resolving concerns which might give rise to requests for euthanasia, and that they ensure that appropriate techniques are available to patients when there is a good chance of providing an extension of life with the quality the patient seeks. The perception of being a burden on carers might be eased by "medical friendship" (see chapter 5, section 5:3.3), by the support and understanding of other carers and, if possible, by making the patient's overall situation more tolerable, for example, by encouraging the patient to investigate additional sources of practical and moral support. There are, however, no easy solutions and society as a whole must be involved in the search for morally acceptable remedies.

The BMA considers that whilst there are many cases where a doctor should accede to a request not to prolong the patient's life, a doctor should not actively intervene to end that life. We also recognise the vital contribution the hospice movement has made, in giving greatly valued practical and spiritual support to terminally ill patients and their families.

In brief, a line is drawn between an active decision not to continue with futile treatment and so allow a patient to die as "nature takes its course" on the one hand, and any affirmative action undertaken with the intent of ending life, on the other. The former, unless an omission resulting from negligence, is both ethical and legal, whereas the latter is most certainly both illegal and ethically unacceptable.

## 6:9 Summary

1    In the BMA's view, liberalising the law on euthanasia would herald a serious and incalculable change in the ethos of medicine.

2    Effective management of pain and distress which has the side effect of curtailing life, is a necessary form of treatment.

3    The Association advises doctors to consider their own views and inform patients at the outset of any absolute objection they might have to the principle of limiting treatment at the patient's request.

4    Treatment decisions regarding severely incapacitated people must be based on what is best for that individual and not on avoiding a burden to the family or to society.

5    When a decision is reached that it would not be in the interests of the patient to give life prolonging treatments, the withholding of certain treatments is ethical, provided that caring attention to the patient's comfort is sustained.

6    Patients can only make valid choices on the basis of shared information about diagnoses, prognoses and realistic treatment options.

7    It is unethical to force reluctant patients to exercise all of their acknowledged rights of self determination at the end of life, whether they like it or not. But an indication must be sought regarding the patient's attitude to discussion of death.

8    When a patient refuses life-prolonging treatments, the health care team should seek to explore the patient's reasons and to correct any misunderstandings. Alternative measures which might be acceptable to the patient should also be discussed.

9    A potentially self-damaging decision by the patient should not in itself lead to a conclusion of incompetence. In cases where any doubt exists, it is vital and proper to take steps to verify that patients are competent when they choose options which appear to be clearly contrary to their interests and survival. An emergency psychiatric assessment could be arranged.

10    The BMA strongly supports the principles underpinning advance directives which represent the patient's settled wish regarding treatment choices when the patient is no longer able competently to express a view.

11    When preparing an advance directive patients are entitled to receive balanced counselling on the medical issues from their doctor. Discussion between patients and doctors of the specific terms of an advance declaration should be a continuing dialogue.

12    The BMA is not in favour of legislation on advance directives.

13    It is the responsibility of the patient to ensure that the existence of an advance directive is known to those who may be asked to comply with its provisions. Doctors, having been notified that an advance directive exists, should make all reasonable efforts to acquaint themselves with its contents. In cases of emergency, however, necessary treatment should not be delayed in anticipation of a document which is not readily available.

14    It is strongly recommended that patients review their advance directives at regular intervals (at least once every five years).

15    The Association encourages doctors to raise the subject of advance directives in a sensitive manner with patients who may be thought likely to have an interest in the matter or who are anxious about the possible administration of unwanted treatments at a later stage.

16    Late discovery of an advance directive, ie after life-prolonging treatment has been initiated, is not sufficient grounds for ignoring it.

17    The BMA recognises that the nomination of a health-care proxy by the patient may be another helpful development in communicating the patient's views when the patient is no longer capable of expressing these. Where such a person has been nominated by the patient, the criterion to be followed in decision-making should be that of "substituted judgement", with the agent acting as a sympathetic interpreter of the patient's own values, rather than attempting to judge the patient's best interests.

18    The patient's refusal of specific treatments should be respected but it neither implies nor justifies abandonment of the patient.

19    Patients cannot insist on the provision of treatments which clinical experience indicates to be futile for their condition and which diverts resources from other patients.

20    The views of competent patients should be sought with regard to do-not-resuscitate decisions when such a decision may arise for that patient.

21    Cardiopulmonary resuscitation should be routinely undertaken in patients who suffer cardiac or respiratory arrest except:
      a)  Where the patient's condition indicates that effective CPR is unlikely to be successful.

b) Where this is not in accord with the recorded, sustained wishes of the patient when mentally competent.

c) Where successful CPR is likely to be followed by a length and quality of life which would not be acceptable to the patient.

22 The overall responsibility for do-not-resuscitate decisions rests with the consultant in charge of the patient's care. This decision should be made after appropriate consultation and consideration of all aspects of the patient's condition.

23 Doctors should not give treatment simply because it is available but in cases of doubt about the best interests of the patient, the presumption should be in favour of prolonging life, with a regular review of the situation.

24 No ethical difference is perceived between initial non-treatment and withdrawal of a treatment which is shown to be unsuccessful in achieving the desired effect. When in doubt, the BMA believes that treatment should be given, although this may be eventually modified or even withdrawn, as clinical prognosis becomes clearer.

25 The BMA believes that artificial feeding is a medical treatment which cannot be implemented contrary to the wishes of a patient who refuses consent. Such refusal can be expressed through a competent advance directive.

# 7 Treatment and Prescribing

*Prescribing criteria; clinical responsibility and clinical freedom; liaison between doctors; doctors working for private facilities, including weight-loss clinics; nurse prescribing; complementary practitioners; patient addiction; summary.*

## 7:1 Introduction

Treatment follows the establishment of a working diagnosis. It may be undertaken directly by the doctor, such as a surgical operation, or through the agency of other health professionals, such as nurses and pharmacists. All treatments carry elements of risk and some of these are involved in the administration of the procedure itself. As is discussed more fully in chapter 10 (section 10:1.2), doctors have an ethical and legal responsibility to ensure that they are competent to carry out the procedure they judge to be necessary.

In an emergency all doctors would be expected to offer assistance, but the extent of care provided will depend on the nature of the emergency; the likely availability of more expert help; the degree of immediate threat to the patient's life; and the doctor's willingness to tackle procedures outside his or her usual clinical experience.

## 7:2 Surgical procedures

In the case of pre-planned surgical procedures, doctors must be satisfied that they are competent to carry out the procedure to a successful conclusion and to deal with any complications which may arise. Inexperienced doctors may find themselves asked to carry out surgical procedures which they have not previously undertaken and for which they have received no directly relevant training. These doctors must call in a senior colleague when they know they have not obtained sufficient experience to carry out the proposed procedure alone. The BMA has undertaken to support any doctor who refuses to perform a task which he or she has not been trained adequately to fulfil. Similarly, experienced doctors may be given the opportunity to undertake surgical procedures which they would like to perform, but which they may not have carried out for a number of years. All medical techniques change over time and even a high level of competence achieved some years previously may not be in accordance with current clinical standards and practice. It is the doctor's responsibility either to decline the request, or, preferably, obtain some refresher type training which will restore the level of competence to its previous level (see also chapter 10, section 10:1.3).

Equally, it is encumbent upon health authorities and other employers, which create such opportunities, to ensure that the training facilities which doctors consider that they need, are actually available to them. Once the necessary level of competence has been achieved it is the responsibility of the doctors to ensure that they carry out sufficient procedures to maintain the required level of competence. Regular participation in medical audit and appropriate continuing education are obviously ways of retaining such standards.

In an emergency doctors may be confronted with a situation which they have never previously encountered. If the doctor is prepared to undertake the procedure and judges that the patient will die without it, the doctor is unlikely to be criticised as long as he or she displays the ordinary skill that any other doctor might be expected to show[224] (however, see also chapter 10, section 10:1.2). Similarly, with other emergency situations the doctor must assess the likelihood of access to appropriate specialist expertise against the immediate risks for the patient. Doctors need to recognise their limitations and call for help as appropriate.

## 7:3 Medical treatments

### 7:3.1 Invasive procedures

Doctors in a number of specialties, and particularly general medicine and radiology, are acquiring skills in a wide range of invasive procedures. Usually a training programme is devised and the operator is carefully supervised until the requisite standard of competence has been achieved. Again doctors are expected to judge their level of competence and to ensure that it is adequate to undertake the procedures proposed. As a general rule no doctor should undertake the procedure for the first time without the supervision of an experienced operator in the field.

### 7:3.2 Drug administration in hospital

Those who accept inexperienced doctors for training have an ethical responsibility to ensure that such doctors are adequately supervised and trained in the procedures which the unit undertakes. This particularly applies to the administration of drugs by doctors themselves. There is a basic requirement for all doctors supervising medical training to create a clinical environment in which junior doctors are encouraged to seek help in the acquisition of relevant clinical skills and to share their uncertainties with more senior members of the team.

181

Protocols should be prepared, setting out clearly the clinical policy concerning the re-constitution of drugs and the checking procedures which must be followed to ensure that the dose and strength of the drug are those prescribed and that the drug is administered to the correct patient. Such procedures may well be carried out in conjunction with a nurse. They in no way restrict the doctor's freedom to prescribe a different dose to that commonly recommended. It is bad practice for doctors to seek direct access to the drug cupboard, in order to administer to the patient the drugs they consider necessary. In such ways mistakes are made.

The speed and timing of administration may be as vital as the dose and the preferred route. Again it is sensible to check the procedures with the British National Formulary or the manufacturer's instructions using the checking procedures described above. For some drugs, such as the newer heparins, and in some forms of practice, such as paediatrics, dosages must be based on body weight rather than predetermined formulae. The advice of the pharmacist should be sought and if one is not immediately available, the urgency of the procedure should be carefully reviewed.

In all these procedures inexperienced doctors need to recognise that they are carrying out an unusual and unfamiliar procedure. The patient may well be the only one on the ward requiring this particular form of treatment. Simply because it is unusual the doctor needs to exercise special care about the method of administration and the correct procedures to be followed. Unless the doctor has considered all these points it is unethical to proceed and the doctor should seek advice from a more experienced member of the clinical team.

### 7:3.2.1 Chemotherapy

Particular problems arise in relation to chemotherapy. Because of the potency of the drugs involved it is assumed that doctors will normally administer the drug personally, even though they may have had no previous experience of the procedure. Safety at work procedures require that the doctor is trained to make up the drugs, and understands the nature of the agents including their danger to the doctor and other employees. Protective clothing may be required. Special storage arrangements may be necessary, together with special procedures in the event of spillage or a failure in clinical technique during administration. Careful preliminary preparation will be necessary and consultation with the pharmacist is essential. Supervision and advice must be available from a more senior colleague and the doctor must not be afraid to seek it. The doctor is also responsible for ensuring the safe disposal of any unused drug and the containers and instruments used in administration. This can only be achieved if there has been an adequate level of training for all the personnel involved. Again it is the doctor's ethical responsibility to be satisfied that he or she has the necessary competence and support to undertake the procedure.

# 7:4 Prescribing

Choosing the drug to offer to a patient in a particular situation is a matter of clinical judgement and so this chapter should not be seen as an attempt to lay down rules but rather as an attempt to enlarge on some of the general principles as they relate to prescribing. The principles apply equally to other aspects of providing treatment but they bear reiteration in this specific context.

In addition to the information given here, the General Medical Services secretariat of the BMA can advise GP members on the contractual aspects of prescribing. Dilemmas about prescribing for minors (in particular with regard to contraceptives) is discussed in chapter 3 on children and young people (section 3:3.1.1).

### 7:4.1 *Prescribing criteria*

Prescribing decisions are governed by some basic tenets. The widely accepted definition of good quality prescribing is that which is based on the criteria of appropriateness, effectiveness, safety and economy. Implicit in the assessment of appropriateness is the principle that medicines should only be prescribed when they are necessary. In all cases the benefit of administering the medicine should be considered in relation to the risk involved. Sometimes it may seem easier for a doctor, and more acceptable for a patient, to write a prescription than to spend time assessing the root of the problem and other options. Patient demand and the placebo effect have been put forward as a justification for prescribing drugs acknowledged by the doctor to be pharmacologically ineffective. This is not good practice. It also undermines the ideal of a doctor-patient relationship based on honesty.

Regarding the doctor's assessment of effectiveness, it should be borne in mind that the effectiveness of conventional treatments has not always been scientifically proven. With regard to safety, prescriptions should not be provided in over-large quantities, which could lead some patients deliberately, or inadvertently, to misuse the product. The indiscriminate and routine long-term prescribing of benzodiazepines is perhaps the best recent example of this but the BMA also receives reports of some doctors in slimming clinics giving patients quantities of appetite suppressants in excess of the manufacturers' recommendations.

The prescribing decision must be based on the medical interests of the patient. Again with regard to slimming clinics, some appear to have a pre-defined policy as to the product which doctors should offer to any and all patients. Prescriptions must not be influenced by factors such as the convenience of the clinic management or the prospect of improper financial benefit to the doctor when, for example, the doctor owns the pharmacy nearby. The equitable distribution of resources is another issue raised regularly in relation to prescribing decisions and this is discussed further below in 7:5.1.4

### 7:4.2 Information to patients about medicines

As with the seeking of consent to the provision of any treatment, when prescribing there is an ethical duty to provide patients with information about the products prescribed, including information about side-effects. There is a duty to make sure that the patient is aware of the risks of treatment and any alternatives available. It is up to the doctor to use clinical judgement when deciding how much to tell the individual patient about risks, and the degree of disclosure necessary to assist the particular patient in making a choice about treatment. Provision of information is discussed in chapter 1, section 1:1.2.4

The primary responsibility for informing patients about prescribed medicines rests with the prescribing doctor, although pharmacists now share that responsibility. Pharmacists also have a central role in providing information about "over the counter" medicines available from pharmacies. Increasingly, the provision of written information to patients in the UK will be influenced by EC legislation and soon package leaflets for patients on medicines will become standard practice.[225] The BMA strongly emphasises, however, that written information does not diminish the duty of doctors to discuss the medication to the patient's satisfaction. The information should be comprehensible to the patient, with special attention being given to the needs of groups such as the elderly, the blind and speakers of other languages.

## 7:5  Responsibility for prescribing

### 7:5.1 Independence in prescribing matters

Doctors are individually responsible for the products they prescribe and must be able to justify, if necessary, the prescribing decisions they make. In its publication "Professional Conduct and Discipline: Fitness to Practise", the General Medical Council states that:

> "prescribing doctors should not only choose but also be seen to be choosing the drug or appliance which, in their independent professional judgement and having due regard to economy, will best serve the medical interests of the patient" (para 119 in January 1993 edition).

#### 7:5.1.1 Financial involvement of doctors in external health-related services

Doctors often raise questions about the ethics of their financial involvement in health-related services outside their particular surgery or hospital. The BMA would be concerned about doctors being involved in

184

any business ventures which might give rise to doubt about their prescribing independence. In circumstances where the doctor has a role both as the purchaser and provider of a service or product, such concerns arise. The importance of not only acting, but being seen to act, independently, in the matter of treatment and prescribing is emphasised by the BMA.

Common enquiries in this area concern the propriety of doctors prescribing for their patients medicines marketed by companies in which the doctor or the doctor's family has a significant financial interest. Sometimes the financial interest is acquired after patients have been prescribed a long-term course of drugs which suits them. In such cases, it has been thought unlikely that any objection would be raised to the doctor maintaining the patients' prescription, since the prescribing decision pre-dates the financial incentive.

On the other hand, most doctors would think it unethical to consider changing a patient's medication from an already established pattern to a new medicine in which they have financial interests. It would certainly be unethical to do so if the doctor's decision was influenced by any financial connection. Dilemmas arise, however, if the doctor becomes convinced of the superiority of the product with which he or she has a financial connection. Such cases have been raised with the BMA, which recognises that genuine concern for the patient's benefit can easily be confused with self interest. For such reasons, the Association believes it is generally unwise for doctors to form a business connection with companies producing, marketing or promoting such products.

For other aspects of this issue of financial interest in health-related services, such as doctors having a stake in private nursing homes or clinics, it is considered sufficient for the doctor to make the patient aware of the doctor's financial interest in the matter, and of alternative options (if available), in which the doctor has no special financial interest. The general advice on declaring a financial interest is given in chapter 10 (section 10:2.7). This advice to declare an interest does not provide sufficient safeguard, however, in the case of prescribing, since the patient is usually not in a position to exercise an informed choice about other medicines available as suitable alternatives to the one in which the doctor has a financial interest.

### 7:5.1.2 Ownership of pharmacies

The topic of doctors' relations with pharmacists is discussed in chapter 11 (section 11:6, see also chapter 10, section 10:2.8). For many years, the BMA advised against GPs owning a pharmacy within their practice area on the grounds that the patients might think that the doctors' prescribing would be influenced by financial considerations. In 1992 the Association revised its advice, recognising that many aspects of the delivery of health care were changing. Like the GMC, the BMA reminds doctors that prescribing decisions must be based on the interests of the patient and that GPs should inform their patients of any financial interest they hold in a pharmacy.

### 7:5.1.3 Acceptance of gifts from pharmaceutical companies

Questions are often raised in connection with relationships between doctors and the pharmaceutical industry. The acceptance of gifts, loans or hospitality is discussed in chapter 11 (section 11:7.1). The BMA does not approve of doctors demanding a fee before they will agree to see a pharmaceutical company representative.

### 7:5.1.4 Pressure from patients

It is usual for doctors to be influenced by colleagues, the medical literature and established guidelines in arriving at prescribing decisions. Patient preference too must be considered. Ethical dilemmas may arise, however, when substantial additional expenditure for the NHS results from acceding to such preferences and this affects resources for other patients.

The BMA considers that it is the doctor's ethical duty to use the most economic and efficacious treatment available when the patient is receiving treatment within the NHS. Therefore, choosing a costlier product is unethical unless it can be expected to produce a superior outcome. Patient preference and compliance may be elements which constitute superior outcome. Implicit in this view is the assumption that objective assessment should be made of the elements which might justify prescribing the more expensive product. When patients are being treated privately, there can be no objection to them choosing a more expensive option which they prefer and are prepared to pay for. However, private insurance schemes may not be willing to cover options which are more expensive than they consider necessary.

Other dilemmas arise from patients insisting on the continuation of a prescription which the doctor feels can no longer be justified. Common examples include hypnotics and anxiolytics which may have been prescribed to enable the patient to deal with a painful situation such as a bereavement. Similarly, amphetamine-type appetite suppressants are often sought by patients who desperately want to lose weight. Patients may underestimate or disregard the possibility of creating a physical or psychological dependence, particularly when they are feeling in control of their drug use. Dealing with the situation requires time for doctors to listen to patients' views and for doctors to explain their clinical understanding of the situation. Some doctors have proposed that if counselling fails to convince the patient of the undesirability of the requested treatment, the patient should be asked to sign a document accepting responsibility for insisting upon a prescription. Such a document is unlikely to carry any weight in law. Ethically, it would not justify doctors who make such a prescription, contrary to their own judgement, at the patient's request.

### 7:5.2 *Clinical freedom and resources*

Doctors can prescribe whatever approved medicine they consider appropriate for a patient but, in practice, clinical autonomy is not absolute. Within the NHS, the state takes an interest in prescribing habits and studies have identified tremendous variations in the volume and cost of prescribing between different geographical areas and between individual prescribers.

For ethical, as well as practical reasons, doctors need to be aware of the implications of their prescribing habits. Measures are available to assist the development of such awareness. Prescribing Analysis and CosT (PACT) reports automatically produced by the Prescription Pricing Authority (PPA) in varying levels of complexity indicate trends in costs, and prescribing patterns. They can be used as a teaching tool for trainees and can also be used as a doctor's formulary. Indicative prescribing amounts (IPAs), introduced by the Department of Health in 1991 are supposed to encourage GPs to examine the cost of prescribing in a considered and deliberate way and thus develop rational prescribing policies. Since the new GP contract was introduced in April 1991, general practitioners have therefore received monthly budgetary information. Concerns have been expressed, however, that IPAs may exert a downward pressure on prescribing costs which may not necessarily be in patients' best interests.

### 7:5.2.1 *"Uneconomic" patients*

Some NHS GPs have considered removing a patient from their lists for so-called economic reasons, such as the patient's need for expensive drug treatment. The BMA considers this to be unethical. The GMC restated its position in January 1993.

> "Patients have a right, enshrined in law, to choose their family doctor. Doctors have a parallel right to refuse to accept patients, or to remove them from their lists, with no formal obligation to give reasons for their decision. These rights flow from the belief that a satisfactory relationship between patient and doctor will arise only where each is committed to it; consequently, if either party believes that the relationship has failed, they have a right to end it.

> Given this, family doctors, as the professionals involved, have special responsibilities for making the relationship work. In particular, it is unacceptable to abuse the right to refuse to accept patients by applying criteria of access to the practice list which discriminate against groups of patients on grounds of their age, sex, sexual orientation, race, colour, religious belief, perceived economic worth or the amount of work they are likely to generate by virtue of their clinical condition."

187

## 7:6 Shared responsibility for prescribing

It is preferable for one doctor, the general practitioner, to be fully informed about, and be responsible for, overall management of the patient's health care. In some circumstances, two or more health professionals may be responsible for different aspects of care and this is increasingly the case. In any situation where responsibility is shared, liaison between the health professionals is essential. It is unethical for doctors to hold back from an appropriately accredited health professional information necessary for proper care of the patient unless the patient refuses to allow the disclosure. (Explicit patient consent for disclosure to other health professionals is discussed in chapter 2, section 2:1.5.) It is also unethical for doctors to encourage patients to hold back from their GP important medical facts. Doctors have a duty to tell patients why it is important for them to share such information with their GP. Such problems can arise when care is shared between GPs and doctors employed by private clinics. In recent years the BMA has received many complaints that some slimming clinics fail to mention to patients the importance of informing their GP about their medication.

### 7:6.1 Prescribing shared between GPs and doctors employed by private clinics

General practitioners sometimes unwillingly, and often unwittingly, share responsibility for the clinical management of a patient with private clinics. Patients often self-refer to facilities which offer treatments to reduce weight, restore hair or remedy sexual dysfunction. The BMA issues an advice leaflet[226] for doctors employed by private organisations providing clinical, diagnostic or medical advisory services. This deals with issues such as referral, follow-up, commission and product liability as well as prescribing.

Private slimming clinics are the focus of much correspondence to the BMA. In some of these clinics, centrally acting appetite suppressants are provided routinely as part of clinic policy, as is often made clear in the advertisements to the public. In some cases, prescribing of these products is initiated without enquiry as to the possibility of pregnancy, clinical contra-indications or psychological disturbance and without mention of liaison with the patient's GP. The BMA considers that the use of centrally acting appetite suppressants in weight-loss treatment is to be deprecated and that it raises ethical concerns. Attitudes to such products have hardened since modern research has found that they often give little benefit because tolerance develops, and also because the drugs may undermine the efficacy of behaviour therapy. Doctors prescribing these preparations are advised to bear in mind the opinion of the British National Formulary which states that "use of amphetamine-like drugs is not justified as any possible benefits are outweighed by risks involved".[227]

A doctor employed by a private organisation bears responsibility for prescribing and must be able to exercise independent clinical judgement, regardless of the policies of the clinic's management. The doctor must ensure that the prescription is appropriate for the patient's needs and does not conflict with other treatment provided by the patient's general practitioner. This requires liaison with the patient's GP, with the patient's consent, before any prescribing is done by the clinic doctor. There is an ethical duty to draw to patients' attention the advantages of involving their GP, and the risks of conflicting treatment or misdiagnosis when the GP is not informed.

### 7:6.2 *Prescribing shared between GPs and consultants*

Sometimes GPs have not been informed - either by patients or specialists - when patients have sought help to conceive. For a time, concern about patients' sensitivity regarding their infertility led to the legal prohibition of liaison between the specialist and the GP, even with the patient's consent. This was changed in 1992 by an amendment to the Human Fertilisation and Embryology Act 1990 which allowed specialists to communicate directly with a patient's GP regarding her treatment, with the patient's consent.

Shared prescribing can also cause problems in the context of fertility treatment. It is accepted that a doctor who has clinical responsibility for a patient should undertake the necessary prescribing for that patient. Within the NHS, difficulties have arisen in cases where prescribing responsibility and costs have been transferred inappropriately to the general practitioner when the patient's (NHS or private) treatment is being supervised by a hospital consultant.

GPs are thus placed in the invidious position of either appearing unsupportive of the patient or accepting legal, financial and ethical responsibility for a course of prescriptions which they have not initiated and which they sometimes feel inappropriate for that patient. Where the product is of a very specialised nature they may feel they have insufficient expertise to supervise its provision.

The GMC's statement of January 1993 on "Contractual Arrangements in Health Care: Professional Responsibilities in Relation to the Clinical Needs of Patients" makes reference to this:

"In the Council's view the question is one of professional practice. In general doctors are expected to take account of appropriateness, effectiveness and cost when prescribing any drug. Where there is shared care doctors responsible for the continuing management of the patient must be fully competent to exercise their share of clinical responsibility and have a duty to keep themselves informed of the drugs that are recommended for their patients. Specialists, for their part, should not put general practitioners under pressure to take responsibility for their prescribing recommendations. Rather, there should be full consultation and agreement between general practitioners and hospital doctors about the indications and need for particular therapies. Where such agreements are reached doctors should have no inhibitions about prescribing on the basis of the patient's need; such agreements would be the basis for justifying cost."

The Department of Health, in consultation with the medical profession, has also provided guidance on the transfer of prescribing responsibility.[228] The guidance is helpful in clarifying responsibilities so that GPs can decide under what circumstances to accept prescribing responsibility, and hospital consultants can assess whether transfer of responsibility is appropriate.

The following basic points should be borne in mind:

- Legal responsibility for prescribing rests with the doctor who signs the prescription.

- Hospital consultants have full responsibility for prescribing for in-patients and for specific treatments administered in hospital out-patient clinics.

- Responsibility for prescribing should rest with the consultant if the drugs are included in a hospital-based clinical trial and when it is more appropriate for the consultant to monitor the medication because of the need for specialised investigations, or where there are supply problems with the drugs.

- When a consultant considers a patient's condition stable, he or she may seek the agreement of the GP concerned to share care. In proposing a shared-care arrangement, a consultant may advise the GP which medicine to prescribe. Where a new or rarely prescribed medicine is being recommended, its dosage and administration must be specified by the consultant so that the GP can monitor and adjust the dose if necessary. When a treatment is not licensed for a particular indication, full justification for the use of the drug should be given by the consultant to the GP. Where a hospital drug formulary is in operation and a recommended treatment is not included, the GP must be informed and given the option of prescribing alternatives.

- When an in-patient is discharged from hospital, sufficient drugs should be prescribed and dispensed by the hospital pharmacy for at least a seven-day period. The GP to whose care the patient is transferred, should receive notification in good time of the patient's diagnosis and drug therapy in order to maintain continuity. If that information cannot be transferred to the GP within the timescale, drugs should be prescribed by the hospital for as long a period as is necessary.

- When clinical, and therefore prescribing, responsibility for a patient is transferred from hospital to GP, it is of the utmost importance that the GP feels fully confident to prescribe the necessary drugs. It is essential that a transfer involving drug therapies with which GPs would not normally be familiar should not take place without full agreement between the hospital consultant (or any transferring doctor) and the GP, who must have sufficient information about the drug therapy. When drawing up protocols, or where there is a professional disagreement over who should prescribe, it may be necessary for local discussion to take place between district health authorities, hospital managers and medical staff and the relevant local medical committee as a prelude to establishing agreement with individual GPs. A GP is only obliged to provide treatment consistent with the GP terms of service.

- When a GP takes responsibility for prescribing or dispensing drugs which have not normally been dispensed in the community, there should be liaison between the transferring hospital and the community pharmacist to ensure continuity of supply.

### 7:6.3 *Prescribing shared with a doctor in another country*

A very difficult question, which arises frequently, concerns prescriptions for patients who live in other parts of the world. Relatives in this country often approach their own GP with a request for medication for a seriously ill patient abroad where appropriate drugs are unobtainable. Many doctors do not wish to be involved in such cases because of the obvious risks of prescribing for a patient they have not seen. It is also clear that while doctors here have no ethical obligation or duty of care regarding the sick person, they may feel impelled by humanitarian considerations to look into the case. Doctors particularly seek advice about the ethical considerations when it is a case of life or death for the person abroad. Such situations are fraught with difficulty, but if doctors are willing to pursue the matter, after considering the risks for the overseas patient, and for themselves as prescribers if harm to that patient should result, the BMA gives the following advice.

It is unwise to rely solely on the relatives' account of the patient's condition. Often the patient's own doctor abroad is willing to give a clinical account of the condition and recommendations for medication, as well as confirming that the medication is necessary and unobtainable by other means. Such cases virtually amount to a situation of shared prescribing with the doctor who writes the prescription relying heavily on the medical opinion of the examining doctor. Some lives are probably saved by this arrangement and this is usually the factor which persuades

191

the prescribing doctor to co-operate, on the grounds that in the particular situation the risks of not obtaining treatment at all are likely to be greater than the risks of prescribing error. We have not heard of any cases where a prescribing doctor subsequently suffered legal repercussions, although the possibility of erroneous prescribing in such situations cannot be ruled out.

Even where the prescribing doctor is willing to participate in such an arrangement, there are a number of further hurdles to be overcome and these may influence the doctor's view of the practicality of the proposal. For example, relatives have to consider how the drugs will be transported, including the rules governing the export and import of drugs which are not for their personal use.[229] As a final minor point, such prescriptions must be paid for privately as they are not covered by the NHS.

### 7:6.4 *Prescribing shared with nurse prescribers*

There has been much debate about empowering suitably qualified nurses, such as district nurses, health visitors or paediatric community nurses, to prescribe items necessary for the care of patients with conditions for which such nurses take independent clinical responsibility. Many doctors welcome the principle of nurse-prescribing in clearly defined circumstances and within a set protocol. A cost-benefit study commissioned by the Department of Health revealed that, even prior to legislation, a number of flexible arrangements already existed, which virtually gave nurses the de facto power to "prescribe". As in any other circumstance where prescribing responsibilities are shared, good communication between health professionals is essential.

### 7:6.5 *Practitioners in complementary therapies*

An area of concern about shared prescribing arises in connection with the treatments recommended by complementary practitioners to whom patients self-refer. Anxiety is often expressed by doctors about patient decisions to suspend or postpone scientifically proven treatments in preference for other remedies. In this context, however, we would note again that not all conventional treatments have been so proven and, indeed, many complementary therapies are in the process of being scientifically assessed. When patients attempt to combine two systems of treatment this may well leave doctors unclear about the extent to which they may co-operate with a non-medical practitioner. General guidance on such liaison is given in chapter 11, section 11:3. Discussion of the potential risks and benefits of particular treatments may help doctors and patients decide on a mutually acceptable course.

Whereas some doctors have little sympathy with complementary therapies and regard them as potentially dangerous because, for example, vital time may be lost in postponing effective orthodox treatment or the practitioner may be unregulated, other doctors see the public's interest in

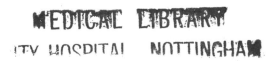

such therapies as an indication of patients seeking to control their own health management by self-help and preventive measures. Some argue that the profession should accept the trend for patients to consult complementary practitioners, since to do otherwise is to risk losing contact with such patients altogether. Individual doctors will have to decide within the context of the particular case and the liability involved, whether they are able to share the patient's management with such practitioners. Many general practitioners are now employing complementary therapists such as hypnotherapists or acupuncturists in order to broaden the range of services which they offer to their patients. Overall clinical responsibility rests with the doctor. In 1993, the BMA published a report[230] on complementary therapies which further explored some of these issues.

## 7:7 Dependence and misuse

### 7:7.1 *Responsibilities of the prescriber*

The prevalence of drug dependence and misuse in Great Britain, particularly amongst young people, gives rise to concern amongst doctors, other health professionals, teachers, social workers and the police. Doctors should be familiar with the regulations[231] concerning controlled drugs and the notification of addicts. Prescribers have three main responsibilities concerning drugs likely to cause dependence or misuse:

a) To avoid creating dependence by introducing drugs to patients without sufficient reason. In this context, the proper use of the morphine-like drugs is well understood. The dangers of other controlled drugs are less clear because recognition of dependence is not easy and its effects are less obvious. Perhaps the most notable result of uninhibited prescribing is that a large number of patients take tablets which do them neither much good nor much harm, but to which they are committed indefinitely because the tablets cannot readily be stopped.

b) To see that a patient does not gradually increase the dose of a drug, given for good medical reasons, to the point where dependence becomes more likely. This tendency is seen especially with hypnotics and anxiolytics, where patients may accumulate stocks from family or friends.

c) To avoid being used as an unwitting source of supply for addicts, whose methods include visiting more than one doctor, fabricating stories and forging prescriptions. Doctors should be wary about prescribing for strangers. The BNF advises that doctors may be able to obtain information about suspected opioid addicts from the Home Office and lists a number of precautions to minimise the likelihood of misuse or theft of prescriptions pads.

193

## 7:8 Summary

1    Medicines should be prescribed only when necessary.
2    Prescribing should be rationally based on what is appropriate, effective, safe and economic.
3    Doctors are individually responsible for the products they prescribe and must be able to justify, if necessary, the prescribing decisions they make.
4    There is an ethical duty to provide patients with information about the products prescribed, including information about side-effects.
5    Written information does not, and never should, replace the need for doctors or pharmacists to discuss the medication to the patient's satisfaction.
6    The prescribing decision must be based on the medical interests of the patient and not dictated by the policies of the doctor's employers.
7    Doctors should avoid accepting any pecuniary or material inducement which might compromise, or be regarded by others as likely to compromise, the independent exercise of their clinical judgement in prescribing matters.
8    It is generally unwise for doctors to form a business connection with companies producing, marketing or promoting pharmaceutical products which the doctor may wish to prescribe.
10   Doctors must take into account the responsible distribution of resources.
11   Where prescribing responsibility is shared, liaison between the health professionals is essential and the effective management of the patient's condition must be the prime consideration.
12   Prescriptions should not be provided in over-large quantities or over an excessive period of time, both of which might encourage the patient to abuse the product.
13   Doctors have an ethical duty to keep abreast of new developments in medicine and prescribing, without seeking financial inducement to do so.

# 8 Research

*In this chapter we look at the potential conflict of interests which arise in research and how attempts are made to achieve balance between the rights of individuals and the needs of society. The definitions of therapeutic, non-therapeutic research and innovative treatment are briefly examined. Consent is discussed, particularly in relation to randomised trials and vulnerable subjects. Confidentiality and ownership of material are discussed. The work of local research ethics committees is discussed. The legislation on embryo research is mentioned and the moral arguments surrounding such research are touched upon. Published guidelines are noted. Reference is also made to financial considerations connected with research. Summary.*

## 8:1 Introduction

### 8:1.1 *Seeking balance*

As members of society, we all benefit from advances in medical knowledge and have an interest in seeing research promoted within an acceptable framework. In elaborating such a framework, ethicists have sought to balance the desire of researchers to extend knowledge with the rights of research subjects. In this chapter, therefore, we aim to discuss the balance between the benefits society derives from research and the interests of individuals. Central topics are the themes of consent and confidentiality raised in chapters 1 and 2.

Another aspect of balance concerns the patient's right to autonomy and the doctor's duty to act in the patient's best interests. Patient autonomy and choice in the context of research is a much debated issue. In the past the doctor's disclosure of information to patients was dominated by the beneficence principle. A prime objective was to maintain the patient's morale and sense of hope. Medical uncertainty was hidden from the patient. In 1803, Percival offered the advice that "the balance of truthfulness yields to beneficence in critical situations".[232] This guidance set the tone for more than a century and a half and still reverberates, particularly in discussions about research. The so-called doctrine of informed consent is an American concept, introduced into medical practice in the USA in the late 1950s and into clinical study a decade later[233] following Beecher's study (see 8:4.2 below). From the outset, however, questions have been regularly raised about the possibility of determining whether research subjects can ever give true consent based on full information. This also is discussed in this chapter.

The task of ensuring balance by assessing research projects is given to local research ethics committees (LRECs) who weigh the information about possible risks against potential benefits. Not all research, however, is undertaken solely to benefit patients. Research projects may be carried out to generate income for further research or as part of medical training or to further the researcher's career. This highlights the need for well informed ethics committees, who have clear ideas of what society expects.

Yet there is no legal obligation for researchers to obtain independent ethical approval for studies. In practice, it is virtually impossible to obtain financial support for a study which does not have approval by an ethics committee but there are no binding rules to govern the work of such committees nor are there minimum legal criteria for their constitution. There have been persistent calls for regulation in this area. In addition to the scrutiny of trained LREC members and peer review, many believe that research should also be subject to specific legislation, to examination by an overall monitoring body and to an independent investigatory mechanism for fraud. All of these points are discussed further below.

### 8:1.2 *Limits on experimentation*

Some argue that all advancements of medical science inevitably entail a benefit to mankind and that there is a moral imperative to pursue them. However, for moral or pragmatic reasons, there are limits beyond which society is not willing to allow researchers to go. The Warnock Report[234] argued for "barriers that are not to be crossed, some limits fixed, beyond which people must not be allowed to go. The very existence of morality depends upon it." In response, Parliament specified statutory limits on experimentation on embryos.

Pragmatic reasons given for drawing boundaries are that unless some experimental therapies are controlled, the cost of the research distorts health funding so that many people suffering from easily treatable complaints are deprived of help. (Issues relating to resources are discussed in general terms in chapter 12).

### 8:1.3 *A legislative framework*

Attention is often drawn to the fact that, as a nation, we have regulated research on animals by law for over a century (since the Cruelty to Animals Act 1876) but no specific legislation covers research on humans subjects, apart from that regulating embryo research. At present, most research on human subjects is covered primarily by the vaguely defined common-law concept of consent which does, however, recognise limits to the degree to which people can consent to potentially damaging measures (see 8:2.2 below). Safeguards are also provided by the statutory framework for drug licensing by the Committee on the Safety of Medicines. The

Human Fertilisation and Embryology Act 1990 brought research on embryos within statutory supervision but other difficult areas such as research on children, prisoners, mentally incapacitated people and the elderly remain as yet unregulated by law. The confusion experienced by some LRECs about the ethics of such research was reflected by the 1992 report of the King's Fund Institute.[235]

The report echoes long felt dissatisfaction about the lack of a clear public policy, expressed through statute. Others have also pointed out that doctors carrying out research are at least bound by the rules of the General Medical Council, in contrast to other practitioners whose research work is largely unregulated. A persistent fear is that if the issues surrounding so-called "informed" consent are not clearly ironed out, a cause celebre will eventually be fought through the courts and lead to tough restrictions. To forestall this, many support proposals for the profession to agree in advance a statutory code of practice, to safeguard the interests of research subjects and ensure the continuance of properly regulated research. Others maintain that law should only be a final safety net and that standards should be set by bodies such as the Royal Colleges, the BMA and the Medical Research Council. The arguments may soon be resolved, since Great Britain's membership of the European Community is likely to change the current situation with the harmonisation of national legislation.

There is no shortage of guidance, however, and in the absence of statute, there is a plethora of published guidelines. The most important of these is the World Medical Association's Declaration of Helsinki most recently modified in 1989.[236] The BMA supports this declaration, which specifies that the design and performance of each experimental procedure must be subject to independent review.

## 8:2 Definitions

It may be useful to define the parameters of discussion before we proceed to analyse the issues. Confusion sometimes arises from the wide range of procedures covered by the term, "research". Research which consists of analysis of identifiable or non-identifiable data without any patient contact or change of medication stands at one end of the spectrum. Studies which involve changing a patient from a proven treatment to a different regime, the benefits and risks of which are not fully known, stand at the opposite end of the spectrum.

It may be helpful to look at how the topic of research is often divided into the categories of therapeutic and non-therapeutic. It is important to see if and how these differ from innovative treatments, since often the guidance offered depends on the category, as do the legal implications.

### 8:2.1 *Therapeutic research*

The World Medical Association first published its code of ethics on human experimentation, the Declaration of Helsinki, in 1964 (modified 1989). This states:

"In the field of biomedical research a fundamental distinction must be recognised between medical research in which the aim is essentially diagnostic or therapeutic for a patient, and medical research, the essential object of which is purely scientific and without implying direct diagnostic or therapeutic value to the person subjected to the research".

This indicates that the clinician's ultimate aim is as significant as the procedure, since it is the doctor's intention which allows the label of "therapeutic" or "non-therapeutic" to be applied. Despite the implication in the Declaration of Helsinki, the distinction between therapeutic and non-therapeutic research is often not at all clear, with a consequent blurring of the moral focus.

### 8:2.2 *Non-therapeutic research*

Non-therapeutic research can be defined as treatment whose principal intention is to extend knowledge of the particular condition in a way which will benefit future patients. Some see this activity as "real research" and clearly it must be subject to full ethical review by LRECs. It may either involve healthy volunteers or patients but is undertaken with the purpose of testing a hypothesis and contributing to general knowledge. The subject's consent must be based on adequate information but, even so, given the lack of benefit to the individual, the law is likely to set limits on the risk of harm that an individual may agree to. Some legal experts envisage that a court would only accept the validity of consent to what is frequently called "minimal risk". (A list of definitions of various degrees of risk is given at the end of the chapter).[237] While some expected or unexpected benefit for the research subject may result from the treatment, this does not alter the status of the project as research.

### 8:2.3 *Innovative treatment*

It is often unclear how new treatments and techniques fit into the framework of ethical review. At present they are sometimes seen as an extension of the usual treatment, even though such treatments may expose the patient to more than a minimal risk of harm. However, they are often classified as research. Where the digression from usual practice is small and designed merely to deal with the particular circumstances of an individual patient, it is argued that it is justifiable to classify this on an extension of usual treatment. An experienced surgeon, for example, may modify the approach to a particular surgical procedure for an individual patient. The procedure remains essentially the same but the surgeon anticipates a superior outcome from a relatively minor modification. If the modified procedure works well, it should then be submitted to further scrutiny, including a clinical trial. What begins as treatment becomes research.

In the eyes of many people, innovative treatments straddle the gap between research and medical practice. Doctors, it is argued on the one side, have always modified methods of investigation and treatment in the light of experience. Thus, some people say innovative treatments are a standard feature of medical practice; they regard the fact that useful information is gained as a by-product as largely incidental to the intention of effectively treating the patient. Others, including some eminent researchers,[238] totally reject this notion, seeing the "trial and error" formula as offering no protection to the public. They refute the idea that innovative treatment is different from research, particularly if it involves an unknown or increased element of risk for the patient. They believe that efforts to differentiate between the two suggest a double standard which is scientifically and ethically unacceptable since it would permit untried remedies, including new surgical techniques, to be applied without ethical restraint or independent assessment. Thus, the implementation of innovative therapies has given rise to many anxieties. In particular, innovative therapies may be repeated without being subject to the formal scrutiny of an LREC.

Some have seen an answer in dividing innovative treatment into the same previously stated categories of therapeutic and non-therapeutic. They propose that if the motive for the modification of treatment is to choose the best possible course of action for the individual patient, even though it is unconventional, it should be viewed as treatment rather than research. The patient, of course, should be informed of how and why the proposed treatment differs from the usual measures and give consent after deliberation on the information. The degree of digression from usual practice is also an important consideration. Ethical committee approval should be sought for any measures which involve more than a minimally greater risk than the usual treatment. Conclusions reached from the implementation of changes in treatments should be shared with others and such practices must also be subject to peer review.

It is clear that where the clinician's intention is to acquire new knowledge rather than solely to care for the patient, the constraints applicable to the conduct of research should apply. Thus, in cases where a doctor proposes, for an individual patient, a course of action which diverges substantially from normal medical practice, with the intention of gaining information which might help future patients, the activity must be subject to review by a local research ethics committee and possibly further review as well, if the implications are particularly significant and clearly extend beyond the interests of the locality (see 8:5 below).

199

The BMA considers that in cases where the proposed treatment diverges radically from accepted practice and has wide implications, expert scrutiny, in addition to that of the local committee, is desirable.

### 8:2.4 *Areas of overlap*

As has already been mentioned, some projects overlap from one category into the other but where the focus of attention is not solely the best interests of the individual patient, treatment must be subject to the rigorous standards required for research projects.

Projects which begin in one category may drift into another. Thus, what starts out as treatment may turn into a research project. In 1975, for example, when John Lorber published the Milroy Lecture on "Ethical Problems in the Management of Myelomeningocele and Hydrocephalus",[239] he reported how a pattern of treatment changed radically without public debate of the implications. Beginning from a position of uncritical enthusiasm for surgically treating all infants born with myelomeningocele (but, according to Lorber, without adequately consulting parents), "accepted" treatment options passed through four different phases until Lorber, himself, established a set of criteria for selective non-treatment. (Non-treatment decisions in general are discussed in chapter 6, section 6:3 and decisions regarding treatment of severely malformed infants in chapter 3, section 3:3.6.1).

The criteria for decision-making in such cases, and the introduction of radical changes in practice further to this, must be subject to public debate.

## 8:3 Medical practice

Having identified broadly different categories, we need to look at each of these in greater detail. In accordance with the definitions above, we exclude accepted medical practice from the realm of research. It is interesting to note, however, that within the conduct of normal medical practice, it is well established that doctors are not free to press ahead in an unconstrained manner. Traditionally it has been accepted that reference should be made to the opinion of the peer group and this was accepted practice at the time of Thomas Percival, who wrote in the early 19th century:

> "It is for the good of patients, and especially the poor, that new remedies and new methods of chirugical treatment should be devised. But in the accomplishment of this salutary purpose the gentlemen of the faculty should be scrupulously and conscientiously governed by sound reason, just analogy or well authenticated facts. And no such trials should be instituted without a previous consultation of the physicians or surgeons according to the nature of the case".[240]

In the UK, the importance of peer concurrence has been emphasised in recent times in a number of legal cases, which can be traced back to the Bolam judgement of 1957, which established that "a doctor is not guilty of negligence if he has acted in accordance with a practice accepted as proper by a responsible body of medical men skilled in that particular art".[241]

In 1803 it was not expected that patients should, or probably ever would, have any voice in the matter and, since the central issue in the Bolam case was the matter of patient information and consent (which was judged to be necessary to the degree which the profession saw appropriate), it is clear that this was the view which prevailed until relatively recently. Bolam still sets the legal standard, but there is ever-increasing acknowledgement that the patient's views dictate what are judged to be appropriate levels of information, not only for research, but also for activities which clearly fall within the scope of accepted practice. This is discussed further in chapter 1 (section 1:2.4) on consent.

## 8:4 Research

### 8:4.1 *The need for research*

In past centuries attitudes towards medical experimentation were very different. In the early 18th century, "condemned prisoners in Newgate Gaol who volunteered for experimental variolation in return for their freedom (if they survived) probably had few second thoughts".[242]

In principle, a general need for research is usually conceded to be beyond argument. Nevertheless, criticism is rightly levelled at particular research projects which ignore patient rights or whose methodology, execution or utility is suspect. Patients and doctors worry that some research projects have not been properly thought through and are flawed from a scientific perspective, are not properly monitored or are undertaken unnecessarily in order to promote some researcher's career prospects, perhaps duplicating previous projects.

### 8:4.2 *Flawed research*

Historically there have been very good grounds for such concerns, as is discussed further below. Even in comparatively recent times there have been well documented examples of severely flawed projects. In the United States in 1966, Beecher[243] identified 50 unethical studies, and referred to a further 186 likely examples. The examples given by Beecher make chilling reading and range from the withholding of known effective treatment, resulting in one case in at least 23 potentially avoidable deaths in a group of 408 patients, to scientifically dubious experiments, such as the transplantation of a melanoma from a daughter to her volunteering mother in the hope that the production of tumour antibodies might help the daughter. In the latter case, Beecher comments that "the hope expressed seems to have been more theoretical than practical". The daughter died on the day after the transplantation of the tumour into her mother and the mother died a year later of diffuse melanoma that metastasised from a small piece of the transplanted tumour.

In 1967, in England, Pappworth published his influential study, Human Guinea Pigs,[244] which laid the groundwork for the establishment of regional committees to supervise research. It was hoped that by subjecting each research project to the scrutiny of these committees blatantly unethical practices would be eliminated. Unfortunately, the efficacy of the review system has often been questioned. A notable example of its ineffectiveness was provided in 1981 when an elderly widow died from the effects of an experimental drug used in a trial which had the approval of eleven ethics committees. Her death was caused by bone marrow depression induced by the drug. The patient had been included, without her knowledge, in a randomised controlled clinical trial of the new drug. At her inquest, attention was drawn to the fact that patients could be subjected to a risky procedure without their knowledge or consent. The chairman of one of the committees which had approved the trial argued that the patient's consent to surgery for cancer extended to related, albeit experimental, treatment and that seeking informed consent would involve "unacceptable psychological trauma". The Lancet strongly condemned the study procedure, stating:

> "The fluoroucil trial, involving a portal catheter and a toxic drug, should - on the criteria of both variance from standard procedure and degree of risk - have had special consent... If the patient is not capable of understanding the basic plan of management, he or she should not be included in the trial. No one pretends that these matters are easy for doctor or patient, but it is important that the clinical research exercise remains a partnership built on trust".

Such trust depends upon the observing of high ethical standards which give due prominence to the duties owed to research subjects (see 8:8 below).

### 8:4.3 *Achieving good standards*

It is not difficult to understand the apprehensions of patients regarding research. Society and the profession must concentrate on building an ethical framework which permits research activities to progress, while at the same time maintaining the public's confidence that individual autonomy is respected. Various measures have been set in train to achieve this. The Department of Health has, for example, commissioned specific training materials for members of local research ethics committees. The King's Fund report[245] draws attention to the confusion experienced by some committees about their role and has given detailed recommendations on both the work of LRECs, and on measures to facilitate good ethical practice.

The various guidelines (mentioned in 8:12 below) also set high standards but do not have the force of law. Nevertheless, influential research bodies have made considerable efforts to promote good practice. The Association of the British Pharmaceutical Industry (ABPI) has, for example, voluntarily adopted as policy the European Commission's principles of Good Clinical (Research) Practice in advance of this being mandated by an EC Directive. (These principles are discussed further in 8:8 below.)

Efforts have also been made to eliminate fraud in research. Until recently only one case of clinical research fraud appeared to have been reported, although many in the field believed that some of the data supplied by UK clinical investigators was fraudulent.[246] Common-sense principles for the detection of fraud have been set down by the ABPI, which recommends that any investigator found to have submitted fraudulent data be referred to the General Medical Council or prosecuted for the criminal offence of fraud. The BMA also emphasises that fraud is totally unacceptable and supports such measures to detect and eliminate it.

All recognise that particularly vulnerable groups require special consideration when research is proposed but there is still disagreement about whether and how members of such groups should be included in research. We consider below (8:8) the involvement of minors, the mentally handicapped, psychiatric patients and prisoners in research projects.

## 8:5 Innovative treatment

Although in the past fears have been expressed about the lack of review or limitation of innovative treatments, nowadays, local research ethics committees are usually asked to approve innovations but may be faced with requests to approve activities which have far wider implications than a merely local application. Examples of this type of activity have included the transplantation of fetal tissue for treatment of Parkinson's disease, intubation of moribund patients for the purposes of organ transplantation and the transplantation of animal organs into human beings. Many would say that such important issues should be aired in public and fear that there may be inherent risks in relying solely on local committee approval. Anecdotal examples can be found of innovative techniques being approved by committees whose membership includes individuals who might be personally interested in promoting the project.

The BMA supports the elaboration of public policy on such issues through debate in a public forum which includes both experts and non-experts.

## 8:6 Consent

Research brings the risk of causing harm, in the practical sense of possibly damaging or disadvantaging a patient, and of doing wrong, in the

203

moral sense of ignoring the autonomy of that individual. People are wronged if they are deprived of choice or their values are transgressed on the assumption that the best clinical outcome is necessarily what is best for them. The possibility of harm cannot be entirely eliminated from research but by insisting that patients have adequate information and choice about participation, we minimise the possibility of wronging them.

### 8:6.1 *Background to the emphasis on voluntary consent*

Following World War II information came out about the atrocities, conducted in the name of scientific experimentation, in concentration camps. This led to serious international concern about the use of non-consenting subjects and has lent a very emotive undertow to the discussion about research, particularly in Europe. Since the Nuremberg Trials, the issue of consent and the amount of information required to make such consent valid, has received more attention than any other ethical issue in biomedical research involving human subjects. The Nuremberg Code and WMA Declaration of Helsinki[247] arose from this concern.

#### 8:6.1.1 *The Nuremberg Code*[248]

Rule 1 of the Nuremberg Code states:

"the person involved should have the legal capacity to give consent; should be so situated as to be able to exercise free power of choice, without the intervention of any element of force, fraud, deceit, duress, over-reaching, or other ulterior form of constraint or coercion; and should have sufficient knowledge and comprehension of the subject matter involved as to enable him to make an understanding and enlightened decision. This latter element requires that before the acceptance of an affirmative decision by the experimental subject there should be made known to him the nature, duration and purpose of the experiment; the methods and means by which it is to be conducted; all inconveniences and hazards reasonably to be expected; and the effects upon his health or person which may possibly come from his participation in the experiment".

Most people will strongly refute the existence of even the ghost of a connection between the criminal acts of wartime and present-day research and see no analogy between the two. Nevertheless, this is clearly not an issue for complacency. As a 1991 Lancet editorial indicated:

"Like other self-evident truths, the need for informed consent has not been universally recognised, even after the Nuremberg judges stated it so plainly. The columns of the Lancet bear witness to research by fraud and research verging on common assault in which patients participated in pure research disguised as clinical investigation or treatment".[249]

It is important, therefore, to reiterate the general principles which govern the seeking of valid consent to research.

### 8:6.2 *General principles*

Fundamental principles of consent are discussed in chapter 1 where it is seen that the BMA generally lays great emphasis on valid patient consent, freely given after the patient has received as full an explanation as the doctor thinks appropriate, giving due regard to the individual needs of the patient and the Bolam principle (see chapter 1, section 1:2.4). The researcher should inform the subject about potential benefits and risks of the procedure, why it is proposed and the significance in terms of advancing knowledge and the researcher's own stake (if any) in proposing the procedure. Where patients are offered choices, they need information about the alternatives to the treatment recommended by their doctor. When a clinical study is proposed patients need to know about the advantages and shortcomings of conventional treatments as well as the options in the trial. In any situation, the more risky or invasive the procedure, the greater attention must be paid to the patient's understanding of it and consent to it.

There are problems with applying such a view to randomised trials, which are sometimes seen as very stressful. Such trials, by their impersonal nature, take no account of the therapeutic effect of the patient having confidence in the doctor's advice. Given the clinical uncertainty which justifies the trial and the fact that some treatment options may only be available as part of the trial, there is often little meaningful freedom of choice for patients about participation. In any situation, however, treatment decisions are not dictated by clinical reasons alone and patients may have preferences for one treatment rather than another, for personal reasons. Clearly, patients who have such preferences should not participate in any study where their treatment will be randomised. This is discussed further in 8:7.3 below.

As previously mentioned, the BMA supports the general tenets of the Helsinki Declaration. An exception is made in the Declaration of Helsinki to an absolute requirement for patient consent in therapeutic trials but the researcher must justify to the ethical committee the reasons why patient consent should not be sought.

The Department of Health advises that written consent should be required for all research, except where the most trivial of procedures is concerned, and that in cases of therapeutic research, patient consent should be recorded in the patient's medical records.

### 8:6.3 *Information and information sheets*

#### 8:6.3.1 *Informed consent*

It is necessary to examine what type of information is needed in order to obtain valid consent. Informed consent is an American rather than a British preoccupation but even so, it is often said that this is a fashionable shibboleth to which the medical and legal professions pay lip-service while neglecting other ethical values. In the context of cancer research in particular, some feel that the requirement to explain fully the limits of medical knowledge undermines patient confidence and may retard the validation of new and possibly more effective treatments by making patients reluctant to participate in trials. Therefore some doctors feel that the duty of beneficence obliges them to conceal uncertainty. The BMA believes that doctors should be frank with patients when there is uncertainty about the merits of various treatments.

Research subjects must be told that they are free to withdraw without explanation or hindrance at any stage of the procedure and, if a patient, with no detriment to their treatment. Patients must know not only the details and risks of the treatment(s) proposed in the trial but also the alternatives open to them if they do not choose to participate in the study. Since much routine research, particularly in general practice, is undertaken at the behest of the pharmaceutical industry, it is important that patients have an accurate perception of their contribution and are not given a false impression of the nature of the study.

#### 8:6.3.2 *Full information*

In general terms, we talk about giving patients full information and doctors often ask the Association for guidance about what that means. It is clearly impossible for a health professional to convey to the patient a summary of all available information. The Helsinki Declaration requires that every subject "must be adequately informed of the aims, methods, anticipated benefits and potential hazards of the study and the discomfort it may entail". What is adequate information, will clearly vary with the requirements of the individual patient, the complexity of the procedures proposed and the capacity of the researcher to get across that information. As previously mentioned, patients also need information about the advantages and disadvantages of the alternatives, including those of the conventional treatment and no treatment.

Talk of the duty to provide full information or full disclosure of risks does not advance our understanding of what doctors must tell research subjects. In some cases, one risk may give rise to a host of sub-risks of varying likelihood and one possible outcome of treatment may give rise to a legion of other events, whose statistical predictability is subject to almost infinite variability. It would be entirely inappropriate to say that doctors should draw the line at mentioning a risk which is one in a hundred or a thousand or one in ten thousand. Common sense must prevail and what is adequate will be interpreted in different ways by different people. What is certain, is that sufficient time must be taken and sufficient skill used, to establish beyond doubt that the research subject understands what is being proposed and freely consents to it.

### 8:6.3.3 Information sheets

Information sheets are sometimes used as a way of providing research subjects with detail. The BMA supports this practice of providing documentary material but emphasises that written information should be in addition to, not in place of, the opportunity for the individual to pose questions. The King's Fund report[250] sets out criteria for good information sheets. They should deal straightforwardly with the patient, and with the nature of the research, making it clear that the best treatment is not known since if it were, the research would be unjustifiable. It should be made clear that the patient can withdraw and any risk involved by being in the study, however minimal, should be clearly spelled out. The report also maintains that information sheets should mention financial aspects of the project, noting, however, that while some LRECs consider patients might feel pressured to participate if aware that this would attract funding, others feel that patients should be in a position to question the money-making aspect of their participation.

In the United States, patients are often provided with very substantial background documentation, covering not only the possible risks and side-effects relating to the present trial but containing also frank discussion of the sometimes poor results obtained by the conventional alternatives. Some[251] have pointed out the terminology and legal precision of these documents indicate a greater interest in protecting the researcher from a potential lawsuit than empowering the patient. In our view, the aim should be to inform the patient in as much detail as the averagely prudent person might be expected to require and such documents must be combined with the opportunity for further questioning.

Other forms of conveying information to the public, such as books and videos have been proposed and many would welcome further educative work in this area.

### 8:6.4 Voluntariness

Reference to consent is often prefixed by qualifiers such as "real" or "informed". We have discussed what might be understood by informed consent but have greater difficulty in envisaging how "real consent" can be obtained. All acknowledge that such consent is highly desirable but there is considerable scepticism amongst patients and doctors about whether it can be obtained. The balance of power in the doctor-patient relationship and the vulnerability of patients ensures that patients are influenced by doctors' choices. Indeed, many commentators draw attention to the fact that patients may submissively agree because they wish to please the medical team, to appear co-operative and to be "good patients" or because they have not initially understood fully their options, including the option to say "no". It is important that patients should be helped to feel comfortable about saying "no" when they feel this is the right choice for them. Such problems do not apply only to research but to treatment in general, but may be more acute in the case of research.

### 8:6.4.1 Pressure

Pressure on patients to participate may be unintended and not perceived as such by the researcher seeking to explain how the study is in the interests of society and future patients. Nevertheless, patients sometimes report that they are left feeling guilty or uncaring if they refuse. Certainly patients should know the reason for the research and its likely future benefits but care must be taken to avoid the impression of direct or indirect pressure to participate.

It is often suggested that the patient's consent should be witnessed or that a person other than the researcher should seek patient consent in order to ensure that no pressure is brought to bear. It is generally envisaged that this role be undertaken by nurses but it is sometimes argued that this simply extends the chain of implicit pressure so that nurses feel obliged to cajole patients on behalf of the doctor. The BMA rejects this argument and sees the independence of nurses as a valuable asset in ensuring that pressure is avoided. It is inappropriate for anyone, including a nurse, to be asked to approach patients about consent unless that person has been trained to do so.

### 8:6.4.2 Healthy volunteers

In the context of research on healthy volunteers, medical students and others may be pressured by financial considerations or hopes of advancement. Members of the armed forces may also have little option but to agree. In practice, healthy volunteers are often recruited from the researcher's own students or nursing staff. The risk of pressure has led many to believe that the use of medical students and junior staff from the researcher's own department should be discouraged and that stronger guidelines should be brought in to achieve this. The risks and safeguards for healthy volunteers are discussed further in 8:8 below on vulnerable subjects.

### 8:6.5 A trusting relationship

Despite the role of medical students and nurses, the vast majority of research subjects are lay people. Since the 1960s, a heightened awareness of both civil and consumer rights have firmly and rightly brought in the lay person as partners in decision-making, both as informed subjects and as members of ethics committees. Attitudes about the doctor-patient relationship have changed dramatically over the past 30 years. Patients rightly expect both information and support. The fact that this is not easy for either side is frequently evident but it must remain the goal. A patient's perspective is described by Faulder:[252]

> "Doctors do not like to confess their own doubts and worries; indeed they regard such revelations as a sign of weakness, a threat to the patient's morale and a major offence against the canon of trust in the patient-doctor relationship. But who has established this canon of trust? And why is it that the trust is almost uniquely discussed in terms of the patient's confidence in the doctor? Seldom do we hear about doctors trusting their patients... Trust between two people, if it is to mean anything, must be reciprocal."

This involves health professionals trusting that patients will voluntarily support research if they do not feel suspicious about being entered for trials without their knowledge. Veracity, we believe, is an essential element throughout medicine but particularly so in the difficult area of experimentation. The problems associated with telling patients the truth - that of undermining patient morale and confidence, or of introducing difficult decisions at a vulnerable time, are often laboured but evidence suggests that uninformed patients may also be alarmed, anxious and subject to considerable stress, precisely because they are being kept in the dark.

## 8:7 Randomised controlled trials (RCTs)

### 8:7.1 *Background*

At the beginning of this century, controlled clinical trials began to be accepted as a proper method of scientific evaluation. Randomisation was introduced into medical research by Sir Austin Bradford Hill in 1946 with the trial of the antibiotic streptomycin for treatment of tuberculosis. In the early 1970s Dr Archibald Cochrane contributed greatly to the spread of RCTs, seeing them not only as a way of evaluating new treatments but also as an important method for testing traditional procedures seen by some as illogical or outdated.

### 8:7.2 *Randomisation and the double-blind technique*

Despite their wide use, RCTs remain the most fiercely argued aspect of research and much has been written on the subject. Within the medical profession, there are those who maintain that RCTs are the only effective way to validate treatment options and that it is unethical to subject patients to invalidated procedures, while others question the methodology and ethical basis of RCTs.

Randomisation, as its name implies, works on the "toss of a coin" principle. Patients suffering from a particular disease - at the same stage - are randomly allocated to separate groups. Different treatments, sometimes including placebos, are given to each group, which is then carefully monitored to assess the efficacy and drawbacks of the treatment. Randomisation can be accompanied by the "double-blind" technique, which eliminates the subjective preferences of doctors by keeping the assigned therapeutic groups secret from the doctor as well as the patient.

It is often said that randomised clinical trials can never be reconciled with the best treatment for the patient because of the element of random selection but unless RCTs are conducted, it is impossible to ascertain with confidence what is the best treatment for the individual patient or for patients in general.

### 8:7.3 *Uncertainty and equipoise*

The prerequisite for establishing RCTs is the lack of a recognised optimum treatment for the condition. The principle is embodied in the maxim "only randomise if uncertain" and is sometimes called the uncertainty principle.[253] Alternatively, the clinician may be described as being in equipoise.[254] Thus, randomisation is only ethical if there is substantial uncertainty about the best treatment for that patient. If the doctor considers that one of the treatments in the study is appropriate or inappropriate for a particular patient for any reason, (including that patient's irrational fears or subjective preferences) then randomisation would be unethical and the patient should be offered the options which the responsible clinician considers appropriate.

Similarly, to be equipoised, the clinician should be indifferent to the choice of treatment because he or she has no knowledge to indicate that one option is better than another. Many suggest that doctors can never be genuinely indifferent for a number of reasons, including the fact that they must also take into account the patient's preferences, which may be based on values other than purely clinical considerations. Once there is unequivocal evidence of the superiority of one treatment, it is unethical to deprive a patient of that treatment. What one patient considers to be a superior outcome may be based on different values to that of another patient. The example given by Botros[255] concerns a patient with breast cancer for whom the options are mastectomy which she is told offers her an 80 per cent chance of surviving more than five years and lumpectomy for which she is told there is no assured survival rate. The personal values of some patients may lead them to see the lumpectomy and avoidance of disfigurement as a superior outcome for themselves even though it offers no surety of prolonging life.

Patients are often alarmed at the prospect of deliberate randomisation, even though variable and unknown bias has long been a feature of medical practice. In any area of treatment where there are divergent views within the medical profession, the individual patient's health-management will depend to some degree on the particular preference of the medical team consulted. Baum, discussing breast cancer treatments, raises this point:

"Until ten years ago we truly did not know whether the disease could be adequately treated by breast conservation (that is lumpectomy and radiotherapy), or whether in preserving the breast we risked the woman's life. But although the experts did not know, there were many surgeons who thought they knew with absolute confidence. The curious thing is that the surgeons who had all the answers had different answers and ten years ago you would have surgeons who confidently believed that mastectomy was the best treatment, whereas you had an equal number of surgeons who confidently believed that lumpectomy and radiotherapy was the best treatment, and their behaviour was judged completely ethical. And yet it was a 50-50 chance whether you turned left or right in Harley Street, or whether you went to King's College Hospital or 'St Elsewhere', whether you had a mastectomy or a lumpectomy".[256]

When preferences are being discussed and there is no one treatment recognised as superior to others on offer, then the patient's preferences are the more important ones, and should be accorded "due weight".

### 8:7.4 *Problems arising from RCTs*

Randomisation is said to be poorly understood by the public and various models to make the concept more accessible have been put forward. These usually include some element of pre-randomisation before the matter is discussed with the patient and probably have as many disadvantages as advantages in their potential for confusing patients and undermining confidence.

It is often argued[257] that since the subjects are able to exclude themselves from randomised trials, the final self-selected group are not representative of the total population. Measures can, however, be taken to compensate for any bias evident in the self-selected group. If this is not addressed, the conclusions cannot be generalised to apply to particular patients outside the trial group except by the processes of inference which RCTs are designed to replace. Kennedy picks up this point, saying that if this is recognised as a valid argument "it deals a death blow to RCTs, since if they are not scientifically valid, they are necessarily unethical".[258]

Practical problems arise if the doctor considers that the appropriate treatment for a patient is a new product only available in a trial since randomisation may deprive the patient of it. There is also a problem when patients wish to continue, after the end of the study, treatment which has proved beneficial to them in the trial but the product involved in that treatment is not yet licensed for general use. In exceptional cases, treatment can be provided on a named patient basis, or by means of a doctor's exemption certificate from the Medicines Control Agency.[259]

There is an ethical imperative to ascertain that the treatments doctors provide are effective. RCTs provide a means of scientifically assessing the effectiveness of treatments but they involve uncertainty for the patients who participate in them. These patients cannot know whether the treatment given to them is the most effective until the trial is over and the results assessed. Some doctors are afraid that by attenuating our commitments to present patients in favour of benefits to those of the future, we may lose overall more than we gain.[260] These doctors also believe that the view that we should curtail the primary interests (in more than a strictly medical sense) of our current patients in exchange for future certainties is ethically dubious. Other doctors try to resolve the dilemma by stating it as a duty that they remove uncertainty for this patient and for future patients.

In the BMA's view, RCTs are ethical when the trial subjects receive thorough information, counselling and support at all stages where a choice is open to them. The main choice they must make, of course, is whether to participate or not, since after an initial decision to do so, subsequent treatment will be given in accordance with that offered by the branch of the trial to which the patient is allocated. At any stage, however, the patient may have doubts or want to discuss further the treatment allocated by the study. At any stage, therefore, patients must have a choice to withdraw and should be supported if that is their decision.

## 8:8 Research subjects

### 8:8.1 *Vulnerable subjects*

To some extent, almost all research subjects can be said to be vulnerable for one reason or another - patients by reason of their illness, and healthy volunteers because of employment considerations. There are, however, special factors which must be borne in mind regarding research on subjects who cannot consent, such as young children or mentally incompetent people. People in a situation of dependency are capable of giving valid consent but precautions to avoid coercion or inducement must be considered. In this country, prisoners do not participate in research but people detained in other circumstances, such as under the Mental Health Act 1983, may. All research projects should be subject to LREC approval and committees should give particular consideration to those involving subjects unable to consent. The degree of risk in any such project should be the object of particular scrutiny.

The accepted principle applied to all of the groups discussed below is that no research that could equally well be carried out on competent adults, should be carried out on individuals whose comprehension is limited, whether by reason of age or of mental disability. Some have argued that individuals who cannot give consent should not be involved in any research. Others argue that research on such groups is ethical if it is not contrary to the individual's (see 8:16 below) interest, if it poses only minimal risk and if it benefits others in the same category. This is broadly the view taken by the BMA, but see also the discussion on research in children in chapter 3, section 3:7.

It should be noted that the European Commission has issued Guidelines on Good Clinical Practice for Trials on Medicinal Products in the EC. These are more restrictive than presently accepted practice and require that research which is intended to be carried out on subjects incapable of giving personal consent, should be to "promote the welfare and interest of the subject".

### 8:8.1.1 Research involving minors: consent

Research on children and young people is discussed in detail in chapter 3 (section 3:7). The legal and ethical validity of minors' consent is also discussed in the same chapter. It may be sufficient to note here that, in the view of some commentators, parents or guardians cannot in law consent to any treatment or procedures which are contrary to the child's interests. The point remains to be clarified in the courts but it is the opinion expressed in guidance issued by the Department of Health in 1991. This states:

> "Those acting for the child can only legally give their consent provided that the intervention is for the benefit of the child. If they are responsible for allowing the child to be subjected to any risk (other than one so insignificant as to be negligible) which is not for the benefit of that child, it could be said that they were acting illegally."

In the BMA's view, the consent of a competent child or young person to therapeutic treatments intended for that person's own benefit is sufficient from an ethical viewpoint. It would be prudent, however, to seek young people's permission to involve their parents. The British Paediatric Association,[261] (BPA) draws attention to the fact that many children are vulnerable, easily bewildered and frightened, and unable to express their needs or defend their interests. Potentially with many decades ahead of them, they are likely to experience, in their development and education, the most lasting benefits or harms from research. Consent is not a single response but involves a continuing commitment. The BPA also states that "A research worker must recognise when a child is very upset by a procedure and accept this as genuine dissent from being involved." The

213

prospect of blood sampling or injections, for example, upsets many children and the BPA sees a child's refusal on that score as no different from an adult's refusal to join a research project because of an extreme dislike of venepuncture.

### 8:8.1.2 The interest of minors

Research projects involving minors must have an identifiable prospect of benefit to minors. Procedures should first have been tested on consenting adults before they are carried out on children. Children and very young people are individuals with variable responses so that generalisations about risk tend to be controversial. A procedure which does not bother one individual arouses severe distress in another. "Researchers sometimes underestimate high risk of pain if the effects are brief, whereas the child or parents may consider the severe transient pain is not justified by the hoped-for benefit. There is evidence that tolerance of pain increases with age and maturity when the child no longer perceives medical interventions as punitive".[262]

### 8:8.1.3 The mentally disordered

Included within the scope of the term "mentally disordered" is a group of individuals with widely varying and significant differences in their capacity to understand. The Medical Research Council,[263] for example, adopts a definition which includes the mentally ill, the mentally handicapped, the demented and the unconscious. Some of these persons will never have the capacity to give consent, some will lose it irrevocably and in some it will be present at times but not at others. We have attempted to demarcate within this range of conditions.

Many patients with a mental disorder are able to consent, if care is taken in explaining the procedures and therefore consent should be sought to the extent that the individual is capable of providing it. The general advice on consent to treatment is fully explained in chapter 1. Therapeutic research (to the extent that this may be distinguishable from treatment) should not proceed if the individual appears to object either by words or actions. The proxy consent of carers carries no legal weight and cannot take precedence over any apparent objection by the patient. The Law Commission is considering this issue and proposes that participation in research by people with a mental disorder should fall within a special category of treatments which require court authorisation.[264]

### People with learning disabilities

We believe that research involving procedures which are not contrary to the interests of people with learning disabilities, which exposes them to only minimal risk and which may potentially benefit others in the same category is not unethical but must be carefully scrutinised by LRECs. We foresee no ethical problems with research which simply involves monitoring some normal procedure, such as testing of the subject's hearing or colour discrimination.

**Mentally ill people**

Many drug trials are carried out on anti-depressants and other products for the mentally ill. Apart from those patients suffering from severe conditions such as dementia, the vast majority of mentally ill people will be able to give valid consent, as is emphasised by the Royal College of Psychiatrists.[265] This includes patients detained in psychiatric hospitals under the Mental Health Act 1983, whose consent should be sought. It is unlikely that non-therapeutic research on such patients would be ethically acceptable, since although they may understand the procedures, the very fact of their detention means they cannot be said to give free consent.

**Demented and unconscious patients**

It is questionable whether such patients should be exposed to any procedure not designed for their own benefit. Our general view is again that measures which are not contrary to their interests, involve only minimal risk and may potentially benefit others in the same category are not unethical but must be carefully scrutinised by LRECs.

*8:8.1.4 The elderly*

The case detailed in 8:4.2 above shows that the elderly may be at special risk because of general health concerns, because they are hospitalised, because they may be residing in an institution where they feel they must conform with the views of others or, because, whatever the actual circumstances, they are in a position of dependency. Studies aimed to benefit elderly people often cannot be carried out on other sections of the population since reactions or metabolism may be different in the elderly. In such cases, the use of elderly volunteers may be justified, subject to the provision of valid consent and LREC approval.

*8:8.1.5 Embryo research*

Embryo research stands out as the only research area where there is clear legislation and a statutory monitoring body. For many years, the ethics of conducting research on embryos was the subject of heated debate, much of which continues even though such research is now governed in law by the Human Fertilisation and Embryology Act 1990 (see also chapter 4, section 4:8, on embryo research).[266]

*8:8.1.6 Research involving fetuses or fetal material*

Research involving fetuses is governed by widely accepted guidance rather than legislation. The Review of the Guidance on the Research Use of Fetuses and Fetal Material[267] (otherwise known as the Polkinghorne Report) was published in 1989. This proposes that:

215

"All research, or therapy of an innovative character, involving the fetus or fetal tissue should be described in a protocol and be examined by an ethics committee. Projects should be subject to review until the validity of the procedure has been recognised by the committee as part of routine medical practice. The ethics committee has a duty to examine the progress of the research or innovative therapy (eg by receiving reports). It should have access to records and be able to examine the record of any financial transactions involving fetal tissue. Before permitting the research the ethics committee must satisfy itself:

a)    of the validity of the research or use proposed;

b)    that the objectives of the proposed use cannot be achieved in any other way;

c)    that the researchers or clinicians have the necessary facilities and skill."

As noted in section 8:2.3 above, the BMA considers that in cases where an innovative treatment diverges radically from previously accepted practice, it is desirable to have additional expert opinion to supplement the views of the local research ethics committee. (Maternal consent to the use of a fetus or fetal tissue is discussed in chapter 1, section 1:7.1.6, on consent).

### 8:8.2  *Healthy volunteers*

*8:8.2.1 Definition*

Healthy volunteers are defined as individuals who do not suffer from any significant illness relevant to the proposed study. They may not be entirely "healthy" in that they suffer from disabilities which are irrelevant to the study in question. On the other hand, individuals who are temporarily "healthy" but are only in remission from a relapsing condition cannot be healthy volunteers for a study related to that condition.

*8:8.2.2 Safeguards*

In 1984 and 1985 two apparently healthy young medical students died in the course of clinical trials of new drugs. The incidents aroused great public concern. Furthermore, unease was expressed in several quarters in the 1980s about growing commercial interest in the establishment of drug-research units in university and NHS premises as well as private institutions and it was felt safeguards should be drawn up. Bodies such as the Royal College of Physicians and the Association of the British Pharmaceutical Industry (ABPI) published guidelines for medical experiments in non-patient human volunteers.

The principal safeguards for the healthy volunteer concern selection, consent, conduct of the research and compensation for injury. As mentioned previously (8:6.4.2 above), the recruitment of students and junior staff from the same department as the researcher should be avoided. In principle, no study on healthy volunteers should involve more than minimal risk and, of course, all studies must be subject to the scrutiny of an appropriate ethics committee. Subjects should not participate in more than one study at a time, although it is notoriously difficult to monitor such participation and it is often suspected that volunteers are involved simultaneously in several projects.

Some have called for independent, external scrutiny of the clinical research departments of commercial organisations and for a register of approved institutions. Unfortunately as yet, there is no indication when such measures are likely to be implemented and it has not been specified who might take on these responsibilities.

### 8:8.2.3 *Why use healthy volunteers?*

It can be argued that it is more ethical to test drugs on patients who might stand to benefit from them rather than on healthy volunteers but there are undoubted advantages to doing initial (Phase 1) studies on healthy people. There is less physiological variation in healthy responses and ethical dilemmas about starting treatment with an inadequate dose or of withholding potentially effective treatment do not arise.

It is unethical to use healthy subjects when harmful drug effects can be expected at therapeutic dose levels. With certain drugs, such as those used for cancer or leukaemia, it is more ethical to undertake initial studies on patients who may stand to benefit.

### 8:8.2.4 *Financial inducements*

Payments to healthy volunteers should never be for undergoing risk and the payments should not induce subjects to volunteer more frequently than is advisable for their own good. The BMA recommends the monitoring of financial, as well as other, aspects of research on healthy volunteers.

Many students - and others - who participate in healthy volunteer research, do so for financial reasons. Like all other subjects, they must be free to withdraw from the trial at any time. It is sometimes said that subjects feel pressured to continue because they do not want to lose all their financial rewards by withdrawing from the trial. The ABPI recommends that if a volunteer withdraws for medical reasons related to the study, full payment should be made. If the volunteer withdraws for any other reason, a proportional payment may be made. Other financial considerations relevant to research are considered in section 8:13 below.

### 8:8.2.5 *No fault compensation*

Healthy volunteers who develop illness as a result of participating in a research project are only legally entitled to compensation if they can show negligence on the part of the investigator, the host institution, the sponsor

217

of the research or their respective staff. Volunteers have no legal redress if they are unable to show negligence. However carefully a research project is executed, the possibility of injury resulting from a cause other than negligence cannot be eliminated. In such a case the volunteer participating in NHS hospitals, MRC establishments and universities is dependent upon ex gratia payments. The BMA considers this lack of automatic compensation measures unacceptable and has called for more formal compensation arrangements.[268]

## 8:9 Confidentiality

### 8:9.1 Epidemiological research

A central question concerning the use of medical records in research is whether the patient must give consent to this. Many have argued that it would be impractical to demand that researchers obtain individual consent, although a variety of ways have been suggested to try and facilitate such a procedure. It has been proposed, for example, that whenever a new medical record is opened, the patient - either in the GP-surgery or hospital context - be asked to sign a form saying he or she is willing/unwilling for information to be used for research purposes. Whatever system is adopted for seeking patients' consent, the BMA's general view is that such consent should be periodically reviewed every five years or so and should not be regarded as indefinitely valid without further consultation with the person concerned. Whenever patient-identifiable information is used for research purposes, adequate safeguards for confidentiality must be built into the research programme.

### 8:9.2 GMC guidance

The GMC's guidance on confidentiality states:

"Medical teaching, research and medical audit necessarily involve the disclosure of information about individuals, often in the form of medical records, for purposes other than their own health care. Where such information is used in a form which does not enable individuals to be identified, no question of breach of confidentiality will usually arise. Where the disclosure would enable one or more individuals to be identified, the patients concerned, or those who may properly give permission on their behalf, must wherever possible be made aware of that possibility and be advised that it is open to them, at any stage, to withhold their consent to disclosure".[269]

This begs the question of "who may properly give permission" on patients' behalf. In the BMA's view, patient consent should generally be sought to the release of information for research purposes. If the patient has died, consent should be sought from the patient's representative. If an adult patient is unable to consent by reason of mental disorder, no other person can give consent for that person in law (except perhaps in Scotland if a tutor dative has been assigned powers to cover this eventuality). In practice, carers and those close to the patient are often asked to give proxy consent and their views are often accorded moral rather than legal weight.

There may be exceptional or particularly sensitive areas where patients or patients' representatives should not be approached, for example in studies concerning childhood illness where information may concern children who have died. In such circumstances, it is essential that a local research ethics committee has satisfied itself that the balance of public interest and individual privacy justifies dispensing with patient (or relatives') consent.

### 8:9.3 *Responsibility for data*

Where medical records are to be used in research, a medically qualified person should be identified who will undertake responsibility for ensuring that the medical records are handled responsibly and no breach of confidentiality occurs.

### 8:9.4 *Liaison between practitioners*

When a patient or healthy volunteer is involved in a research programme which may have a bearing on other medical treatment provided to that person by another doctor, the subject's consent must be sought for information to be shared between the relevant clinicians. Clearly both the subject's health and the conclusions of the study may be affected by non- complementary prescribing in the absence of liaison between practitioners. Some believe that the onus is entirely on patients to ensure that any doctor treating them is aware of their participation in research. In our view, the researcher also bears a responsibility for making sure that subjects know the importance of informing other health professionals who are treating them.

## 8:10 Monitoring and approving research

As previously noted, local research ethics committees (LRECs) are the mechanism for monitoring and approving research but are often hampered by factors such as the lack of any legal requirement which obliges researchers to consult them. In the past, LREC members also often lacked training for the job but this is now increasingly provided by various bodies.

The BMA is often asked whether GP studies should be subject to LREC approval, because committees are often seen as having a remit primarily for hospital-based research. The question also arises, whether only NHS-based research must be subject to LREC scrutiny. The BMA takes the view that all research conducted within a particular locality should be submitted first to the relevant LREC, since it is important for the LREC to be aware of all clinical trials in its district. Approval by a research ethics committee, not only of protocols for clinical trials, but also of investigators conducting trials, protects both the subjects of research and the investigators.

### 8:10.1 *Functions and composition of local research ethics committees*

The 1992 King's Fund Institute Report on these committees produced 12 detailed recommendations as to their constitution and working. These complement and build upon the earlier recommendations of the BMA, the Department of Health and the Royal College of Physicians. Some core points, identified in various guidelines, should always be considered by LRECs:[270]

- whether the scientific quality of the protocol has been properly assessed. Studies which are unscientific are also unethical;

- whether the investigator and any others involved in the trial are competent and have adequate facilities;

- possible hazards to trial subjects and precautions taken to deal with them;

- measures for providing information and seeking appropriate consent;

- whether adequate compensation arrangements are in place in case of any harm arising from the trial;

- methods of recruitment and any payments to subjects;

- payments to investigators;

- storage and use of subject-identifiable information.

The BMA guidance on the ideal composition of LRECs was drawn up in 1983 and revised in 1986.[271] There is widespread agreement[272] on the composition of LRECs, which should be drawn from both sexes and include senior and junior hospital doctors, GPs, nurses, lay members including community health council representatives. Some specify that a pharmacologist, pharmacist or pathologist should be included. The BMA's view is that it would be valuable to have a panel of experts in various fields who could be called upon when required.

The reality has often fallen short of the ideal. Questionnaires circulated by the BMA to 138 local committees in 1980 showed that there was no set pattern of LREC membership and that efficacy was variable. In the years that followed, correspondence to the BMJ consistently raised concerns about inadequacies in LREC composition, function and efficiency. The implementation of guidelines issued by the Department of Health and the Royal College of Physicians in 1991 was subsequently monitored and reported on by the King's Fund, which remarked on the dominance of hospital doctors, who constituted more than half of the total membership of 222 LRECs, and the under-representation of lay people, who made up less than 20 per cent of the overall membership. Women were found to be significantly under-represented, many committees had no GP and most had no psychiatrist member, even though many of the protocols concerned trials of drugs for psychiatric patients. Some LRECs had no nurse, and most had only one, although the report commends the valuable role played by nurses in drawing other non-doctors into discussions. A third of LRECs had only one lay person and some of these members were not truly independent outsiders but members of the DHA; there also appeared to be no clear route for selecting lay people.

It was shown that some LRECs had no constitution and those who did have, omitted from it the purpose of the committee, how it worked and how researchers could make applications to it. It is not surprising, therefore, that the King's Fund Report also noted some confusion among LREC members as to their role and whether public expectations of LRECs were being met.

### 8:10.2 *Training and support*

LREC members' perceived lack of training and sense of isolation have long given cause for concern. This was reiterated by the BMA in 1991[273] when it called for training and support for local research ethical committees to be introduced nationally. The Department of Health has undertaken to distribute training packs, which include internationally agreed codes and other guidelines. Conferences for chairmen and members have provided fora for the exchange of ideas and dissemination of good working methods. The BMA, with its long history of support for the concept of a national research agency (see 8:10.4 below), believes that this would provide additional support and information. It is envisaged that the national agency would act as a repository of information about all research, promote good practice and by collecting the annual reports of local committees, assist in raising standards.

Possible lack of adequate expertise to deal with special circumstances, such as "first-time" drug studies (Phase 1 studies) in human subjects, lead some to support examination of such protocols by research ethics committees set up by drug companies. All agree that such company-based committees must include highly qualified and truly independent members if the committee's views are to have credibility. Such review does not negate the need for local opinion by means of LREC scrutiny.

#### 8:10.2.1 *Disease-specific liaison committees*

Disease specific research liaison committees are a measure which attracts support as a means of helping LRECs. It is proposed that such committees would have responsibility for coordinating and monitoring multicentre national trials related to their sphere of expertise in conjunction with LRECs. Supporters of this proposal argue that such liaison committees will be able to submit protocols to rigorous scientific scrutiny.

### 8:10.3 *Independent local research ethics committees*

The BMA receives both enquiries and complaints about research approved by self-appointed bodies outside the NHS, known as "independent" committees. Complaints include allegations that such committee decisions are biased, dominated by one interest group or reflect perfunctory consideration of some aspects of the research. In essence, many of these complaints about "independent" committees are identical to those sometimes raised about LRECs. The latter, however, are subject to DHA monitoring and control whereas "independent" committees appear free from supervision and sometimes unwilling to explain their procedures or conclusions. After consideration, the Association sees no place for independent local research ethics committees in the assessment of research involving patients.

### 8:10.4 *A national research ethics committee*

In its early attempts to improve the network of LRECs, the BMA identified a need for a further committee at national level which could co-ordinate and advise on research but which would have no power to interfere with local autonomy. In cases where one LREC had thoroughly investigated the local aspects of a nationwide study, the national agency could make that information available to other LRECs considering the same trial. Such a national committee would complement the information about all published trials held in the National Library of Medicine (in Bethesda, Maryland, USA) and help overcome publication bias. Local research ethics committees have supported the idea in principle, as have many other bodies concerned with research. Discussions with the Department of Health and the RCP have continued over recent years. Funding and the manner of dealing with heavy demand are seen as problems to be resolved.

In 1990 the BMA made the following recommendations regarding the composition of a national body:

a) That the chairman be appointed by the Secretary of State in full consultation with the Presidents of the GMC, Medical Research Council and Conference of Medical Colleges.

b) That membership should include at least two lay people nominated by the Secretary of State; two members nominated by the Conference of Medical Colleges; one nominee of the MRC, Social Science Research Council, UK Central Council for Nursing, Midwifery and Health Visiting, Council for Professions Supplementary to Medicine and Association of the British

Pharmaceutical Industry (in consultation with other groups in the pharmaceutical industry).

c)   The Department of Health should fund the committee.

d)   The committee should be primarily accountable to the Secretary of State but also accountable to some degree to the nominating bodies.

e)   It should meet at least four times a year.

### 8:10.4.1 Multicentre research

The difficulties researchers have faced in obtaining approval for multicentre research is one of the principal reasons why the BMA has supported the concept of a national body concerned with research.

In the absence of such a national body, some multicentre research is currently evaluated centrally. For example, a committee of the RCGP deals with research protocols involving general practitioners. Local research ethics committees can legitimately have confidence in the views of such a body when they come to evaluate protocols it has approved. It is sometimes erroneously thought that the BMA's Medical Ethics Committee fulfils a similar function. While the Committee receives many applications, apart from a long-standing agreement regarding approval of protocols submitted by the Office of Population and Census Surveys, it is unable to "approve" them and they should be directed to the relevant local research ethics committees.

Although only local committees can be expected to be aware of local circumstances, ethical approval of multi-centre projects can be facilitated if a single LREC, with a good range of expertise, examines the protocol in depth and shares its views with other LRECs. A group of LRECs may agree to such a mechanism whereby one committee is selected to analyse the ethics of the protocol, leaving the other LRECs to concentrate on local aspects, such as the suitability of the investigator.

### 8:10.5 *Monitoring embryo research*

The principal conclusion of the Warnock Report was that human embryos should have special status but could be used for research, subject to stringent controls. The Human Fertilisation and Embryology Act 1990 introduced statutory control, taking over from the previous Voluntary Licensing Authority. Issuing licences for research and monitoring compliance with the provisions of the Act is undertaken by the Human Fertilisation and Embryology Authority (HFEA). Each research protocol must relate broadly to one of the stated categories of research aims. These are:

a)   promoting advances in the treatment of infertility;

b) increasing knowledge about the causes of congenital disease;

c) increasing knowledge about the causes of miscarriage;

d) developing more effective techniques of contraception;

e) developing methods for detecting the presence of gene or chromosome abnormalities in embryos before implantation;

f) for the purpose of increasing knowledge about the creation and development of embryos and enabling such knowledge to be applied.

### 8:10.6 *Monitoring the ethics of gene therapy*

In response to the rapid advances in genetic modification in recent years and the prospect of gene therapy being introduced into medical practice, in 1989 the Government established the Committee on the Ethics of Gene Therapy, under the chairmanship of Sir Cecil Clothier. Its remit was to draw up ethical guidance for the medical profession on the treatment of genetic disorders by genetic modification; to consider proposals from doctors wishing to use such treatment on patients and to provide advice on medical developments which bear on the safety and efficacy of human genetic modification. The Committee reported in early 1992.[274]

It concluded that the development and introduction of safe and effective means of gene modification to alleviate disease in an individual patient, and that individual alone (somatic cell gene therapy), was an appropriate goal for medical science and recommended that the necessary research in this area should continue. Such research, the Committee considered, should be subject to the same exacting requirements which apply to all other types of medical research involving human subjects. However, because the Committee expected such research would necessarily require an uncommon degree and range of scientific and medical expertise it recommended the establishment of a non-statutory supervisory body to oversee and monitor research proposals. Proposals would not only need to be approved by the new body but also by a properly constituted local research ethics committee. (At the time of writing the Committee's recommendations were still being considered by the Department of Health, following a public consultation exercise).

Genetic modification of the germ line (germ line gene therapy), the Committee considered should not yet be attempted. Indeed, it is currently outlawed under the Human Fertilisation and Embryology Act 1990. (See also chapter 4, section 4:9.1).

## 8:11 Ownership of research

### 8:11.1 *Ownership of results*

It is generally recognised that while financial sponsors have a right to receive the full results of research, LRECs have a responsibility to ensure that patient research is free from commercial bias. In studies which involve sustained patient co-operation, the patient, as well as the sponsor, should be informed of the outcome.

A problem which may arise when sponsors "own" trial results is that these are only likely to be published if publication is in the sponsor's interests. The National Library of Medicine collects all published studies but no systematic monitoring occurs of studies which have been carried out but not published. As mentioned above, a national research agency could monitor such research by collecting together the annual reports of all LRECs and comparing the number and type of trials approved with those whose results are published. This would provide a record of research which has been conducted but not published and also help to reduce duplication of the same research, since it would be possible to discover when a project has been carried out already although its results were not published.

### 8:11.2 *Ownership of tissue for research*

It has been widely debated whether expressed patient consent, or merely implied patient consent, is necessary for research on therapeutically removed tissue. The BMA's views on this matter are noted in chapter 1 (section 1:4.1.3). The principal recommendation is that patients should be specifically informed when material excised during the course of investigation or treatment is to be used for any purpose, including research or commercial development. The wishes of patients who object for cultural, religious or other reasons should be respected. The ownership and use of fetal tissue are also discussed in chapter 1 (section 1:7.1.6).

## 8:12 Guidelines on research

In Britain, research, apart from that on embryos, is not governed by legislation. In some other countries regulation is tighter. In France, for example, a law of 20 December 1988 is "relative a la protection des personnes qui se pretent a des recherches biomedicales" (for the protection of human research subjects). Many people see a need for statutory regulation in Britain and the continuing harmonisation of EC legislation is likely to facilitate this. Some measures, such as the European guidelines on good clinical research practice, are already having effect and pharmaceutical companies which do not comply with them are likely to find it increasingly difficult to have new products licensed in EC countries.

The absence of legislation means there is no legal requirement for LRECs to be established in all health districts although it is Department of Health policy that such committees should be established and that all research carried out in the NHS be subject to their scrutiny. The BMA considers that all research, both within and outside the NHS, should be subject to LREC approval.

There is a wide range of guidance relating to research. The most widely known statement is the World Medical Association's Declaration of Helsinki. Particular attention is given to how the Helsinki Declaration is applied internationally and in developing countries through the guidelines on biomedical research and ethical review of epidemiological studies, produced by the Council for International Organisations of Medical Sciences (CIOMS).[275] A wide variety of other international and national guidance has been published.

## 8:13 Finance and research

### 8:13.1 *Disclosure of financial information to LRECs*

The BMA considers that the protocols submitted to LRECs should contain details of the financial arrangements of the study. The GMC also supports the inclusion of full financial details as an appendix to the research protocol.

### 8:13.2 *Per capita payments*

The ethics of per capita payments have been debated in various fora. Some bodies see per capita payments as potentially unethical since doctors may be influenced by the prospect of personal gain to put pressure on patients to participate in a trial. Others maintain that it is not the existence of payment but the level of payment which is crucial. The BMA's view is that any payments to doctors carrying out research should be the subject of assessment by the LREC and should not exceed a "reasonable estimate" of the cost of studying the patient together with any legitimate profit. What constitutes legitimate profit should be considered by the LREC on the basis of accepted practice. The BMA does not consider per capita payments unethical, per se.

### 8:13.3 *Acceptance of hospitality*

The BMA takes the view that there is an ethical imperative for doctors to keep abreast of new developments in medicine, including information about new drugs and the conclusions of recent research. Attending presentations by pharmaceutical representatives is one means of doing this and should not be the subject of payment to the doctor.

## 8:14 Fraud in clinical research

The BMA has expressed concern about the absence of an independent mechanism for investigating possible cases of fraud in clinical research. The Association sees value in the establishment of such a mechanism. The BMA supports the efforts of the Association of the British Pharmaceutical Industry in encouraging all its member companies to introduce standard procedures for investigating suspected cases of fraud and implementing appropriate action.

## 8:15 Summary

1. A fundamental tenet of the Declaration of Helsinki is that the patient's interest must come first. The Declaration also stipulates that potential research subjects must be adequately informed of the aims, methods, anticipated benefits and potential hazards of the study and the discomfort it may entail.

2. Having been informed about the procedures involved in the research, the subject has the absolute right to decline to participate without detriment to his or her care.

3. No direct or indirect pressure should be used to obtain the potential subject's consent. If healthy volunteers are required, it is advisable that these are not recruited from among the junior staff or students of the researcher's own department.

4. If the research is non-therapeutic, it should involve no more than minimal risk.

5. The riskier or more invasive the procedure, the greater the attention that must be paid to the subject's understanding of it and consent to it. Truth-telling is an essential element of all medicine but should be particularly emphasised in the difficult area of experimentation.

6. Innovative treatments which diverge substantially from normal practice, with the intention of gaining information to help other patients and which involve more than a minimally increased risk, should be reviewed by an ethics committee. In cases where the treatment is radically different from normal procedures and has wide implications, additional expert scrutiny is desirable.

7. No research which could be equally well carried out on competent adults with their consent, should be carried out on people who cannot give valid consent.

8. Research on children cannot be carried out if contrary to the interests of the individual child.

9. Young people of sufficient maturity can consent on their own behalf. In cases of doubt, the young person's permission should be sought (if appropriate) to consult parents.

10. Research involving procedures which are not contrary to the interests of people with learning disabilities, which exposes them to no more than very minimal risk and which may benefit others in the same category is not unethical but must be carefully scrutinised by LRECs.

11. Many mentally disordered people are able to give their valid consent to participation in research. This applies to people detained under the Mental Health Act 1983.

12    All clinical research must be approved by an LREC. Studies which fall into the grey area between therapeutic and non-therapeutic research should be subject to the constraints of the latter; they require LREC approval. It may help an LREC to reach a decision about the acceptability of a protocol if a central body such as the research ethics committee of the RCGP has previously expressed its views on the protocol or if one LREC has examined general ethical aspects of the protocol in depth.

13    Patient consent should be sought to the release of identifiable information for research purposes, unless the LREC has dispensed with this requirement. Doctors should be responsible for ensuring the confidentiality of data.

14    Consent to participate in research should be witnessed to ensure that no pressure is being put on the subject. It may also be advisable for another person, such as a nurse, rather than the researcher, to seek the consent of a patient who is also being treated by that researcher. Written consent should be required for all research (except where the most trivial of procedures is concerned). In cases of therapeutic research, patient consent should be recorded in the patient's medical records.

15    Patients should be specifically informed when material excised during the course of investigation or treatment is to be used for research or other purposes. The wishes of patients who object for cultural, religious or other reasons should be respected.

## 8:16  Tables of Risk Equivalents

Two different ways of assessing risk are mentioned here as useful guides.

I

|  | Negligible | Minimal | More than Minimal |
|---|---|---|---|
| Risk of Death | Less than 1 per million | 1 to 100 per million | Greater than 100 per million |
| Risk of Major Complication | Less than 10 per million | 10 to 1000 per million | Greater than 100 per million |
| Risk of Minor Complication | Less than 1 per 1000 | 1 to 100 per 1000 | Greater than 100 per 1000 |

## II

Assessment of risk when children participate in research.

**Minimal** (the least possible) risk describes procedures such as questioning, observing and measuring children, provided that procedures are carried out in a sensitive way, and that consent has been given. Procedures with minimal risk include collecting a single urine sample (but not by aspiration), or using blood from a sample that has been taken as part of treatment.

**Low** risk describes procedures that cause brief pain or tenderness, and small bruises or scars. Many children fear needles and for them low rather than minimal risks are often incurred by injections and venepuncture.

**High** risk procedures such as lung or liver biopsy, arterial puncture, and cardiac catheterisation are not justified for research purposes alone. They should be carried out only when research is combined with diagnosis or treatment intended to benefit the child concerned.[276]

# 9 Doctors with Dual Obligations

*Introduction: medical examinations for insurance and employment: occupational health: community physicians: police surgeons: prison doctors: doctors in the armed forces: doctors as company directors: media doctors: summary.*

General principles behind the issues raised in this chapter are also discussed in chapters 1 and 2 on consent and confidentiality.

## 9:1 Introduction

### 9:1.1 *Implications of the dual obligation*

The doctor-patient relationship is not always based on the usual model of partnership recommended in previous chapters. Over a wide range of very differing circumstances, doctors have to balance their concern for the individual patient with other considerations. It may be that the doctor is not acting primarily or solely in a therapeutic role vis-a-vis the patient and has an obligation to another party, such as the doctor's employer or to a court of law. Or the patient may be part of a special community, such as the armed forces or the prison population, where modification of individual rights is an accepted fact. The common factor in the situations explored below is a dual duty on the doctor's part and a potential limitation to some degree of the patient's usual rights, particularly the right to confidentiality. Or there may be pressure of some sort upon the patient to accept treatment or procedures, for instance the assessment of mental capacity or HIV-testing, which in all other circumstances patients would be free to decline.

There is a danger that any responsibilities owed to the patient in such circumstances might be left vague and unspecified, while the doctor's duties to the employer or body paying for the medical report are more clearly defined. In all cases where the doctor is acting for another party, he or she has an obligation to ensure that the patient understands that.

### 9:1.2 *The role of the medical expert*

In many instances where doctors have a dual role, one facet of their work is to act as a medical expert.

### 9:1.2.1 Impartiality

In all circumstances the doctor must take an impartial role and attempt to provide objective advice, based upon clinical and professional experience. It would clearly be improper for doctors to act in a partial way which is detrimental to the patient solely because this supports the interest of the body which has commissioned the doctor's services or because the doctor identifies with colleagues whose aims are contrary to those of the patient. Such potential conflicts are present in many everyday situations but are highlighted in a very dramatic way if the doctor concerned is a forensic specialist, an expert legal witness or a doctor in the armed forces. It is unethical for a forensic doctor or psychiatrist to withhold evidence solely because, for instance, it contradicts the aims of the police who are seeking a conviction. Similarly, overt or implicit pressure might be brought to bear on a doctor asked to give an independent expert opinion in a legal case, or on a doctor in the armed forces who does not want to be isolated from other members of the unit by taking a stand about behaviour he or she considers inappropriate.

Conversely, a doctor might compromise objectivity by unreasonably favouring the patient's viewpoint and this is equally unacceptable. Cases are sometimes referred for medical examination by solicitors who consider that there may be medical evidence to support their client's claim on some issue such as industrial injury. The doctor may be asked to prepare a report outlining what, if any, injury has been sustained, the role of pre-existing or coincidental factors and some form of prognosis. Since the solicitor is representing the client's best interests, he or she will be concerned to present such evidence as will assist in advancing the client's case. The solicitor is under no obligation to inform the doctor of any facts adverse to that case. The doctor must not therefore assume that the solicitor has related all of the material facts. The onus is upon doctors to discover and report upon any material features which they consider may be adverse to the case of the party instructing them.

Doctors who are asked, for example, to provide a medical report to the Home Office on a person seeking political asylum should be clear that an objective medical assessment is required. This entails indicating, where appropriate, that there are possible causes other than political maltreatment for the subject's symptoms. Doctors who undertake this form of work invariably build up expertise in the patterns of maltreatment or torture common to the regions of the applicant's origin. They may offer an opinion as to the most likely aetiology of the asylum applicant's condition, based upon observed facts but should not speculate more widely. This is discussed further below in 9:8.

### 9:1.2.2 Medico-legal reports

Such medical reports should be factual, detailed and carefully worded,

231

avoiding assertions that cannot be defended. Unlike the provision of information for colleagues, this type of report is mainly read by non-medical officials and so abstruse medical terms should be avoided, or if they must be used, defined.

## 9:2 Medical reports for insurance

One of the most common situations in which a doctor has a duty to another party concerns the completion of medical reports for the patient to obtain insurance cover. This situation is not like some others explored later in this chapter, in the sense that the patient seeking insurance is under no obligation to accept either examination or the release of personal medical information. Nevertheless, doctors frequently fear that financial constraints pressurise their patients to agree to forms of testing about which the doctor and patient are unhappy and which are not clinically indicated, but which the doctor has been paid to undertake. Most commonly, the testing concerned relates to HIV status, which is discussed further below in 9:3.2, and more extensively in chapter 1 (section 1:5.1). There is, however, little that doctors can do in such situations after impartially counselling the patient. Ultimately it is for the patient to decide whether or not to accept the terms laid down by the company or to consider other alternatives.

### 9:2.1 *Purpose of insurance medical reports*

The purpose of the medical report is to permit the insurance company to assess the individual's risk factors in order not to disadvantage other clients of the insurance scheme. Although such reports are often undertaken by the patient's own practitioner, the doctor is working exclusively for the insurance company in this case. This should be made clear to the patient. Some have suggested that insurance medical reports should be undertaken, wherever possible, by doctors who have no clinical responsibility for the patient, thus avoiding a conflict of interest. This is a matter for individual patients and doctors to decide.

### 9:2.2 *Patient consent and access*

No report can be provided without the patient's written authorisation and if a report is sought from the patient's own GP, the patient has a statutory right to see it under the Access to Medical Reports Act 1988.[277] Patients do not always exercise their right of access and the BMA considers it wise for doctors to advise them to do so if the disclosure is clearly disadvantageous to their patients so that the latter can consider their course of action. Clearly, it is improper for doctors to change any detail in the report which is factually correct but details which the patient points out are incorrect, must be removed. Patients have a right to append comments on any disputed information which the doctor believes to be correct. The Act does not apply to reports written by doctors who are not responsible for the patient's treatment. Therefore the patient has no statutory right to see such reports or append comments to them. (The lack of a statutory right does not mean that the examining doctor cannot show the report to the patient. It simply means that the doctor is not obliged to comply with the patient's request to see it. Some insurance companies prohibit the examining doctor from showing such a report to the individual it concerns). Nevertheless the BMA recommends frankness in these situations and considers that such doctors have a duty to act in the patient's interests. Upon discovering a significant abnormality requiring investigation or treatment, of which the patient and the patient's GP may be unaware, examining doctors should liaise with the insurance company's medical officer to ensure that the condition is brought to the notice of the individual or his or her GP. Patient consent must be obtained for liaison with the GP.

Part of the rationale for the distinction in the Act between reports produced by the patient's own doctor and other doctors is the need to draw attention to patients' right to control information about themselves. The independent examining doctor has only the information obtained from the examination but the GP has the entire medical history of the patient and family upon which to draw. It was considered incongruous for patients to be asked by insurers and employers to authorise the company's access to such potentially wide-ranging information in the medical report, while the individual patient remained unaware of what would thus be revealed. In some cases, erroneous information may have inadvertently been placed on the patient's GP file and would, in the past, have been passed on unchallenged. It was felt that the patient should have a legal mechanism for challenging any of the information given in the medical report by his GP. The Act provides such a mechanism.

### 9:2.3 *Lifestyle questions*

In the past, doctors have sometimes objected to certain questions on the medical report form, particularly questions which seemed to imply that the patient's lifestyle could be judged from the individual's appearance and demeanour. BMA members have expressed concern that in some instances they were apparently being invited to speculate about the patient's potential risk of disease on the basis of subjective or non-medical information. The acceptability or relevance of some information asked of doctors has therefore been a subject of long discussion between the BMA and the Association of British Insurers, who have now agreed joint guidance for doctors completing medical reports for life insurance and permanent health insurance purposes.[278]

Insurers consider questions about the individual's lifestyle to be an important feature when assessing that person's insurability. Within the category of "lifestyle" questions the doctor may be asked to comment about the patient's alcohol or drug abuse and/or smoking habits. The doctor may well have factual medical information on such matters. Risks likely to give rise to HIV infection, such as patients having unprotected sexual relations with multiple partners are less likely to come within the scope of the doctor's knowledge. The BMA recognises that it is appropriate for queries on such matters to be put to the individual applying for insurance but considers that it is inappropriate for doctors to comment on matters which are not medical. Whilst it is acceptable, therefore, for doctors to respond to factual questions such as "Has the patient ever had treatment for alcoholism?" or "To your knowledge, has the patient had an HIV test?", the BMA believes that doctors should decline to answer questions which draw them into speculation. Such questions might be framed in terms of asking the doctor if he or she considers there to be factors in the patient's lifestyle which might lead to an increased risk of disease. Unless there is factual data in the record, doctors should avoid answering such questions. Doctors should not be drawn into conjecture based on hearsay on matters of which they do not have certain knowledge.

### 9:2.4 *Assessment of risk*

A doctor should also not be asked to give an opinion as to whether a patient's condition merits the application of a "normal" or "increased" rate of insurance. The doctor's concern is to record the facts and give an opinion as to the patient's medical condition, not to form an opinion about actuarial risk. In cases where doctors consider it inappropriate to answer a question, they should say so rather than leaving it blank, which will simply result in the report being returned for completion.

### 9:2.5 *Confidentiality*

Often reported to the BMA are patient concerns that information provided to doctors for health care purposes may be disclosed later for other purposes because the patient is under pressure to agree. This is discussed in 9:3.1 below and in chapter 10 (section 10:2.4.1). BMA members also frequently express concern about the confidentiality of information they have supplied to the insurance company on the patient's behalf. (Further issues of confidentiality are discussed in chapter 2.) Questions arise, for instance, when the examining doctor has returned the medical data to the chief medical officer of the company in an envelope marked "confidential", in accordance with BMA advice, but is subsequently contacted by an underwriter or other non-medically qualified employee for further details. The BMA emphasises that medical information should be submitted to the chief medical officer or senior medical adviser, who then bears responsibility for its confidentiality. The insurance company CMO may delegate further enquiries to non-medical employees but will remain ultimately responsible for confidentiality and medical decision-making.

### 9:2.6 *Genetic testing for insurance purposes*

The debate on genetic testing for insurance purposes is only just beginning but there is already public concern that insurance companies may make genetic testing for certain diseases, or predispositions to disease, a compulsory component of an insurance application. In the publication "Our Genetic Future",[279] the Association comes out strongly against compulsory genetic testing. It is of the opinion that it would be better for everyone to pay higher premiums than to oblige people to find out information about their health status which they may not wish to know.

Relevant genetic information already known to a person before applying for insurance would be expected to be revealed, as the insurance industry sees such information as being no different from any other medical information which companies use in underwriting health insurance. In principle, this is acceptable to the BMA, providing that such information is meaningful and interpreted correctly. However, because this is such a newly developing area of health policy the Association would like to see guidelines drawn up which will protect insurance applicants' interests and ensure scrupulous practice on the part of insurance companies.

## 9:3 Pre-employment reports and testing

### 9:3.1 *Doctors' concerns*

Employers and prospective employers have no right to medical information about an individual without that person's consent. They have a right to know whether, in the doctor's opinion, the individual is fit for certain duties.

Some of the same concerns that arise with reports for insurance are evident in queries from BMA members about pre-employment reports, which are also covered by the provisions of the Access to Medical Reports Act 1988. GPs sometimes question the extent of medical information which potential employers seek and point out that although the patient gives consent, in areas of high unemployment, for example, the individual has little free choice in the matter. The BMA notes the call from some doctors for a boycott of reports which require detailed past histories of the patient's physical and mental health and that such reports are increasingly required for teaching or other stressful posts. It is argued that patients will decline to inform their doctors of certain episodes of illness if they believe that later a potential employer will oblige the patient to authorise disclosure of it. Despite the arguments presented, the Association considers that it would be incorrect for doctors to pre-empt patient choice and to assume it is necessarily contrary to the patient's interest to provide information. The decision about whether to authorise disclosure must ultimately rest with the patient. Again, patients should be encouraged to exercise their right of access to the report before it is submitted, if it might be detrimental to their interests.

Often patients only give consent for the release of information to their employer or to an insurance company because if it is withheld the employer or insurer will draw adverse conclusions.

The general view is that it is not for the doctor to enquire into the motives or constraints that underlie a consent freely given in full knowledge of the implications. Therefore provided the statutory requirements relating to consent for insurance or employment medical reports have been complied with, the doctor ought to accept the consent given.

There is another point of view which, although a minority point, deserves acknowledgement both because it is carefully argued and also because some of the medical advisers to the trade union movement have urged it upon their trade unions. This view argues that the purpose of confidentiality is to secure a free flow of information between doctor and patient and that this flow is inhibited just as much by the fear that the patient may be placed under constraints requiring consent to disclosure as by the fear of unauthorised disclosure.

Accordingly it is argued that those who seek medical information about an individual should primarily obtain it through an examining doctor relationship and that consent to the release of information given in a therapeutic relationship is only an acceptable alternative where the patient has chosen that option, having had the genuine alternative of being examined by a doctor with whom no previous therapeutic relationship has existed.

### 9:3.2 *HIV-testing*

Questions are sometimes raised about the inclusion of HIV-testing in pre-employment medical examinations, and discriminatory practices arising against applicants who either decline to be tested or test positive. The BMA is, in principle, opposed to coercive measures being applied to people to oblige them to accept any form of treatment, particularly measures which do not bring benefit to the individual but which might, on the contrary, be extremely disadvantageous. It also condemns employment discrimination based solely on an applicant's HIV status. This practice cannot be justified by reference to the risk of transmission (although the GMC recognises that HIV-positive individuals employed in some areas of the health care sector may represent a hypothetical risk to patients). Nor is it necessarily the case that HIV-positive workers will be incapable of carrying out their jobs solely by reason of their HIV status.

With the exception of sexual, racial and, in Northern Ireland, religious discrimination, the law does not provide a remedy to an individual refused employment on the basis of some discriminatory views of the employer. Employers can therefore refuse to employ applicants who refuse to submit to tests such as that for HIV.

In all circumstances, doctors who carry out HIV-testing have an ethical duty to provide pre-test counselling and to recognise that the applicant may also require post-test counselling, for which arrangements must be made. Further discussion of such testing is included in chapter 1 (section 1:5.1).

### 9:3.3 *Genetic screening for employment purposes*

As genetic predispositions to disease are increasingly identified it is expected that employers may wish to introduce screening of employees and prospective employees in order to identify those most at risk of developing adverse reactions to hazards in the workplace. Such screening, if implemented with appropriate safeguards, can have benefits for both employers and employees alike. For this to be so, the screening must be optional and should be offered to inform employees about the health risks they may run if they are employed in particular types of work. If an employee is found to have an increased susceptibility to certain occupational illnesses the decision whether or not to accept the risk should be left to that individual. The purpose of the test should not be to exclude people from employment who are considered by the company to be an economic risk, or to avoid the implementation of safer working conditions or practices which would be of benefit to all employees. Furthermore, employees or prospective employees must have the right to refuse genetic screening without prejudice to their employment prospects.

Because of the sensitive nature of genetic information and the possibility that employers might interpret wrongly the significance of such information, the use of genetic screening in the workplace should move forward only very slowly and guidelines or legislation may be required to bring appropriate control to this area.[280]

## 9:4 Occupational health physicians

### 9:4.1 *Objectives*

Occupational medicine deals with the effects of work on health and the implications of the employee's health on his or her performance and that of others in the workforce.

The objectives of an occupational health service can be summarised in five points:

- to promote and maintain the health and safety of employees;

- to provide immediate treatment for the sick and injured;

237

- to advise on rehabilitation and suitable placement of employees who are temporarily or permanently disabled by illness or injury;

- to promote safe and healthy conditions by informed assessment of the working environment and by providing advice or educative material;

- to promote research into causes of occupational diseases and means of prevention.

The occupational physician must act as an impartial professional adviser, concerned with the health of all those employed in the organisation. Such responsibilities can lead to very real dilemmas, for example, when the doctor believes that the working environment may exacerbate health problems of certain employees or applicants for employment. Also, statutory and other periodic medical examinations may affect continued employment. Pilots, workers in the atomic energy industry and medical staff developing allergies to drugs are examples of difficult cases. Occupational physicians must then be careful not to take over the role of the line manager in deciding whether such an individual should be offered employment or advised to leave. The patient must be reminded of the doctor's role as the agent of a third party. The doctor's role in such cases must be to advise the employer, with the subject's consent, of possible health problems which could arise.

### 9:4.2 *Consent to examination*

In some companies, employees are required by statute or their contracts to undergo medical examinations. Examples of examinations of fitness required by statute include drivers of heavy goods or public service vehicles and airline pilots. Industries such as those concerned with food handling usually have contractual examinations. It could be inferred from the subject's attendance that he or she agrees both to the examination and to the disclosure of the result. Nevertheless, the doctor should ensure that the employee understands the context in which the examination will take place, the nature of the examination and the need for disclosure of the significance of the findings. These should also be set out in the contract, or in the corresponding reference documents.

The Association is sometimes asked to comment upon schemes for doctors to conduct random drug-testing, or other testing, among applicants for employment or current employees. Although this is not, as yet, a widespread practice in this country, such testing is sometimes justified by the argument that the applicant appointed may endanger the lives of others if impaired by drugs or alcohol. The advice which the BMA has given is that applicants and employees should be informed in advance that testing is required on a regular or random basis. It is not acceptable for identifiable samples obtained from the subject for other purposes, to be tested without the individual having been told of this possibility.

238

### 9:4.3 *Confidentiality*

Although paid by the management, the occupational physician's duties concern the health and welfare of the whole workforce, both individually and collectively. In English law no privilege is attached to the information which a patient gives to a doctor but the usual ethics of confidentiality, discussed in chapter 2, are relevant in the occupational health situation. The fact that a doctor is a salaried employee gives no other employee of that company any right of access to medical records or to the details of examination findings. With the subject's consent, the employer may be advised of information relating to a specific matter, the significance of which the subject clearly understands.

If an employer explicitly or implicitly invites an employee to consult the occupational physician, the latter must still regard such consultations as confidential.

Individual clinical findings are confidential but their significance may be made known to an appropriate third party such as the employer or health and safety representatives. Thus, while an individual reading of a laboratory result is confidential to the individual it is proper to disclose to those with a responsibility for overseeing safety that a group, or an individual, shows, for example, a significant degree of exposure to a potentially toxic hazard.

### 9:4.4 *Sickness absence*

The occupational physician does not usually have to confirm or refute that an employee's absence from work is due to sickness or injury. If the occupational physician wishes to assess the fitness for work of an employee who is still absent for health reasons, he or she should consult the general practitioner, with the patient's written consent.

On an employee's return to work the occupational physician is responsible for advising management on the worker's fitness for the job and may be asked to assess whether temporary or permanent modifications to the work are necessary. Doctors should inform employees of the advice they intend to give management and seek the employee's consent to discuss with the employer any important changes required by the employee's present health.

In cases where an employee's record of sickness absence is very prolonged, the occupational physician may be asked to advise both employee and employer about future employability. While the employer has no right to clinical details of sickness or injury, it is reasonable for employers to expect the doctor to give an opinion about the anticipated date of the employee's return to work, the employee's work-capacity, the likely degree and duration of any disability, and the likelihood of future absences. It is the prerogative of management to take action against an employee who is excessively absent from work. In such cases, the

239

occupational physician may be called upon to give evidence to an industrial tribunal. This subject is discussed further in 9:4.5 below.

### 9:4.5 *Medical records*

Legal concepts of ownership of medical records are generally under-developed in Britain. Occupational physicians sometimes claim ownership of records which they have generated, but the importance of making past records available to succeeding doctors is usually acknowledged. In the absence of any contractual agreement which specifies ownership of the record, the doctor should ensure that at the termination of his or her contract, it will pass to another doctor or occupational health nurse. Transfer of records is discussed further in 9:4.6 below.

The occupational health physician and nurse are responsible for ensuring the confidentiality of clinical records. Under the supervision of the occupational health team, clerical support staff may see clinical records in the same way as many staff in a general practitioner's surgery. The occupational physician must ensure that such staff understand the need for confidentiality and that they have a contractual obligation to preserve it. Neither employers nor their representatives have a right to examine the records.

In cases where an employee has incurred injury or illness at work, the occupational physician may, with the subject's consent, provide the legal advisers of both sides with factual information about attendance at medical departments, first aid and other treatment. In all questions of litigation, clinical records or abstracts from them, should not be released without the subject's written consent. A court or industrial tribunal may, however, order disclosure.

### 9:4.6 *Transfer of records*

Arrangements must be made for the proper transfer of medical records to another doctor or occupational health nurse when the occupational physician leaves the company. In some cases, where the doctor does not have a clear contract or agreement, supervision of the records is left in doubt when the doctor moves on. In some cases, doctors have attempted to take records with them in the belief that they own them but, as mentioned above, the position in law is unclear. The BMA believes that if no other doctor or nurse has been appointed to succeed the occupational physician, the latter retains responsibility for the custody of those records. If it is proposed to close an occupational health department, the medical records should be transferred to the care of medical staff on another site in that organisation. Alternatively, the records may be offered to the part-time doctor if there is one, or to a suitably qualified nurse who has responsibility for workers. In the absence of occupational health staff, it is acceptable for medical records to be kept securely locked, within the organisation, as long as they can only be accessed by a registered medical practitioner. When the continued security of medical records cannot be guaranteed, the destruction of the records may be considered.

### 9:4.7 *Intra-professional liaison*

The occupational health practitioner deals constantly with other doctors' patients and, in order to ensure the best management of the patient, should generally only provide treatment in co-operation with an individual's own doctor, except in an emergency. Similarly, in an emergency, the occupational physician may refer a patient to a hospital or to a specialist, informing the patient's usual doctor of the action taken. Patient consent must be obtained for liaison between the occupational physician and the general practitioner. In a non-emergency situation, the occupational physician should urge employees to consult their general practitioners if referral is necessary, or arrange referral in agreement with the GP.

### 9:4.8 *Commercial secrecy*

Employers and manufacturers are required by the Health and Safety at Work etc. Act 1974 to disclose information about any process or product which may constitute a risk to health in the workplace. In the course of work, an occupational physician may become aware of confidential information about a commercial process or product. If the doctor believes that the process may be harmful to health but cannot persuade the employer to disclose that information, the doctor's responsibility for the health of workers exposed to the hazard should take precedence over the obligations to management. The doctor should, however, inform management of the steps he or she intends to take. In the last resort, the occupational physician may have to warn the workers and face the consequences.

Further advice for occupational physicians is given in a BMA booklet, produced by the Occupational Health Committee, entitled "The Occupational Physician".[281] The code of practice of the Advisory, Conciliation and Arbitration Service (ACAS), should be followed as laid out in its publication, "Disciplinary Practice and Procedures in Employment".

## 9:5 The public health physician

### 9:5.1 *Duties*

The public health physician is employed to advise upon the health of the local community and to make recommendations, about the ways in which this may be improved, to the health authority, other statutory bodies and the community at large. Doctors undertaking such a role are also expected to recommend how health care services should be modified to meet these needs. The local community normally indicates its wishes through its leaders who, for economic, political or other reasons, may either wish to limit the public health physician's role or oppose his or her recommendations. To maintain an ethical stance public health physicians must retain a right to make a direct appeal to the community and not just to its leaders. They must be able to speak out on public health issues and ensure that health advice is not suppressed but remains a matter for public debate. The annual report produced by the Directors of Public Health must be fully independent. (See also chapter 10, section 10:1.7 on free speech.)

### 9:5.2 *Balancing community and individual interests*

The public health physician will sometimes need to balance the needs of the individual against those of the wider community. An extreme example might be seen in the application of section 47 of the National Assistance Act 1948,[282] which permits the removal from home of individuals who are incapable of looking after themselves or who represent a serious nuisance to others. The person concerned must be suffering from grave chronic disease or be an elderly or incapacitated person unable to cope alone and not receiving attention from others. Not all of the people so removed to hospital are suffering from mental incapacity, although it has been estimated that about half of the people dealt with under emergency powers are mentally disordered.[283]

Immunisation programmes provide a more common example of the tension between the dual obligations of the community physician. A successful programme will depend upon a high level of vaccine take-up being achieved. Unless a certain level is achieved the disease may, if re-introduced, spread within the community. Yet, in some exceptional cases, the vaccine itself may damage an individual. If the risk is widely advertised, the community may decline to take up the programme in sufficient numbers, leaving individuals at even greater risk of damage from the disease itself. If, however, all relevant risks are not fully explained to the individual, can consent in the form required, as described earlier in this book (chapter 1, section 1:2.4) be fully obtained? This dilemma places a particular responsibility on all doctors administering the vaccine to ensure that an individual has no contra-indications to the vaccine, since experience shows that those most likely to be damaged already have contra-indications to its use.

A similar dilemma occurs in relation to screening programmes, many of which are increasingly concerned with modifying the natural history of a disease or pathological process. In some cases the programmes themselves are revealing that these processes are still not fully understood. Most individuals attend a screening programme in the expectation of being proved to be healthy. Some will be disappointed: of these, some will have a serious and potentially fatal condition, whilst others will be found on further investigation not to have the condition for which they had originally proved positive. Again the advantages to the community as a whole must be balanced against the needs of these individuals. Screening for genetic disorders, either within a selected population or more commonly within affected families, also presents potential ethical conflicts, particularly in relation to confidentiality when a member of a family refuses consent for details of his condition to be revealed, or for the family tree to be fully investigated. This is discussed also in chapter 1 (section 1:9.2).

### 9:5.3 *Confidentiality*

Just like any other doctor, public health physicians have a duty of confidentiality. Part of their professional role will involve information about individual patients. While they may interpret and act upon such information, it remains subject to the ethical requirement of confidentiality. This may put such doctors in a difficult position in which they have a duty to disclose their proposed solution to problems, whilst keeping confidential the information on which it is based.

Following the passing of the NHS and Community Care Act 1990, the need to circulate detailed invoices of the health care given to individual patients has caused major and serious breaches of confidentiality. In 1993 the Data Protection Registrar revealed that some purchasers and providers of health services were failing to comply with the Data Protection Principles in their handling of contract minimum data sets. Public health physicians have a responsibility to ensure that procedures are in place within the health authorities to reduce these breaches to a minimum until a more satisfactory system has been developed. They may be asked to approve local procedures designed to avoid inadvertent or malicious breaches of confidentiality. Much of the difficulty could be overcome by a statutory code of practice for all workers within the National Health Service, a reform for which the Association has long campaigned. The matter of such a code is discussed further in chapter 2 (section 2:5).

## 9:6 Police surgeons

Most police surgeons have received specific training for this work. Occasionally, however, the police may need to call upon a general practitioner without special training in the particular types of problems which arise in police work. The following general points are intended to assist such doctors to recognise some of the profound ethical difficulties which may occur.

Police surgeons may have to examine, on behalf of the police, victims of crime and suspected perpetrators, as well as examining and treating people who are taken ill whilst in custody. They see detained people to determine their fitness for custody or interview and may examine people, detained or otherwise, for forensic purposes or to obtain forensic samples. In whichever category the individual falls, the doctor should be clear about his or her responsibilities to that person and ensure that the appropriate guidelines regarding consent and confidentiality are applied.

### 9:6.1 *Consent to examination*

In any case where patients are conscious and competent, their consent to examination must be sought. Written consent is recommended, although verbal consent, freely given on the basis of information, is adequate. Verbal consent should be witnessed. In most cases, the individual also has a choice as to whether examination is provided by the police surgeon or by another doctor of the patient's choice, although obviously this may result in some delay which, depending on the circumstances, could either be prejudicial to the subject's health or to the presentation of that person's case in court.

Police surgeons should identify themselves to the person to be examined. In seeking the person's consent to examination, the doctor should clearly explain the purpose of the examination and of any specimen requested. Problems sometimes arise when the doctor begins an examination, with one purpose in view, which is duly explained to the individual, but the information obtained may later be wanted for another purpose which has not been mentioned to the person. A patient with minor injuries, for example, may be examined to see if he or she is fit to be held in custody but it may later be found that the individual sustained the injuries in a serious assault on another person. A police surgeon may well not know of any changed circumstances, when called upon to make a report for which the patient's consent was obtained weeks or months earlier. For the doctor to refuse to provide impartial medical evidence in such cases (except where consent was not given at the time of examination because, for example, the patient was incapacitated or where consent has subsequently been withdrawn) may not be in the examinee's interests in some cases or in the interests of justice. The detained person, therefore, should be advised before giving consent to the examination that there is no absolute privilege and that information obtained during an examination may later be sought by the police or by lawyers.

### 9:6.2 *Examination in support of a complaint*

Police surgeons should be particularly aware of the case law covering the examination of an individual who makes a complaint against the police and undergoes medical examination in support of that complaint. Following a 1981 Appeal Court ruling,[284] it is generally held that written disclosure of any findings of such an examination to anyone other than representatives of the Police Complaints Authority cannot be made except by leave of a court. Thus the person examined is also excluded from access to the report of the examination. In the original case, the plaintiff sought disclosure of the report about himself for later use in a civil action. Disclosure was denied. A series of cases[285] followed, involving access to material gathered in police disciplinary hearings but parties to those investigations were excluded from the information on grounds of public interest immunity. Thus in law complainants who provide information for such an investigation are not entitled to a copy of their own statement. The significance of this situation is that a police surgeon, when seeking the complainant's consent to examination, should include an explanation of the possible constraints placed upon him or her with regard to disclosure of the results of that examination. Although this may represent the current law, the BMA supports the view of the Association of Police Surgeons that it is neither in the interests of the person examined, nor in the interests of justice, for information to be kept back from the person it concerns. The Association believes the doctor should supply the reports to the person's lawyers on written request.

### 9:6.3 *Examination of victims of crime*

Evidential examination is different in aim, and possibly in procedure, from clinical examination. The purpose of examination is to elicit material evidence regarding a possible criminal charge. When the crime is a serious one of rape or assault, there is inevitable pressure on all parties to act quickly to protect others. The time limits for obtaining both the evidence and full information regarding the alleged crime are unlikely to be dictated by the pace the patient finds most comfortable. The police have done much admirable work to address sensitive issues surrounding sexual crimes and many police forces have specially trained officers to provide counselling and support in non-threatening surroundings. Nevertheless, it is most important that the doctor does not assume that the subject's presence implies consent and ensures that the patient does indeed consent to what is entailed by the examination.

In such cases, all those involved should be sensitive to patients' preferences, regarding the gender of the examining doctor and patients should also be aware that they can be examined by their own general practitioner if they prefer.

Similarly, it is important that in cases of suspected child sexual abuse, children should not be subject to unnecessary examination. Repeated evidential examination should be avoided. Discussion of children's consent to examination and treatment is included in chapter 3 on children (see sections 3:3 and 3:4.1).

### 9:6.4 *Examination of people held in police custody*

The examination of people held in custody often concerns possible offences by drivers who may be intoxicated. As is discussed below, blood

245

samples for drug or alcohol estimations cannot be taken from people who are unconscious or feign unconsciousness. Samples taken for diagnostic purposes may later be released to the courts if the person concerned consents, when able, to analysis.

Refusal to provide a specimen by a competent individual charged with a drink driving offence results in automatic disqualification by the courts, who have no discretion in this matter. Even if the court considers the individual not guilty of the offence, disqualification from driving for at least one year is obligatory.

A doctor may be called to examine a person held in custody, either to look for evidence indicating that that person has or has not been involved in a crime, or because the detainee is ill. In either circumstance, an individual held in police custody is not obliged to submit to examination or treatment or to provide specimens for forensic examination and may legally refuse to do so. Such refusal should be respected and the police should only be given such information as is necessary to ensure the person's safety in detention. If ill, the individual may also request to be attended by his or her own doctor instead of the police surgeon. The patient's consent should be sought before examination. As a general point, it should be remembered that any consent given in custody is unlikely to be free from constraint. In the absence of consent, any treatment or attempt to obtain specimens may constitute a battery in law. If a detainee refuses to be examined or to allow a report to be made, a court order may be sought and the doctor must decide whether to comply with it.

If the individual consents to examination, it is advisable for that consent to be witnessed by a third party. A police officer will be present at examination and the patient should be aware that discussion with the doctor may be overheard. It is often impossible for a police officer to be present and out of earshot. Assaults on police surgeons are not uncommon, even when police officers are present. The presence of a third party may prevent later unfounded allegations against the police surgeon. If a woman is examined, a policewoman or other female should be present. If a solicitor wishes to attend the examination, the individual's consent must first be sought. Relatives may be present at the examination of a minor if the young person agrees.[286] For minors, no forensic examination or samples should be undertaken without the consent of the parent/guardian and the young person. It is unlikely that a young person who is too immature to understand what is involved and therefore cannot give valid consent, would be held in police custody. If this were the case, however, parental consent must be obtained.

As in all emergencies, if the patient is unconscious or otherwise incapable of giving consent, examination and essential treatment should be carried out. Other procedures not necessary to protect the subject's life and health cannot be undertaken at the same time. Specimens may be taken for diagnostic purposes but not for forensic tests. The results of diagnostic tests must not be used for forensic purposes without the individual's consent.

### 9:6.5 *Intimate body searches*

The policy of the BMA is that doctors should not carry out intimate body searches without the subject's consent, bearing in mind the possible constraints which may be placed on free consent. The Association has a guidance note for doctors asked to help the police by conducting an intimate search in accordance with section 55 of the Police and Criminal Evidence Act 1984.[287] Intimate body searches are, however, lawful and in some cases may protect other patients, if, for example, the individual is concealing a weapon.

### 9:6.6 *DNA profiling*

The police may seek samples for DNA examination from victims of crime and from suspected perpetrators. A DNA profile (or DNA "fingerprint") can be obtained from very small samples of blood, hair, skin or other biological materials using polymerase chain reaction techniques. Before subjecting the individual to an invasive procedure such as taking blood or even pulling out some hair, the individual's written consent should be sought and the purpose of the specimen explained. Doctors should not participate in any procedure designed forcibly to obtain samples contrary to the subject's wish. To do so might risk an action for battery.

Despite the obvious benefits of DNA profiling, its use still raises concerns regarding the privacy of the individual. Some people fear that information obtained from their DNA may be held for purposes other than those they have been told about, and may, therefore, be reluctant to participate. It has been suggested, for example, that a national database be set up to identify eventually either all members of the population or all males. The BMA considers that DNA profiling must be subject to strict regulation. (DNA profiling in cases of disputed paternity is discussed in chapter 1, section 1:9.4).

### 9:6.7 *The mentally ill*

The role of police surgeons in the initial detection of psychiatric illness is highly important. All police surgeons are expected to ensure that they are fully aware of all the options open to them when dealing with the mentally ill by liaising with police stations, hospitals and social services.

### 9:6.8 *Confidentiality*

The purpose of examinations conducted by a police surgeon is usually to glean information to be used for the purposes of evidence and possible prosecution of either the assailant of the person examined or of the person examined. Confidentiality therefore becomes a difficult issue and in consenting to examination, the individual should be clear about the consequent use which will be made of the information obtained. (See also 9:6.2 above.)

Whether the subject is a victim or a suspected criminal, any information given to the doctor in confidence is subject to the usual rules of confidentiality, which are discussed in chapter 2. The doctor can disclose such information with the individual's consent. Worries are sometimes expressed that police surgeons record details such as the HIV status of detainees on police computers without the patient's consent. This contravenes the duty of confidentiality. Since no privilege is attached to communications between doctors and patients, however, doctors are obliged to disclose information if it is required by a court of law. In some cases, an overriding duty to others in society or risk to others may also make such disclosure essential. As far as the subject's health is concerned only the information necessary to enable the police to take proper care of the individual should be disclosed. In the case of serious illness of a person in custody, information relevant to supervision may be given to the police.

A confidential record of any medical treatment provided, or requested, by the police surgeon whilst the individual is in police custody, should accompany the individual when transferred elsewhere. It should accompany the detainee when he or she first appears in court, in a sealed envelope marked "confidential". The content of this information may be relevant to the granting or refusal of bail and may be used by court forensic psychiatrists or other doctors who later become responsible for the care of the prisoner.

## 9:7 Prison doctors

### 9:7.1 *Dual obligations*

In England, Wales and Scotland, prison medical officers, whether full-time or part-time, are appointed by the Directorate of Prison Medical Services. Their role within the prison, as with any prison staff appointee, is subject to the authority of the prison governor. Since the governor has responsibility for the security of all the inmates, both in terms of protecting the public by securely detaining convicted people and protecting prisoners from one another, doctors are obliged to make medical judgements in the context of maintaining prison discipline. A doctor coming into the prison recognises that such considerations must be respected. The doctor is responsible for the physical and mental health of inmates but his or her relationship with them is not a straightforward therapeutic one, since obligations to patients must be balanced by duties to the employing authority and the need for order.

The BMA supports the view that a distinction should be clearly made between clinical and management roles and that doctors should not be expected to fulfil both functions.

### 9:7.2 *Differences in Northern Ireland*

In Northern Ireland, prison doctors do not have the same dual responsibilities as their colleagues in other parts of the United Kingdom. They are employed by the Northern Irish Department of Health and Social Services (DHSS) and have duties to the prisoners but not to the prison authorities. This situation has arisen because of the political situation in Northern Ireland, where there was a rapid increase in the numbers of people held in custody in the early 1970s. During discussions at that time between the prison authorities and the DHSS, a clear need was seen for an independent medical service in Northern Ireland and this was established in 1974. In practical terms, doctors are recruited for prison medical duties by the DHSS and seconded to individual prisons. By means of this system, an important principle was established in that medical officers remain professionally responsible to the Government's Chief Medical Officer, although operationally accountable to the prison governor.

Prison rules in Northern Ireland reflect these differing responsibilities, although they are derived from the same Home Office Prison Rules operational elsewhere in the UK. It is often thought, however, that the ethical difficulties facing Northern Irish prison doctors are even greater than those encountered by medical colleagues employed by the Home Office, largely because of the way in which the general population is polarised politically on religious lines and because of the extent of violent crime. Of a prison population of less than 2,000, it is estimated[288] that 25 per cent are serving life sentences for murder and 75 per cent have been convicted of terrorist-related offences. The task of maintaining one's independence in prisons and avoiding succumbing to intimidation carries its own particular burdens. The moral dilemmas faced by medical staff in Northern Ireland are highlighted by the statistics of prison hunger-strike fatalities in 1981, when the deaths of 12 prisoners were reported[289] for the whole of Europe (including one in the USSR). Of these, ten occurred in Belfast, with the medical officers providing advice and medical supervision but respecting the prisoners' clearly expressed wishes to continue their fast to the death. Although clearly an extreme example of the stresses and moral tensions with which prison medical officers must deal, the impression that Northern Irish doctors have a considerably more difficult and ethically demanding job than colleagues elsewhere is unavoidable.

It may be noted here that two BMA reports on abuses of human rights[290] gave attention to the situation in Northern Ireland. The later report makes reference to evidence presented in the United Nations by Amnesty International in October 1991, concerning allegations of maltreatment of suspects in the Castlereagh holding centre in Belfast. The report notes that it was prompt action by doctors which first drew public attention to the complaints. This bears out BMA advice that doctors working in prisons have a duty to ensure that any signs of neglect or maltreatment of prisoners are properly investigated. (See also chapter 10, section 10:1.7 on free speech).

### 9:7.3 *Standards of care*

Prisoners are not generally a healthy population and thus there is a higher level of medical need than in the general population. The health care of prisoners is linked to resource questions and to the general state of prisons themselves. These are generally recognised to provide an unwholesome standard of accommodation, with some prison buildings reflecting the austere and punitive approach of their Victorian founders. Prison conditions came under severe criticism in a series of reports in 1991 by both the Chief Inspector of Prisons, Judge Stephen Tumin, and by the European Committee for the Prevention of Torture and Inhuman or Degrading Treatment. Demoralising prison conditions affect not only inmates but also staff.

Imprisonment deprives the individual of many aspects of autonomy. Loss of liberty does not, however, imply the loss of right to medical care of a proper ethical standard. Doctors in the prison service should be in a position to provide the same standards of medical care as is available to the general population. At its annual meetings the BMA has consistently called upon government to ensure that prison health services match care provided in the National Health Service. The Association has particularly identified a need for improved psychiatric services for prisoners.

The Association considers that prison doctors have a duty to draw attention to any inadequacies of the system which may put lives at risk, including the provisions for supervising potentially suicidal prisoners. In the early 1990s, two BMA working parties[291] looked at reports concerning prison working conditions. Despite the faults identified with the system, the reports of both working parties acknowledged the commitment and dedication of most prison doctors whom they saw as sensitive, sensible staff but regretted that workload and conditions necessarily affected both doctors and prisoners.

### 9:7.4 *Consent*

Prison doctors look after the health needs of people held on remand and those who have been convicted. The same general principles apply to both groups with one important difference: remand prisoners have the option of asking to see a doctor of their choice and convicted prisoners have no choice in the matter.

Prison Standing Order section 13.3(1) requires that every prisoner, including those held on remand, be given a medical examination on reception into custody. Prison doctors have a duty to undertake this examination within 24 hours of the prisoner's arrival. The compulsory examination is intended primarily to identify symptoms of physical illness, mental illness or suicide risk and to ensure that prisoners continue to receive medication previously prescribed. The Home Office has produced good practice guidelines but these in themselves cannot be effective unless proper resources allow for all prison inmates to receive adequate initial examination and proper continuous care. The BMA has recommended that hospital officers with nursing qualifications should be allowed to undertake reception assessments. However, overall responsibility for patient care would remain with the doctor who would see appropriate patients and be available to receive any patient who requested a more personal consultation on the following day.

In the late 1970s and early 1980s, the high prescription rate of psychotropic drugs was a particular cause for concern. Some considered that their use on difficult prisoners was primarily for ease of management as was shown by the name prisoners gave this treatment - the "liquid cosh". It was, however, maintained by some doctors that minimising disruption was in the best interests of everyone. Fortunately, this is no longer an issue since prescribing practices have changed but, in all cases, a prisoner's consent to treatment should be free from any form of pressure or coercion. No influence should be exerted through the special relationship between the doctor and the patient whose consent is sought.

### 9:7.5 *Remand prisoners*

Apart from the compulsory reception assessment, individuals held on remand can consult a doctor or dentist of their own choice. This should be arranged through the individual's solicitor and with the assistance of the prison medical officer. A remand prisoner should also be able to see a doctor in private.

Remand prisoners are considered to be at particular risk of suicide[292] and the introduction of screening procedures during reception was intended to identify potentially suicidal prisoners so that their individual needs could be catered for accordingly. The Home Office Circular Instruction 20/1989 provides clear guidance which is designed to recognise and deal with suicidal behaviour in a manner geared to the needs of the individual prisoner. Nevertheless, the BMA considers that lack of psychiatric training among nursing staff, staff shortages and limited prison hospital facilities makes implementation of the Home Office advice extremely difficult. It also considers that therapy or counselling should be an integral part of the care and treatment pattern for "at risk" offenders and supports the move away from solitary confinement for prisoners perceived to be potentially suicidal.

These and other aspects of the provision of health care in remand institutions are discussed in the BMA's published report on the "Health Care of Remand Prisoners". The report proposes practical recommendations for change.

### 9:7.6 Convicted prisoners

Convicted prisoners have no freedom of choice regarding the doctor they see. Nevertheless, the prison medical officer's duty to, and relationship with, convicted patients is the same as for any other doctor.

### 9:7.7 Confidentiality

Prison doctors are faced with a tension between maintaining prisoners' confidentiality and the obligation to assist the governor to ensure the safe and proper management of the prison. When a governor has a need to know certain information about inmates in order to guarantee either the security of inmates or their safety, the doctor is considered to have an obligation as an appointee of the Directorate of Prison Medical Services to divulge that information. Nevertheless, disclosure of personal health information, other than to hospital or nursing officers, should only be made on the strictest "need to know" basis.

Information about treatment provided by a police surgeon should be made available only to the prison doctor and transferred immediately to the prison medical record. It is not acceptable for medical details to be included in the prisoner's main prison record, with the exception of opinions given by the prison doctor concerning the prisoner's fitness for work or comments regarding matters which directly affect the prisoner's management by prison staff.

Doctors working in prisons must be able to keep independent confidential records. In the course of their duties prison medical officers will make written or verbal reports to courts, adjudication boards, prison governors or other authorities. In the case of reports to courts, the prisoner's consent to disclosure should always be obtained. In other cases consent should be sought, but in the absence of consent prison medical officers must be guided by their assessment of the prisoner's best interests.

### 9:7.8 Liaison regarding the medical history of prisoners

One of the most severe problems faced by prison medical officers is lack of accurate medical information about the individual's previous history. The prison medical officer must rely initially upon information provided by the prisoner, which may be inaccurate or incomplete. Prisoners have a right to withhold medical details. Information submitted, however, to the BMA's Medical Ethics Committee suggested that often problems arise not from prisoners' refusal but rather because some prisoners may be confused and/or unable to provide information, or are briefly questioned in

252

situations which do not afford the opportunity for confidential discussion. Prison doctors are therefore encouraged to contact general practitioners directly, with the prisoner's consent, if the prisoner is competent to give consent at the time, in order to obtain confirmation of the prisoner's medical history.

Difficulties arise when inmates are not registered with a GP or, as sometimes happens, when general practitioners request fees before agreeing to release information, thus delaying the delivery of reports. General practitioners have reported that they too sometimes experience delay in obtaining medical information from the prison doctor after the prisoner's release. The BMA has concluded that there is an ethical duty for doctors to provide information promptly, with the individual's consent. In emergencies, information should be provided by telephone. The BMA does not believe that the requesting of a fee for a written report by a GP is itself unethical, but considers that it may be unethical to delay provision of information or make such provision dependent upon payment.

### 9:7.9 *Mentally ill prisoners*

Liaison between doctors is particularly significant when a prisoner has suffered psychiatric illness. The Gunn Report, published in 1990, (revised 1991), found that about one third of a sample of male prisoners and 59 per cent of females suffered some kind of psychiatric problem. At the same time, a study funded by the Home Office put the incidence of psychiatric disturbance at 14,000 of the 38,000 sentenced prison population, with 1,100 so ill that they required immediate treatment. The British Medical Journal has repeatedly expressed concern about such reports. Yet the management of mentally ill prisoners continues to present a severe problem to prison doctors, who do not have the facilities to provide the necessary treatment. They frequently face reluctance from hospitals to accept such patients, despite the provisions of the Mental Health Act 1983, which enable mentally disordered convicted prisoners to be transferred to hospital following medical reports. Nevertheless, prompt diagnosis and referral are essential and this is an area where prison doctors need the assistance of colleagues working in hospitals to ensure that there is minimal delay in transfer.

### 9:7.10 *Control*

Prison medical officers have no role in the control or punishment of prisoners. They are called upon to determine whether prisoners are fit for adjudication, following breaches of discipline by prisoners. Prison hospital staff must remain an exclusive resource to prison medical managers and must not be regarded as an additional resource to prison governors. Prison medical officers must be able to offer independent clinical recommendations for treatment.

253

## 9:7.11 *Hunger strikes*

In some countries, doctors have been pressured by the authorities and not permitted to exercise clinical control in the treatment of hunger strikers. In such cases, hunger strikers have been forcibly fed, either to punish the prisoner or to avoid any possible embarrassment to the prison authorities which the prisoner's death might cause. The BMA strongly urges that in all cases, artificial feeding and the way it is implemented, must be the result of a clinical, and not an administrative, decision.

The BMA supports the principles of the World Medical Association's Declaration of Tokyo.[293] The Association affirms that when a prisoner, whom the doctor considers capable of forming a rational judgement, refuses nourishment in full knowledge of the consequences, he or she should not be fed artificially.

Furthermore, the BMA recommends that doctors make their policy regarding resuscitation during hunger strikes absolutely clear to the prisoner at the beginning of the strike. Doctors who feel unable for reasons of conscience, or for any other reasons, to abide by the prisoner's decision must allow another doctor to supervise care.

A doctor who has any doubt about a prisoner's intention regarding hunger strikes, or who is asked to treat an unconscious prisoner whose wishes the doctor cannot ascertain, must strive to do the best for that prisoner. This may involve resuscitation if the prisoner's views are unknown. If doctors are in no doubt about the prisoner's wish regarding resuscitation and feeding, they must respect it. If it is clear that the prisoner intends to continue the strike until death, he or she must be allowed to die with dignity.

These and other aspects of medical participation in protecting or abusing the rights of prisoners are fully explored in the BMA report, "Medicine Betrayed". The report lists recommendations for the treatment of prisoners and outlines action doctors can take if they suspect maltreatment of prisoners.

# 9:8 Doctors examining asylum seekers

## 9:8.1 *Port medical officers*

People who arrive in the UK complaining that they have suffered torture or maltreatment in their country of origin are examined by medical officers employed by the Department of Health. Some of these new arrivals will later become asylum applicants. It is important that an adequate medical report be made in all cases when an injured person arrives, and when a new arrival requests medical examination of wounds, scars or bruises. The BMA is concerned by some reports it receives that port of entry medical officers do not always note signs such as wounds or recent scars. The BMA recognises that identification of torture sequelae requires particular expertise and training and cannot be done quickly.

Nevertheless, brief but adequate notes of abnormalities noted by port medical officers could be crucial in the later assessment of the validity of an asylum seeker's case. It would also be helpful if any record made by port of entry medical officers could be made available to other doctors who examine the same individual later in connection with an asylum application. Usually, independent doctors providing later reports are denied sight of medical records made at the time of entry to the country. Superficial signs of maltreatment may have disappeared by the time later medical reports are made.

### 9:8.2 *Expert assessment*

Asylum seekers may live in the community pending adjudication, or may be detained in custody. They do not form a homogeneous group but some common health problems have been identified by experienced doctors working with torture victims' rehabilitation organisations. These draw attention to the fact that the full effects of maltreatment which the applicant may have suffered are unlikely to be immediately evident upon initial examination. Conclusive physical signs are apparent in only a minority of cases but predictable patterns of psychological sequelae are common. Medical opinion varies as to the extent to which such sequelae might be categorised as exclusive to victims of certain types of trauma but the evidence points to the probability that such categorisation is possible. While expert opinions differ, it must be pointed out that ultimately psychological assessment, as with all branches of medicine, is dependent upon experienced clinical judgement and international standards established by specialists in this field. Many of the psychological sequelae of torture take a long time to emerge, which can be problematic given the time-limits imposed upon asylum applications. Discussing past physical abuse, particularly if it involved cultural taboos such as sexual humiliation, is likely to be extremely difficult for the subject.

People who have suffered torture, maltreatment and psychological trauma in their country of origin rely partly upon medical documentation of the detectable sequelae to substantiate their claim for asylum. As discussed above in 9:1.2.1, doctors asked to provide a medical report for asylum seekers must ensure the impartiality of their report and each individual application must be subject to careful and impartial scrutiny. It is important that doctors recognise that there are often cultural differences in the way in which patients present medical symptoms and the importance they accord to different types of injury.

The London based Medical Foundation for the Care of Victims of Torture provides volunteer doctors experienced in documenting evidence of torture, who can give a medical assessment. The Foundation has also drawn up guidelines in consultation with the BMA on the examination of asylum seekers making Home Office applications.[294]

## 9:9 Doctors in the armed forces

### 9:9.1 *Constraints on serving doctors*

All members of the armed forces are subject to both civil and military law. A doctor in the armed forces must obey any lawful command. Disobedience is punishable by various sanctions including those determined by court martial. In addition, like all doctors, serving doctors must behave in accordance with professional ethics.

In all three services, serving doctors are responsible for their professional actions to the same extent as are civilian medical officers, and are expected to work within the same ethical constraints as the rest of the profession. The ethical freedom of serving medical officers is supervised by the Surgeon General who has accepted that no medical officer should be required to treat a patient under the constraint of non-medical orders when the doctor believes that treatment is not in the individual's best interests.

The UK Defence Medical Services has also emphasised the fundamental ethical obligations of doctors in the armed services and has drawn attention to the appeal procedures, operating through the medical chain of command, for doctors who consider they are being asked to act unethically. The UK Defence Medical Services considers, however, that it is unlikely that a serious problem will arise in practice, not least because the armed forces are subject to ministerial control and ministers are concerned to ensure that the behaviour of the armed forces is above reproach.

A matter which has been raised with the BMA on several occasions concerns armed forces doctors who object to boxing matches. These doctors, who do not support boxing as a sport, have been required to carry out pre-bout medical examinations. Some have also complained that they had insufficient examination time and facilities adequately to assess the potential risk to each participant. The BMA has advised that a full explanation of the doctor's objections to boxing as a sport should be given to the commanding officer and that the matter should be handled through the recognised appeals procedure. Some doctors who feel strongly on the matter have considered resigning from the Forces, rather than having anything to do with boxing matches. Although this is an extreme measure, it may be the only solution in cases where doctors consider that the examination facilities or the way the sport is practised do not minimise the risk of severe injury.

### 9:9.2 *Confidentiality*

When an individual joins the armed forces he or she tacitly relinquishes some rights and freedoms. One of these is the right to strict confidentiality. There are occasions when a medical officer is required to discuss the personal health information of patients with a commanding officer.

In many cases the liberties which people in the armed forces have given up are also lost to other members of their families, who may find that in practice, they have no choice of medical practitioner and reduced rights of confidentiality, since it is assumed that the health of the family may affect the serviceman or woman and the unit. This raises some very difficult issues for families of serving personnel. If, for example, a child is suspected of having suffered abuse, it would be customary for the officer in charge of welfare to attend the case conference. In effect, this is involving a representative of the employer, and would be unacceptable in other situations. Case conferences are discussed in chapter 3 (section 3:5.1.2).

## 9:10 Doctors with business interests

In some cases, the dual duty owed by the doctor is of a different nature from those previously discussed. Doctors who own companies wish to promote the interests of those organisations but should not use their reputation and standing as medically qualified people to influence potential customers.

For doctors who either direct or hold a financial interest in medical or non-medical enterprises, the main ethical considerations include the function of the enterprise, the manner in which it may generally be promoted and whether the doctor can refer patients to the organisation - if it offers medical or nursing services.

### 9:10.1 *Nature of the enterprise*

Doctors invest in a wide range of medical and non-medical schemes. The BMA advises that sometimes such investment may give rise to a conflict of interest for the doctor. The Association regards with almost equal gravity, situations in which patients believe erroneously that the doctor's judgement is influenced by such financial holdings and situations in which this belief is well founded. In the former situation, patient confidence in the doctor may be compromised just as surely as if the doctor were indeed putting personal financial interests first. For this reason, the BMA advises against owning or holding shares in, for example, a drug company whose products the doctor may wish to prescribe for patients. (See also chapter 7, section 7:5.1.1 and chapter 10, sections 10:2.6.1, 10:2.7 and 10:2.8).

### 9:10.2 *Referral*

It is acceptable for doctors to refer their patients to facilities in which the doctor has a financial interest. Both the GMC and the BMA state that in such cases the doctor must declare his financial interest to the patient.

## 9:11 Media doctors

Some doctors choose to work partly or exclusively in the media. They are employed to provide general medical advice or commentary. For those in specialist practice, care must be taken not to appear to advertise their own services directly to the public.

Only general rather than patient-specific medical advice should be provided through the media. Patients corresponding with or otherwise contacting media doctors must be advised to seek a consultation with their own practitioner for full treatment of their condition.

### 9:11.1 *Medical telephone advice lines*

A number of telephone services have been developed which offer the public advice and information on a range of health questions. Some services provide tape-recorded messages from which the caller receives standard information about the condition in question. Others are in the form of a "helpline", where the caller can discuss a problem with a doctor, nurse or other patient with experience of the condition.

The General Medical Council has warned of the dangers which may arise if a doctor offers advice to a patient whom the doctor has not seen or examined. The Council does not take exception to recorded messages giving standard advice on health matters by doctors or others. Nor does it object to "helplines" giving general information. Nevertheless "phone-in" programmes and "helplines" which attempt to provide individual advice create problems. To provide the type of specific medical advice, usually provided by a patient's own GP, is not appropriate in these circumstances.

## 9:12 Summary

1  In all cases where doctors are acting for another party, they have an obligation to ensure that the patient understands that fact.

2  Even when doctors are appointed and paid by a third party, they retain a duty of care to the patient whom they examine or treat.

3  Medical reports must be objective and impartial. Doctors should not be drawn into speculation. They may be asked to offer an expert opinion of the most likely aetiology of the subject's medical condition.

4  In most circumstances, even when the doctor-patient relationship does not conform to the usual pattern, doctors have a duty to provide information in order to obtain patient consent and they have a continuing duty of confidentiality.

5  Doctors have a duty to investigate and speak out when services with which they are concerned are inadequate, hazardous or otherwise pose a potential threat to health.

# 10 Relations Between Doctors

*Introduction, including professional standards, personal limitations, disciplinary measures, professional etiquette, arbitration of disputes and the importance of good communication. Issues which concern the general practitioner joining a practice including partnership agreements, daily procedures for running the practice, conciliation and dissolution of partnerships. Professional issues applicable to all doctors whether in general or specialist practice, such as advertising regulations, sharing of premises and schemes for sick doctors are mentioned here as are issues relevant to questions of referral and overall management of patients' health. The limits of loyalty, sick doctors, and disciplinary proceedings are covered. Responsibility for prescribing is mentioned, and is further discussed in chapter 7. Doctors' relations with other professions are covered in chapter 11.*

In this section, we discuss doctors' relations with colleagues. This topic raises sensitive and elusive issues, touching upon competition, status and independence. It is the subject of a large number of enquiries to the BMA, particularly from members who want practical advice and interpretation of how ethical theories apply to common dilemmas.

## 10:1 Introduction

### 10:1.1 *Professional standards*

Medical practice in Britain is governed by a mixture of law, ethical guidance laid down by the statutory body, the General Medical Council, agreed standards of good practice and accepted custom. The medical profession is self regulated by means of the General Medical Council, which in its yearly publication, "Professional Conduct and Discipline: Fitness to Practise", sets standards which are effectively obligatory for all registered medical practitioners. The Council has the power to erase from the Register the name of any fully or provisionally registered practitioner judged by the Conduct Committee of the GMC to have been guilty of "serious professional misconduct". This disciplinary function is discussed in 10:1.3 below.

The GMC's guidance must cover the wide spectrum of traditional, ever-present dilemmas and also those which are newly emerging. It is

259

therefore cast in broad terms. The BMA plays an interpretative role in assessing how the basic principles apply to specific cases. Furthermore, the Association receives a large number of varied enquiries from its members and has thus built up a body of experience on the implementation of ethical advice.

The principal focus of the GMC's guidance concerns doctors' relations with their patients and with third parties such as pharmaceutical companies. Some of the advice, however, concerns doctors' relations with their colleagues or combines professional preoccupations with a concern for patients. In the past, the GMC's prohibition on doctors advertising their services was interpreted by many as having such a dual aspect: reflecting both a concern for vulnerable patients and preventing competition between doctors. This continues in the GMC's condemnation of measures which put pressure on members of the public with the aim of recruiting them as patients. If public confidence is to be sustained, it is clearly important that the profession acknowledges self-interest, where it exists, and not only refrains from trying to canvas patients, but also refrains from claiming that any such attempts are aimed solely at benefiting patients.

Many of the complaints raised with the BMA regarding the behaviour of doctors are not unique to the profession, but mirror concerns common in any group of people. Nevertheless, social indiscretions or misbehaviour are considered much more seriously when doctors are involved because of the vulnerability of the patients concerned and the privileged access doctors have to their confidence. Society expects high standards of professional integrity from doctors in return for the privileges accorded to them.

Although much is expected of doctors both in terms of conformity to ethical norms and expertise in the skills they exercise, it is important that doctors themselves should be aware of their own limitations and not be tempted to step beyond those even for well-intentioned reasons.

### 10:1.2 *Recognising one's limitations*

It may be self-evident to state that doctors have an ethical duty to refrain from measures which may expose patients to risk because of the doctor's lack of experience or confidence in a particular technique. Nevertheless, it is clear that some doctors, particularly junior doctors in hospitals, are sometimes called upon to perform, without appropriate supervision, tasks for which they have not been adequately trained. In such cases, junior doctors should decline to carry out such tasks and draw the attention of senior colleagues to the situation. Unfortunately, there is often considerable social and career pressures upon junior doctors to attempt to handle difficult situations without calling upon senior colleagues, especially during unsocial hours. The BMA offers support to any doctor who refuses to undertake a procedure without prior training and adequate supervision.

Neither ethics nor the law[295] recognises inexperience or a desire to please colleagues as a valid defence if doctors undertake a task beyond their competence and by so doing cause patients to suffer harm. The law requires any doctor to possess the degree of skill and experience appropriate to the task, but recognises that junior doctors must gain experience. An inexperienced doctor has a defence in law by seeking and following the advice of a more senior colleague who may then be held responsible for any resulting harm. The seriousness with which medical errors by inexperienced doctors is viewed by the courts was demonstrated in 1991, by the conviction for manslaughter of two junior doctors, after an error in drug administration which caused the death of a leukaemia patient.

In general practice, also, there may be occasions when doctors are requested to undertake procedures, including some forms of specialist counselling, for which they have not received adequate training. In such cases, the doctor should refer the patient to another practitioner, as appropriate. In the past, some therapies were apparently regarded as more accessible to doctors by reason of their general medical background. Thus the view arose that doctors did not require specific training in the same way as non-medically qualified practitioners of that skill would need. Particular examples may be seen in the practice of complementary therapies such as acupuncture. A doctor who causes injury to a patient by undertaking such therapies in the absence of proper training is likely to be vulnerable to disciplinary proceedings.

### 10:1.3 *Disciplinary measures*

The GMC is responsible for medical registration, education and fitness to practise. Its powers derive from the Medical Act 1983. The GMC's professional conduct committee may remove or suspend an offending doctor from the medical register or place restrictions upon his or her practice. The largest category of complaints to be brought before the GMC's concern disregard of professional responsibilities to patients.

The GMC is also proposing new procedures to deal with poor performance by doctors. These cover instances where a doctor's knowledge or skills are seriously deficient, but there is no question of ill-health. The new procedures apply particularly to unacceptable patterns of practice, such as persistently inappropriate prescribing, failing to examine patients or to keep adequate records of home visits. The new arrangements are expected to resolve some of the problems raised with the BMA by doctors concerning colleagues who make mistakes or who persist in using outmoded techniques which are less efficacious than modern ones for the patient. At present, the Association recommends that doctors with concerns about poor performance by colleagues discuss the issues with the colleagues concerned and also use the mechanisms of peer review. Some doctors have found useful a system of "open days", when hospital

261

consultants invite general practitioners, or vice versa, to debate procedures and exchange information. The Association believes such liaison schemes should be encouraged.

In addition to the disciplinary and regulatory mechanisms of the General Medical Council, professional etiquette and accepted practice exert a powerful influence over doctors' behaviour towards colleagues and others.

### 10:1.4 *Etiquette*

The BMA considers that the etiquette involved in the interaction between doctors is an essential aspect of medical ethics, given that ethical behaviour involves truth telling and proper relationships based on respect for others. Questions of etiquette and customary practice are often given less attention than other facets of medical ethics, but they are the subject of many enquiries to the Association. These frequently concern issues such as charging colleagues for the medical treatment they receive (see 10:6.2 below) and liaison between doctors.

Relations with colleagues, if not handled in a satisfactory way, can give rise to serious disputes and it is in the interests of both doctors and patients that such potential disputes between doctors be foreseen and avoided. The BMA offers advice on some of these questions, upon which there is no specific GMC ruling.

### 10:1.5 *Arbitration of disputes between BMA members*

The BMA has an established machinery at local and national level to resolve ethical disputes between doctors who are members of the Association. Preliminary consideration of the dispute takes place at local level and has the advantage of providing a confidential medical forum for adjudicating disagreements between doctors. Both parties to the dispute must agree to be bound by the decision of the local BMA ethics committee. Matters which cannot be satisfactorily resolved at local level are referred to the Assocation's Intra-Professional Relations Committee. Full details of the procedures are circulated periodically to all BMA Divisions, which make them available to Association members upon request.

### 10:1.6 *Communication*

Many disputes could be avoided by effective communication between doctors, sharing of information, with due regard to confidentiality, and early airing of issues of disagreement. Throughout this book, the Association has sought to emphasise the vital importance of doctors being able to communicate in clear terms with patients, colleagues and other professionals. Unfortunately, in the past, doctors were expected to acquire such skills through observation of senior colleagues, but in recent years the profession has given much serious thought to practical measures, such as the use of video-taped consultations, to provide training in listening and responding effectively.

Rapid and clear communication between all health professionals engaged in the care of patients is essential. If continuity of care is to be properly maintained, information must be available to the doctor who becomes responsible for that patient's immediate continuing care. This applies, for example, where a patient under treatment by a medical practitioner moves to another area, or when a patient enters or is discharged from hospital. Children and other dependent people have sometimes suffered neglect when one of their parents has been admitted to a psychiatric facility and the GP, who might be aware of the family's circumstances, has not been informed promptly enough to alert other agencies. General practitioners also sometimes express concern about the time taken for discharge summaries to reach them after patients leave hospital. It is clearly important that information contained in such summaries are made quickly available to the GP, especially if continuing treatment by the GP is indicated. Another particular area of concern relates to delays in information passing between GPs and prison medical officers regarding the medical history of prisoners (see chapter 9, section 9:7.8). The doctor from whose immediate care the patient is passing should decide the best means of communication, having regard to the circumstances and the likely delay in receiving a posted letter.

Treatment frequently requires communication with other professionals, as is discussed in chapter 11. At all times, the doctor has a "duty of clarity" and should aim to eliminate ambiguity and doubt. Issues associated with information-sharing are discussed in chapter 2 (section 2:1.5.1) on confidentiality, and chapter 3 (section 3:5.1.1) on children, but in all circumstances where professionals are sharing care, clear information diminishes the possibility of mistakes and harm to patients. Particularly on difficult issues such as resuscitation decisions (see chapter 6, section 6:6.2), it is essential that all those caring for the patient are informed of all aspects of the case, especially the patient's views, if known, and those of the family.

### 10:1.7 *Free speech*

The maintenance of a free and informed debate on health matters is important if individual patients and the community at large are to be able to exercise appropriate choices.

It is therefore incumbent on the medical profession, and represents an individual ethical obligation on each member of that profession, to do everything possible to ensure the maintenance of the freedom of speech and publication of the members of the medical and allied professions and of the related sciences. There can be no free and informed debate on health matters if those with an expert contribution to make are excluded from the right to contribute.

263

An unfortunate assertion has recently begun to be made that those who work for NHS (including trust hospitals) employers owe that employer a duty of loyalty which precludes them from speaking out in ways which are contrary to the interests of that employer.

The superficial logic of this argument is instantly belied when it is appreciated that free speech in this instance exists not for the benefit of the speaker but for the benefit of the audiences and that what the employer is claiming is the right to obstruct the public interest in the free flow of information to those who pay for, and have every right to expect accountability from, NHS bodies.

### 10:1.7.1 "Whistle-blowing"

In the early 1990s, "whistle-blowing" became an issue for all health-workers. It was brought to the forefront by the sacking for gross misconduct of the nurse, Graham Pink, who publicly voiced concern about the welfare of acutely ill geriatric patients in a ward which he considered to be dangerously understaffed. In 1990, Mr Pink was charged with a breach of confidentiality when he informed the media of the situation, after the health authority said it could not improve staffing levels. The case raised anxieties for all health professionals, particularly since it coincided with the so-called "gagging clauses" introduced into the employment contracts of trust hospitals. The issue is raised in this chapter because it has important implications regarding the way health professionals support or isolate colleagues who "whistle-blow". Since the BMA considers there is an ethical duty for doctors to take action against unsafe standards of care, it follows that they should also support, and not discriminate against, those who are brave enough to speak out about standards which are indeed unacceptable.

### 10:1.7.2 Trusts and secrecy clauses

As competitive enterprises, trusts demand that employees maintain secrecy about any matters which may affect their commercial viability and have introduced contractual terms to enforce this. These employment clauses are the subject of continuing negotiation between the BMA and the Department of Health. The Association maintains that doctors have a responsibility to patients to speak out on issues which may affect patients' welfare. It should be possible to do this within the new NHS, without necessarily disclosing information connected with the hospital's business affairs. While the Association is aware of the need for great sensitivity in matters relating to commercial issues, nevertheless doctors have a primary ethical duty to draw attention to poor standards of care and to ensure that patients are not put at risk. Existing procedures for dealing with complaints about standards should be used as a first measure and doctors should respect patient confidentiality when drawing attention to problems. Doctors cannot, however, permit commercial considerations to override their ethical obligations. As a final option, when the conventional avenues have been explored to no avail, employees must be able to raise genuine issues of public concern with the media without forfeiting their jobs.

### 10:1.7.3 Special hospitals and psychiatric facilities

All doctors carry responsibility for safeguarding the ethical practice of medicine. Doctors employed in closed institutions have a particular duty to be vigilant and aware of the potential for abuse which may occur in institutions. In 1992, for example, Ashworth special hospital was the focus of an independent inquiry which followed allegations of improper patient care, including the alleged beating in seclusion of a patient who later died. A consultant psychiatrist, three psychologists and a social worker employed at the hospital were given special awards for exposing the abuses. The BMA is aware, however, of the risk that staff in closed institutions may become isolated, identifying themselves as the powers-that-be, losing sympathy and respect for their patients, and thus becoming part of a system of oppression rather than therapy. When bad practice is endemic and part of a closed culture, individuals may fear voicing their complaints. In its report, "Medicine Betrayed",[296] the BMA regretted, for example, the diminution in the powers of the Health Advisory Service to carry out inspections.

The BMA also drew attention to the need for standards of care in residential and psychogeriatric institutions be reviewed and monitored. It called for staff aware of abuses to be supported in their attempts to make them known to the responsible authorities.

### 10:1.7.4 Reporting misconduct by professional colleagues

The question of the limits of loyalty to colleagues raises other common questions. General practitioners seek practical advice on how to approach a partner whom they suspect may be too closely involved with a patient, or abusing alcohol. Often they are unsure of the extent of their responsibility to investigate the facts, how much evidence is required to take a case to the GMC, how to confront the partner or, if a colleague poses a potential danger on the roads, whether it is justifiable to report him or her to the vehicle licensing authority. Similar problems with regard to the confidentiality of patients are discussed in chapter 2 (section 2:4.4). Where a person poses a potential risk to others, counselling should be tried, whether the offender is patient or colleague. As a last resort, doctors may decide to breach confidentiality in order to protect other people.

The GMC makes clear that it is "any doctor's duty, where the circumstances so warrant, to inform an appropriate person or body about a colleague whose professional conduct or fitness to practise may be called into question or whose professional performance appears to be in some way deficient."[297]

265

As with all other areas of social and business activity, awareness of the possibility of sexual harassment or molestation is becoming heightened in the medical world too. The BMA's view is that protection of patients or other members of the public must come first, although clearly it would be inappropriate to bring allegations against colleagues in the absence of convincing evidence. Disagreements may arise between colleagues about matters of apparent misconduct or because views differ on what constitutes good practice. The BMA emphasises the importance of doctors agreeing practice guidelines which reflect the profession's perception of good practice (see 10:2.2.2 below). Conciliation procedures for disagreements are discussed in 10:2.2.3 below.

## 10:2  General practice

Many of the issues discussed in this and following sections concern primarily doctors' relations with patients, but they may also have implications for maintaining good relations with colleagues.

### 10:2.1  *Establishing a practice*

Doctors may practise medicine alone or in partnership with others. A doctor working alone is advised to approach colleagues established in the area and inform them of the proposed new practice, as well as consulting the Family Health Services Authority (FHSA).

Purchasing or developing surgery premises represents the most significant financial commitment of a doctor's professional career. For those practising within the NHS, assistance is available through a number of measures, such as the cost-rent scheme. Doctors interested in such measures are advised to consult their FHSA; the General Medical Services Committee of the BMA may be able to provide further guidance.

#### 10:2.1.1  Goodwill

Under NHS regulations the sale of goodwill is illegal[298] and doctors who are in doubt as to whether any particular transaction constitutes a sale of goodwill should clarify the position with the Medical Practices Committee. Private practitioners may purchase the goodwill of an existing practice. In such circumstances, doctors selling their goodwill should be sure that their name has not previously appeared on the list of practitioners willing to provide general medical services under the NHS.

### 10:2.2  *Joining a practice*

#### 10:2.2.1  Partnership agreements

If working in partnership, it is advisable to have a formal partnership arrangement and for all partners to take legal and accountancy advice when drawing up or entering into a partnership agreement.[299] Some experts believe that standard minimum partnership agreements should be compulsory since it is sometimes said that junior partners in particular may not always be treated equitably. In the absence of a written agreement, they may be subject to measures such as not being permitted to see financial records, being excluded from practice decision-making or being assigned a disproportionate share of the partnership's on-call work. Exclusion from information and discussion may mean that a doctor is unable to influence issues which reflect on the ethical integrity of the practice, or which give rise to ill-feeling. A written partnership agreement avoids abuses and provides a mechanism for establishing an equal share in decision-making for all partners.

Doctors with any doubts about joining a partnership should take advantage of all available information, seeking advice from local medical committees and BMA regional offices, before committing themselves. As mentioned previously, they are advised to insist upon a written partnership agreement which sets out clearly the rights and obligations of all the parties. Some commentators have recommended a change in the nature of partnerships, advising that doctors join practices as assistants for a probationary period. This allows for a time of mutual assessment without definite commitment either by the new GP or the established partners, although there are financial disadvantages to a doctor working as an assistant rather than a partner.

### 10:2.2.2 Rules of procedure

The attention of the BMA has been drawn to some acrimonious disputes which have arisen between partners on issues which generally fall outside the scope of partnership agreements. This has prompted the Association to suggest that multi-partner practices draw up guidelines or rules of procedure on the day-to-day running of the practice. It is suggested that these guidelines address issues such as the amount of time partners should spend in the practice in relation to the time devoted to external activities (including committee work or conferences) which bring kudos to the practice. While this is likely to bring potential problems for a very active media GP, for example, it is often better that these are discussed in advance rather than raised when matters have already come to a head. Guidelines might also include matters such as the practice approach to patient care, research involving patients, availability of chaperons for intimate examinations and a conciliation mechanism for resolving disagreements.

### 10:2.2.3 Conciliation

It may be helpful for practices to make provision in advance for the resolution of disagreements which arise, for example, when one partner persistently disregards agreed practice procedures or acts in a manner which might call into question the reputation of the practice. In the latter case, other doctors in the practice may be considered to have an ethical duty to take action if patients' well-being or confidence in the practice is likely to be compromised. Any member of the practice must be entitled to call a practice meeting to address the difficulty frankly and to attempt to resolve it in a manner supportive to all. BMA industrial relations officers, based in the regional offices, have expertise in achieving conciliation and arbitration, with different officers being assigned to represent each party. Depending on the nature of the problematic behaviour, advice may also be sought from the defence bodies and counselling services for sick doctors. Advisory mechanisms for sick doctors are discussed in section 10:6 below.

### 10:2.3 *Dissolving a partnership*

Doctors in general practice should give forethought to the separation of patient lists upon the dissolution of a partnership, as this is a frequent area of disagreement. When partnerships are dissolved in an atmosphere of ill-will, doctors must be careful not to impugn the skill or judgement of colleagues. The GMC advises that as a general principle, in any circumstances, justifiable comment is appropriate when patients seek a second opinion or an alternative form of treatment, but unsustainable remarks intended to undermine trust in another doctor's knowledge or skill are considered unethical. Complaints about such matters sometimes arise as a result of patients seeking advice as to with which partner they should register or wanting to know the reasons for the practice split. Clearly doctors must be sensitive about discussing their colleagues, while at the same time offering a satisfactory explanation. Nor must they allow false information to circulate unchecked, such as rumours that a colleague is intending to retire from practice or move from the area. In this, as in all matters, patients are entitled to receive balanced advice. Such advice should also make clear that the patient has a right to register with any practitioner. Clearly, this right is exercisable at any time, but it is brought particularly into focus when practice lists divide.

Retention by doctors of computer data about patients no longer registered with them, may give rise to confusion and contravenes the principles of the Data Protection Act 1984 (see chapter 2, section 2:2.7.3).

### 10:2.4 *The NHS GP contract*

A new contract for NHS general practitioners came into force in 1990. Traditionally, NHS general medical services have been mostly those services provided by GPs for sick patients, notable exceptions being maternity medical services and contraceptive services. However, the definition of what is included in the category of "general medical services" has been steadily expanded and now explicitly includes health-promotion and illness prevention services. The contractual changes implemented on 1 April 1990 formalised the position that had been reached in many practices, which were already carrying out health promotion work as part of general practice. The emphasis on health promotion within general practice was increased by measures introduced by the Department of Health in 1993.[300]

### 10:2.4.1 Health promotion and target payments

At the time of the contract's introduction in 1990, the BMA was alarmed by some ethical implications regarding the confidentiality of patient health information and the possible pressure which might be brought to bear upon patients in order for doctors to reach certain targets. Some of these questions were successfully resolved by negotiation with Government, although concerns remain, that the considerable financial differences for doctors achieving different levels within the system of target payments, present an inducement to doctors to put pressure on patients.

The new health promotion measures, introduced in 1993, encourage general practitioners to establish programmes to reduce the incidence of illnesses such as coronary heart disease, diabetes and asthma. This entails collecting information about patients' smoking and drinking habits, their family history of disease, their diet and their physical activity. Obviously, such information has long been noted, but current proposals are that it be more systematically collected by doctors in order to help them promote a healthy lifestyle for patients who might be at particular risk of disease. As is discussed in chapter 9 (section 9:3.1) problems may arise if patients fear that details they provide for health care will later be used in reports for loans or life insurance. Clearly, no information can be released to third parties without patient consent but the patient may be in a poor position to choose if the alternative to authorising disclosure is the loss of a loan or an employment opportunity. The fact that the patient may be prompted to participate actively in measures to improve his health, however, may mitigate the possibly prejudicial effect of previously poor lifestyle habits, as far as insurance companies are concerned.

It is to be emphasised that treatment or diagnostic procedures can only be carried out with patients' consent and for their benefit. A persistent ethical difficulty for general practitioners is that the health promotion measures for which they receive special payments are also the measures which doctors would wish to promote even in the absence of any incentive. Thus, a conscientious effort to educate patients about the importance of preventive measures may also be seen as self-serving. In explaining such preventive procedure to patients, doctors should emphasise that the purpose is to bring benefit to the patient, without concealing the financial implication.

### 10:2.4.2 Screening

Screening is the subject of an on-going debate in the profession. Some consider that it is ethically incorrect to offer screening procedures which have not been shown to be scientifically valid, for conditions which the doctor cannot effectively treat. The act of undergoing screening may also give patients a false sense of security about their health. Doctors should make all efforts to prevent this by ensuring that balanced information is given to the patient.

The GP contract obliges doctors to offer screening tests which the doctor may feel are superfluous for particular, individual patients. As is discussed in chapter 1, doctors should discuss frankly with patients why certain treatments or diagnostic procedures are proposed, as a prerequisite to the patient's consent. With such screening, the motivation for offering tests in individual cases may not be related to clinical judgement. It would be inappropriate for the doctor to pretend it is, rather than acknowledge that it is a contractual requirement. In obtaining patient consent, therefore, doctors should be honest about why tests are offered. It is recognised, however, that many people regard routine health checks as beneficial and those proposed in the contract are in themselves neither unpleasant nor hazardous.

The recording and subsequent use of information obtained from routine testing may also give cause for concern. (See chapter 9, section 9:3.1).

### 10:2.5 *Patient participation*

Since 1972, patient participation groups have been established in a few practices throughout Britain. Originally viewed as a means of giving health-care consumers a say in the running of services, in recent years, the perception of the roles played by such groups appears to have changed somewhat. Fundraising activities have become a more prominent feature of these groups' activities. It is in connection with the fundraising role that most doubts about such groups are voiced and this is discussed below.

#### 10:2.5.1 *Planning health goals*

The fundamental purpose of patient groups is to encourage patients to participate actively in the planning and implementation of the provision of health care. It can be seen as part of the wider ethos of individuals taking responsibility for their own health and for preventive measures against disease. Those associated with the patient participation movement define the essence of patient participation as "the belief that patients, doctors and other medical staff can work together to develop the provision of health services and to realise health care goals."

#### 10:2.5.2 *Confidentiality*

Ethical problems can arise in regard to the protection of patient confidentiality and in regard to the possibility of pressure being brought to bear on patients to participate in group activities and, specifically, in fundraising activities. The doctor is responsible for safeguarding confidentiality and must ensure any disclosure by the practice to the patient group is with specific patient consent. Patients must be clear that the practice does not accept responsibility for the actions of individual group members who might choose to provide voluntary services or counselling.

### 10:2.5.3 Fundraising

Fundraising, which appears to be the raison d'etre of many patient participation groups can also raise ethical problems. Such projects should not impose any direct or indirect pressure on patients to contribute. The BMA has previously advised that collecting boxes in the waiting room are not acceptable, nor should patients be given the impression that essential equipment will only be provided by contribution. It is entirely unethical for charities or voluntary organisations to be encouraged to raise money for equipment which forms part of the indirect expenses element of GP remuneration. Many believe that accepting equipment from charitable or voluntary sources is a very questionable practice. Disputes have also arisen during the dissolution of a partnership, regarding the ownership of equipment provided by patients.

Questions arise too about sponsorship by pharmaceutical companies or others of patient participation group events, for example, marathons, swimming and cycling events, which offer publicity to the products of the sponsoring company. Although much sponsorship is seen by the doctor involved as helpful to the practice and harmless to the practice image, this view is not necessarily reflected by patients. Great caution is advised, therefore, regarding the way in which the practice may become associated in the public mind with the sponsoring company. Events which prominently draw attention to pharmaceutical products, as part of the deal which attracted the sponsorship for the event, may compromise the perceived, if not the actual, independence of prescribing in that practice. They should therefore be avoided.

### 10:2.6 Fundholding GPs

The system of GP fundholding is a relatively new one. Concerns have persistently been raised about the emergence of a two-tier system for patients requiring specialist care although some consider that it is still too soon to judge the extent to which such fears may be justified. It is clear that patient needs and not financial considerations alone should determine the speed and provision of services. To try and ensure this, the Government and the profession produced guidance for all provider units, including NHS trusts. This looked at how the principle of treatment according to clinical need should be recognised within the new contractual framework. Particular emphasis was placed on the need for full involvement for hospital consultants in the initial setting of contracts. The following principles were set out:

i)      common waiting lists should be used by provider units for urgent and seriously ill patients and for "highly specialised diagnosis and treatment";

ii)     contract portfolios should be worked out in close consultation with the hospital clinicians who have to deliver them. Waiting-time specifications offered by provider units should be flexible enough to allow for fluctuations in clinical need and patient flow which will inevitably arise as a result of the demands of the different contracts determining the work of a consultant;

iii)    provider units will not offer contracts subject to i) & ii) to one purchaser which will disadvantage the patients of other purchasers. Equally, purchasers creating additional capacity through their contractual arrangements with provider units will be entitled to the consequential level of treatment specified in the relevant contracts. This additional capacity should also offer advantages for other purchasers' patients and the potential for this should be fully explored before contracts are agreed.

As in all other cases where doctors have a financial interest in referring patients to a particular service, this interest should be disclosed to the patients.

### 10:2.6.1 Fundholding GPs provision of secondary care

As a general principle, it is unwise for the doctors to be both the purchasers and providers of a particular service. Some GPs established limited companies in order to provide secondary services to their own patients. The GMC advised that it was not improper for a general practitioner or practice to set up a company, provided always that the medical interests of patients were paramount and patients were made aware of any personal financial interests the doctor had. However, concerns were expressed about the potential for GPs to make excessive profits. The Department of Health subsequently amended the fundholding regulations to allow fundholders to be paid from the fund for treating their own patients but only in respect of certain specified services and then only with the consent of the regional health authorities.[301] This means that contracts between fundholders and third parties (ie limited companies) are no longer necessary and restricted under the revised regulations.

### 10:2.7 Financial interests in health-care facilities

When referring patients to another practitioner a doctor must act, and must be seen to act, in the best interests of the patient. On principle, doctors who have a financial interest in an organisation to which they propose to refer a patient, should always disclose that interest before making the referral and should not attempt to persuade patients to use the facility in preference to equally suitable alternatives. This applies not only to laboratories and facilities providing clinical or diagnostic services, but also to institutions such as nursing or retirement homes. The GMC advises that:

"A doctor who recommends that a patient should attend at, or be admitted to, any private hospital, nursing home or similar institution, whether for treatment by the doctor himself or by another person, must do so only in such a way as will best serve, and will be seen best to serve, the medical interests of the patient. Doctors should therefore avoid accepting any financial or other inducement from such an institution which might compromise, or be regarded by others as likely to compromise, the independent exercise of their professional judgement. Where doctors have a financial interest in an organisation to which they propose to refer a patient for admission or treatment, whether by reason of a capital investment or a remunerative position, they should always disclose that they have such an interest before making the referral."

"The seeking or acceptance by a doctor from such an institution of any inducement for the referral of patients to the institution, such as free or subsidised consulting premises or secretarial assistance, may be regarded as improper. Similarly the offering of such inducements to colleagues may be regarded as improper".[302]

### 10:2.8 Financial interests in pharmacies

Traditionally the BMA has advised that doctors should not own a financial interest in a pharmacy within their practice area. In the past it was felt that a potential conflict of interest could arise if doctors did so and that the desire for more money might influence, or appear to influence, the doctor's approach to prescribing. This advice was reviewed by the Association in 1992 since many thought it inconsistent with current practice. Nowadays, doctors often have a financial interest in a hospital or nursing home to which they may refer patients and this does not present an ethical problem, as long as referral is made in the best interests of the patient and the doctor's financial involvement is disclosed. The BMA recommends that doctors who have a financial interest in pharmacies which their patients might use should disclose that fact to the patients. There should be no explicit or implied direction of patients to that particular pharmacy. In all circumstances doctors must bear in mind the GMC's injunction that the doctor's decision must always put the medical interests of the patient first. Doctors relations with pharmacists are discussed further in chapter 11 (section 11:6).

## 10:3 Advertising

Advertising is an issue which was hotly debated in the mid and late 1980s when the Monopolies and Mergers Commission conducted an enquiry into the distinction between activities which could be termed as disseminating information and those which constituted advertising or self-promotion. The BMA argued against liberalisation of the restrictions on advertising on the grounds that people who are ill or who are seeking medical attention for their families can be particularly vulnerable to influence and that advertising would open the door to competition and consumerist attitudes which sit uneasily with the purpose of medicine. Some of the force of this argument was acknowledged by proponents of advertising, with the result that the extent to which doctors today may advertise their services is subject to limitations. Obligatory standards have been laid down by the GMC. The BMA provides further interpretation of these.[303] It is important for doctors to distinguish between the BMA's advice and the GMC's regulations. Since both are evolving in response to new variations in advertising schemes, doctors are advised either to consult the most recently revised edition of the GMC publication, "Professional Conduct and Discipline: Fitness to Practice", or to write to the Ethics Division of the BMA in any case of doubt.

### 10:3.1 *Services which may be advertised*

In 1990, the General Medical Council amended its rules to allow general practitioners and doctors offering the eye sight-test to publicise "general medical services". The GMC has made it clear that it is the scale of services rather than the category of practitioner that determines whether advertising is permissible. The GMC has not attempted to produce a definitive description of "general medical services". It would be difficult to do so. For GPs practising within the NHS, reference can be made to the NHS contract, but, even so, some practitioners may have additional expertise in complementary therapies which they offer to patients on their own list under the heading of general medical services. Private GPs are at liberty to decide what range of services to offer. The GMC has indicated the types of service provision which are excluded from general medical services and may not be freely advertised. Doctors providing a limited or specialised range of services, even though they may not see themselves as "specialists", are still subject to restrictions.

Therefore medical practitioners who concentrate on a specific group of patients or single specialised treatments may not advertise directly to the public. GPs sometimes consider providing one or two therapies privately outside their main practice. The GMC has considered such advertisements, in which individual services such as hypnotherapy, hormone replacement therapy, vasectomy and acupuncture were publicised by doctors who

274

presented themselves as general practitioners. It confirmed that doctors who wished to offer such a restricted range of specific services should be bound by the guidance currently governing specialists.

On the other hand, some doctors provide an extended range of therapies beyond the usual scope of primary care services through "alternative" or "complementary" medicines and the GMC has also considered their circumstances. It ruled that doctors providing a full range of primary care using such methods and medicines might legitimately advertise the services they offer.

### 10:3.2 *Editorial control*

Factual information about general practitioner services may be placed in the media. Often this is done in the form of an advertisement, but the BMA has no objection to the information being given in the form of a brief article, as long as this conforms to the general advice on advertising and does not imply a superior service to that provided by other doctors. The type of information should reflect that required in practice leaflets and may include mention of health promotion clinics. Although not mentioned in the GMC's advice, caution is advised by the BMA in regard to newspaper features which focus on, and are full of praise for, a new surgery. These may in effect be a form of secondary advertising for local businesses who are named as offering encouragement to the medical practice. The purpose is often to draw attention to suppliers involved in refurbishing the surgery. Doctors usually have no control over the language and format of such articles, which are a way of increasing advertising revenue for the newspaper. The line between editorial and advertising can become very blurred. It is essential that doctors retain editorial control over any material advertising or alluding to their services, as they may be held responsible for the content.

### 10:3.3 *Practice leaflets*

Under their terms of service, NHS practitioners must provide the public with information about their services in the form of a practice leaflet. There is no obligation for private practitioners to do this or to adopt a particular format for any leaflet they choose to produce. Nevertheless, they may find it useful to note the NHS specifications if considering a private practice leaflet.

There are no restrictions as to the size or format of the leaflet. Information about NHS practitioners provided in the leaflet must cover a list of items specified by the NHS, which includes the full name, sex, registration details of doctors and whether the practice is single- handed or a partnership. It must also state the times the doctor is available, whether an appointment system operates and how an urgent appointment or domiciliary visit can be arranged. Deputising and repeat prescription arrangements must be mentioned, as well as the provision of clinics and a description of the roles of practice staff. The leaflet must state whether contraceptive, maternity and child surveillance services are provided and whether the doctor undertakes minor surgery. Also the practice's geographical boundary, suitability for access by disabled patients, teaching arrangements within the practice and how patients can make comments on the practice must be indicated.

Supplementary to the requirements of the NHS terms of service, doctors can also feature, if they wish, a note about the partners' particular interests, such as child health, or their additional expertise, such as acupuncture or hypnotherapy, as well as a general statement about the practice's approach to health care. There is no restriction on photographs in practice leaflets. Leaflets should be freely available within NHS surgeries. They may be placed in libraries and advisory centres where prospective patients might look for health information. Practice leaflets may also be distributed within the area served by the practice to people who are, or are not, patients of that practice. The GMC forbids advertising by means of unsolicited visits and/or telephone calls with the aim of recruiting patients, whether these are carried out by doctors or agents acting for them.

### 10:3.4 *Doctors advertising other businesses*

The BMA, but not the GMC, offers advice about commercial advertising carried by practice leaflets. In the Association's view, advertisements for local businesses should occupy no more than one-third of the leaflet, which should clearly state that the practice is not endorsing the services advertised. The Association counsels against advertising for products which clearly affect health adversely - such as tobacco products - since this might give a mixed message to the public despite the doctor's disclaimer regarding endorsement. Similarly, the BMA advises against advertising health-related services, such as pharmacies, nursing homes and private clinics in practice leaflets. The Association maintains that despite disclaimers from the practice, such advertising may be thought to imply recommendation and be confusing to patients. It sees no problem in doctors listing, for information, all local pharmacies or health facilities, if they wish. The BMA also discourages advertising in practice leaflets for businesses in which a doctor or a near relative has a pecuniary interest.

In general, the BMA does not support the use of the surgery for the promotion of any businesses, either through promotional literature or electronic advertising. It considers the promotion of life insurance or financial services in exchange for a retainer fee to the practice, inappropriate in this context.

The GMC has not ruled on these issues.

## 10:3.5 *Canvassing for patients*

The GMC prohibits doctors or their agents from contacting prospective patients personally, with a view to persuading individuals to join the practice. It is also clearly unacceptable for pressure to be brought to bear upon patients registered with one practitioner to change to another. Such activities may render a doctor liable to disciplinary proceedings by the General Medical Council.

## 10:3.6 *Information to companies, firms and similar organisations*

Doctors who wish to offer services, such as medico-legal or occupational health services to a company, firm, school, club or association may send factual information about their qualifications and services to a suitable person in the organisation and may, where appropriate, place a factual advertisement in a relevant trade journal.

## 10:3.7 *Advertising by specialists*

A specialist's name, qualifications, address and telephone number may be included in local and national directories, but the same details may not be distributed in an unsolicited manner to the public. Associations of doctors are permitted to release lists of their members to the public on request.

In addition, all doctors are permitted to inform professional colleagues of the services they provide and to invite referrals. This is the only way those in specialist practice are allowed to make their services widely known. Specialists are encouraged by the GMC to provide information to general practitioners and managerial colleagues. Such material as these specialists draw up should not claim superiority for the practitioner's personal qualities, qualifications, experience or skill. These principles apply to specialists working in NHS hospitals, NHS trusts and private practice.

### 10:3.7.1 *Trusts*

NHS trusts present hospital specialists with a new dilemma. The financial prosperity of the trust is likely to depend increasingly upon the quality of the staff, particularly the medical staff, whom it employs. The trust will therefore wish to advertise to its purchasers the particular merits of the specialists it employs. Thus, although it is not intended that the doctor should gain any financial benefit, as would be the case if a private institution used similar methods, the opportunity for unethical behaviours is a very real one. Doctors should be vigilant in ensuring that any advertising material circulated by health service trusts conforms both explicitly and implicitly with the GMC guidelines. Similarly, with the increasingly blurred distinction between health care provided for NHS patients within the service and in private hospitals, specialists who work in both the private and the NHS sector need to be vigilant in observing the rules that apply to advertising in the different sectors in which they practise.

### 10:3.8 *Advertising organisations offering medical services*

The GMC recognises that hospitals, screening centres, private clinics, nursing homes and advisory centres may advertise medical services to the general public. The principles laid down by the Council for the advertising of general practitioner services apply. According to the GMC's rules, such advertisements should not make adverse comparisons with the NHS, nor claim superiority for their professional services. A doctor who has a professional or financial relationship with such an organisation bears some responsibility for its advertising. Ignorance of the content of such advertising is no defence, should advertisements breach GMC standards.

## 10:4 Relations between NHS and private practitioners

### 10:4.1 *Patient choice*

Increasingly, premises are shared by NHS doctors and those offering their services privately. Some doctors provide services within both systems of health care. As a general principle, it is important to recognise clearly patients' autonomy and freedom of choice in this matter, as in others. Patients should be aware that they can consult other appropriate practitioners, either privately or under the NHS, in preference to doctors who happen to share the same premises as the doctor currently responsible for their treatment.

Thus, referrals must be made with the interests of the individual patient taking precedence over other considerations. In many cases, patients will welcome the convenience of additional services on the premises, but the terms and extent of what is provided must be clear to all. Patients must know, for example, whether the other services recommended to them are provided independently, without charge, by quite separate NHS practitioners, by employees of an NHS GP, by private practitioners who charge all patients, or by private practitioners who charge patients not on the list of the GP.

GPs must be able to inform patients about alternative services to those provided by the colleagues with whom they share the building. Patients' freedom of choice should not be compromised by any suggestion of automatic direction to other practitioners on the same premises, particularly where it might be thought that the GP could gain financially from such direction.

## 10:5 Specialist practice

### 10:5.1 *Acceptance of patients by specialists*

It is usual for one doctor to be responsible for the overall management of a patient's health. This ensures that the patient is assessed as a whole and a relationship is gradually built up with benefits to both doctor and patient. Such doctors will acquire the basic personal health information about their patients.

The method of referral from a general practitioner to a consultant or specialist has evolved in response to the need to act always in the patient's interests. The GMC, states:[304]

"Although an individual patient is free to seek to consult any doctor, the Council wishes to affirm its view that, in the interests of the generality of patients, a specialist should not usually accept a patient without reference from the patient's general practitioner. If a specialist does decide to accept a patient without such reference, the specialist has a duty immediately to inform the general practitioner of any findings and recommendations before embarking on treatment, except in emergency, unless the patient expressly withholds consent or has no general practitioner. In such cases the specialist must be responsible for the patient's subsequent care until another doctor has agreed to take over that responsibility.

Doctors connected with organisations offering clinical, diagnostic or medical advisory services must therefore satisfy themselves that the organisation discourages patients from approaching it without first consulting their own general practitioners. ...

In expressing these views the Council recognises and accepts that in some areas of practice specialist and hospital clinics customarily accept patients referred by sources other than their general practitioners. In these circumstances the specialist still has the duty to keep the general practitioner informed."

In any context such liaison between practitioners requires patient consent. In general, a doctor in consultant or specialist practice should not normally accept a patient without reference from a general practitioner except in the following circumstances:

a) In an emergency.

b) If a consultant is asked for a confirmatory opinion by the specialist to whom the patient has been referred.

c) If reference back to the GP would result in a delay seriously detrimental to the patient. The specialist should inform the GP as soon as possible of any action taken and the reasons for it.

d) If referred by doctors in the school or other community child services.

e) If it is for a consultation in sexually transmitted disease.

279

f)   If the consultation is for a refraction examination only.

g)   If a patient is formally referred by a doctor from outside the United Kingdom.

h)   If the patient is seeking contraceptive advice and treatment and is unwilling to consult her own GP about contraception, or her own GP does not provide contraceptive services. It should be explained to the patient that it is in her own best interests that her GP be informed that contraception has been prescribed and of any medical condition discovered, which requires investigation or treatment. Every attempt should be made to obtain permission to contact the GP. This is particularly important if the patient is at the same time under the active clinical care of her own general practitioner or that of another doctor.

i)   If the patient is seeking therapeutic abortion and is unwilling to consult her own GP. It should be explained to the patient that it is in her best interests that her GP be informed of the treatment or advice given. Every attempt should be made to obtain the patient's permission for this.

j)   If patients who consider it seriously detrimental to their financial or employment prospects to have details of episodes of psychiatric treatment recorded in their GP notes, self-refer to accident and emergency departments or to psychiatric hospital drop-in emergency centres. The medical advantages of involving the GP should be explained to the patient.

Doctors may have special skills; they may use acupuncture or hypnosis as part of treatment. The use of these skills in relation to a patient for whom the doctor is not the usual GP is in practice analogous to that of a specialist. If such a doctor accepts a patient without reference from a GP other than in the circumstances outlined, the guidance set out above should be observed.

### 10:5.2 *Clinical responsibility*

The sharing of clinical responsibility for a patient between specialists and general practitioner is explored in chapter 7 (section 7:6.2) on prescribing. An important issue which bears repetition is the need for proper communication between professionals for the good of the patient. It is noted that emphasis on professional independence sometimes leads to the opinion that it is not necessary for one practitioner to explain fully the treatment which has been provided for the patient to other practitioners assuming care. It is sometimes implied that such detail should not concern practitioners of other disciplines. This is regrettable.

# 10:6 Sick doctors

## 10:6.1 *Self-treatment*

When doctors require medical treatment themselves, the BMA strongly recommends that they seek an independent professional opinion rather than self-treat. Similarly, the Association also recommends that doctors do not prescribe for themselves or their families.

## 10:6.2 *Charging colleagues*

Charging professional colleagues and their dependants is a matter of etiquette, not ethics. The BMA's policy is to support the tradition of not charging colleagues for medical treatment. Where doctors intend to charge, it is strongly recommended that this be made very clear before beginning treatment.

## 10:6.3 *Confidentiality*

As a general principle, doctors who are ill are entitled to benefit from the same strict rules of confidentiality as other patients. It is regrettable that the confidentiality owed to a patient who happens to be a doctor is sometimes overlooked, particularly regarding doctors undergoing psychiatric treatment. There have also been cases where speculation and discussion about sick doctors have taken place before the doctors themselves have been informed of test results. We therefore thought it necessary to draw attention here to the application of the basic principles of confidentiality discussed in chapter 2, since it sometimes appears to be thought that these do not apply to doctors. As with the general principles of confidentiality, in some circumstances a breach may be justified by the treating doctor's overriding duty to society.

## 10:6.4 *Counselling service*

The conflict between professional loyalty owed to colleagues and the need to ensure patients are protected may pose a dilemma for doctors who believe a colleague is ill and possibly putting patients at some risk. The National Counselling Service for Sick Doctors[305] is a confidential independent service supported by the Royal Colleges, the Joint Consultants Committee, the British Medical Association and other medical professional bodies. The service started in 1985 and since then has been asked to help a large number of doctors whose health is causing concern to colleagues, often because the doctor is not taking steps to deal with the problem. About a quarter of the calls received come from doctors seeking help for themselves, outside the geographical area of their own practice.

### 10:6.5  *GMC procedure*

There are differing procedures for assisting sick doctors who may pose a risk to patients. The procedure introduced by the General Medical Council in 1980 is based in law. The main provisions are set out in the Medical Act 1983 (Part V and Schedule 4).[306] Details of how the procedure works are given in the GMC publication "Professional Conduct and Discipline: Fitness to Practise" (January 1993) Part 4. Many are doctors who go through this procedure suffer from alcohol or drug-related problems, mental illness or a combination of these.

### 10:6.6  *"The three wise men"*

An alternative to the GMC procedure is the "three wise men" procedure, designed to prevent harm to patients by sick medical or dental staff. According to the latter procedure, each health authority is mandated to establish a special professional panel to "take appropriate action on any report of incapacity due to physical or mental disability including addiction."[307] A sub-committee of the panel can make confidential enquiries to verify the accuracy of allegations and can interview the practitioner. If the panel is unable to assure the protection of patients by counselling the doctor, they can inform the regional medical officer.

National Health Service regulations grant powers to FHSAs to take over the running of a practice. These powers may be invoked if a practitioner is too ill or too obdurate to seek medical assistance.

### 10:6.7  *Guidance for doctors suffering from infectious conditions*

The General Medical Council has issued advice on the question of doctors suffering from infectious conditions such as Hepatitis B or HIV infection. It considered it to be imperative, both in the public interest and on ethical grounds, that any doctors who think there is a possibility that they may have been infected with HIV should seek appropriate diagnostic testing and counselling and, if found to be infected, should have regular medical supervision. They should also seek specialist advice on the extent to which they should limit their professional practice in order to protect their patients. They must act upon that advice, which in some circumstances will include either a requirement not to practise, or to limit their practice in certain ways. No doctors should continue in clinical practice merely on the basis of their own assessment of the risk to patients.

It is unethical for doctors who know or believe themselves to be infected with HIV to put patients at risk by failing to seek appropriate counselling, or by failing to act upon it when given. The GMC advises that a doctor who has counselled a colleague who is infected with HIV to modify his or her professional practice in order to safeguard patients and who is aware that this advice is not being followed, has a duty to inform an appropriate body that the doctor's fitness to practise may be seriously impaired.

Appropriate bodies, in this context, include the GMC's health procedures mechanism or the "three wise men" mechanism mentioned in 10:6.6 above. If necessary, the GMC can take action to limit the practice of such doctors or to suspend their registration.

## 10:7 Summary

1   Doctors should not undertake measures that they cannot perform with competence and confidence. A junior doctor should not be asked by a senior doctor to provide treatments beyond the expertise of the junior doctor. Inexperienced doctors who are faced with the necessity of performing treatments beyond their skill must refuse and draw the situation to the attention of their senior colleagues and managers.

2   Doctors have a right of free speech and a duty to draw attention to inadequate standards of care. Colleagues should support "whistle-blowers" when their complaints appear justified.

3   Rapid and clear communication between all health professionals engaged in the care of a patient is essential.

4   The type of information used in advertising should reflect that required in practice leaflets. It is essential that doctors try to retain editorial control over any material advertising their services, as they may be held responsible for the content.

5   The BMA advises against advertising health-related services, such as pharmacies, nursing homes and private clinics, in practice leaflets.

6   Advertisements issued by private facilities should not make adverse comparisons with the NHS, nor claim superiority for their professional services. A doctor who has a professional or financial relationship with such an organisation bears some responsibility for its advertising.

7   Specialists are encouraged by the GMC to provide information to general practitioners and managerial colleagues. Such material drawn up by specialists should not claim superiority for the practitioner's personal qualities, qualifications, experience or skill.

8   If a specialist does decide to accept a patient without a reference from a GP, the specialist has a duty to inform the GP of any findings and recommendations before embarking on treatment except in an emergency, unless the patient expressly withholds consent or has no general practitioner.

9   Doctors connected with organisations offering clinical, diagnostic or medical advisory services must satisfy themselves that the organisation discourages patients from approaching it without first consulting their own general practitioners.

283

10    The Association recommends that doctors do not prescribe for themselves or their families.

11    BMA policy is that doctors should not charge their colleagues for medical treatment. Where doctors intend to charge colleagues or their immediate dependants, it is strongly recommended that this is made very clear before beginning treatment.

12    Doctors who are ill are entitled to benefit from the same strict rules of confidentiality as other patients.

13    Doctors who think there is a possibility that they may have been infected with HIV should seek appropriate diagnostic testing and counselling. They should also seek specialist advice on the extent to which they should limit their professional practice in order to protect their patients. A doctor who has counselled a colleague who is infected with HIV to modify his or her professional practice in order to safeguard patients, who is aware that this advice is not being followed, has a duty to inform an appropriate body.

# 11 Inter-Professional Relations

*In this chapter, we discuss doctors' relations with non-doctors, including other professionals who provide health care, particularly the nursing and midwifery professions and the professions supplementary to medicine. Consideration is also given to relations with complementary practitioners. We consider doctors' relations with other professionals who work outside the health sphere, such as social workers. Attention is also given to the relations between doctors and pharmacists and doctors and the pharmaceutical industry. Summary.*

## 11:1 Introduction

### 11:1.1 *Background*

Sick people have always sought help from a variety of sources. Thus the complementary role of medicine with that of some other professionals has long been acknowledged. The shared responsibility between doctors and pastors for the physical and spiritual care of sick people has been relatively uncontentious, perhaps partly because of a clear demarcation of roles until the growth of psychiatry as a branch of medicine.

By the eighteenth century, three groups of medical practitioners were recognised - physicians, surgeons and apothecaries. Not only was there professional friction between practitioners of each group but also with others outside these groups. The management of pregnancy and childbirth, for example, gave rise to rivalry between medical men and midwives. Thomas Percival sought in his code of medical ethics to encourage co-operation between physicians and apothecaries. He saw such co-operation in the interests of the patient as a moral duty "when health or life are at stake".[308] "Quackery", however, a term applied to any therapies outside the accepted medical field, and to which some patients obstinately made recourse, was firmly deprecated by Percival and his colleagues. Nevertheless, traditional healers, herbalists and others now grouped together as "non-conventional" therapists have long provided a variety of treatments outside the scope of conventional medicine.

Over the last two centuries, power struggles developed between doctors and other people providing services, as health care became increasingly regulated. Traces of past battles can still sometimes be seen in uneasy aspects of the relations between the professions even though the emphasis nowadays is on patient choice in health care and liaison between professionals for the good of the patient.

The British Medical Association was established in the mid-nineteenth century and arose partly from a concern to protect the public from "quacks" and to promote good medical practice and partly with the aim of binding together the "fraternity" of doctors, excluding all outsiders. It sought to safeguard the honour of the profession and promote good communication between members.

One of the first activities of the Association was to produce a report on "quackery", by which was understood the treatments offered by practitioners who were not medically qualified. It was subsequently, at the instigation of the BMA, that the General Medical Council was established under the Medical Act 1858. The principle of the Act was "that persons requiring medical aid should be able to distinguish qualified from unqualified practitioners". Under the terms of the 1858 Medical Act, a doctor could be removed from the register for sending a patient to a non-medically-qualified practitioner. Therefore the tradition of medical practice as a discrete body with its own sphere of knowledge was established.

The dominance of the medical profession was further strengthened at the beginning of this century. Government concern about the poor quality of volunteers for the army during the Boer War led to measures such as the establishment of the inter-departmental committee on the Physical Deterioration of the Population, which reported in 1904. Infant mortality was seen as an issue which Government had to address if the country's defences were not to be jeopardised.[309] Control of midwifery[310] was tightened and the role of doctors and hospitals in childbirth expanded. There have been trends recently, however, to reverse this, by emphasising the combined role of a variety of health professionals to allow more care to be provided outside the hospital setting.

These trends have also focused attention on the many roles undertaken by nurses, who are the largest single group of staff working in health care in Britain.[311] New categories of nurses, such as nurse practitioners and nurses who can prescribe from a limited formulary, are recognised as working autonomously in liaison with doctors.

Gradually, other professional groups have also gained statutory recognition. Independent professional associations govern their behaviour and maintain high standards by issuing agreed codes of professional ethics and regulating practice.

Relationships with other professional groups have been a continuing preoccupation of BMA ethical guidance, although the focus has changed with time. For various reasons, present day ethical guidance is more likely to deal with the difficulties of liaising with the social worker and the complementary practitioner rather than with the pastor and the pharmacist.

### 11:1.2 *Changing practice*

Recent decades have seen a shift in emphasis regarding the way health care is provided. There has been considerable discussion in many countries about changing the locus of care from institutions to the community, where emphasis is placed on a multidisciplinary approach to health management. Medicine has also seen a decline in its traditional monopoly on health matters in favour of an interdisciplinary or team approach and a consumer-led interest in the potential of other therapies. As with nurses, the independence of other health professionals has become increasingly recognised and respected.

Within multidisciplinary teams, all professionals have responsibility for ensuring the competence and proper functioning of other team members. The whole team works together to ensure the avoidance of any inadequacies or mistakes which might put patients at risk. Good communication is vital. It is recognised that all team members have a duty to raise problems for discussion. Emphasis is placed on the need for moral support of colleagues who draw attention to bad practices. Most people agree that mutual support measures for "whistle-blowers" throughout the health service should be established. The BMA endorses calls that have been made for confidential counselling for any health professionals concerned about standards.

It is often said that difficulties arise when conflicting values and goals are espoused by professionals with differing codes of practice. In the BMA's view, however, some of the apparent differences in ethos are superficial rather than deep-seated. Some suggestions for addressing them are discussed in this chapter.

## 11:2 Inter-professional relations

The part played by non-medically-qualified health care workers is now well recognised. In recent years, the General Medical Council has consistently welcomed "the growing contributions made to health care by nurses and other persons who have been trained to perform specialised functions".[312]

In the health care team, the doctor is responsible for medical treatment and overall management of the patient but must recognise that other team members have skills which they can exercise without reference to the doctor. In exercising these skills, they are professionally responsible for their own actions.

### 11:2.1 *Professions supplementary to medicine*

Under the Professions Supplementary to Medicine Act 1960, each of the professions has a board and a disciplinary committee. The professions include chiropodists, dietitians, medical laboratory scientific officers, occupational therapists, orthoptists, physiotherapists and radiographers. When working with members of these professions the doctor has overall responsibility for treatment but not for the fine details, which a reasonable doctor would not be expected to check or supervise. The individual therapist is independently responsible for the details of treatment.

The Disciplinary Statement of each board underlines the maintenance of high standards of professional conduct. Doctors should make sure that the people to whom they refer patients are professionally registered. The doctor should also ensure that patients are referred in a "proper" manner and understand that the doctor retains final authority for the continuation or otherwise of therapy.

### 11:2.2 *Nurses, midwives and health visitors*

Nurses, midwives and health visitors are personally accountable for their practice. In the past, these professionals have often felt that their role and independence was not adequately recognised. This was, undoubtedly the case.

The code of practice of nurses, midwives and health visitors obliges them to acknowledge any limitations in their knowledge and to decline to undertake any duties or responsibilities unless they are able to perform them well. It is for the individual nurse or midwife to decide what procedures are within his or her competence. Obeying an instruction from a doctor to undertake some procedure about which a nurse does not feel competent is no defence for the nurse if harm results. Nurses may be removed from the register in such cases.

Although nurses must decide for themselves whether they are competent to undertake a requested procedure, doctors must also ensure that nurses are not required to undertake a task beyond their experience or ability. This is usually adequately established by asking the nurse's opinion. The nurse has a reciprocal duty to ensure that the doctor is competently carrying out treatment and, in any case of doubt, to check that prescribing and other procedures for which the doctor is responsible conform with accepted practice.

Nurses may be particularly aware of patient needs because of the substantial amount of regular contact they often have with patients and those close to patients. Specialised nurses such as Macmillan nurses, and others who work in the community, may have opportunities to develop an insight into the overall situation and problems of patient and family. GPs may have a different perspective, having often been responsible for the family's treatment over a prolonged period. It is clear that nurses and doctors should respect each other's area of expertise and benefit from the particular insights of each. Patient wellbeing and confidence may be jeopardised by overt disagreements between professionals responsible for their care.

*11:2.2.1 Nurse prescribing*

There is great value in empowering suitably qualified nurses, such as district nurses, health visitors and community nurses to prescribe those items necessary for the basic care of some conditions. As in all other cases, where more than one health professional looks after the patient, it is essential that there is good communication on the different facets of care. This issue is discussed in chapter 7 (section 7:6.4) on prescribing.

*11:2.2.2 Nurse practitioners and junior doctors*

The entrenched concepts of the roles of both doctors and nurses are increasingly being challenged as the distinction between junior doctors and experienced nurses becomes less well defined.

In hospital practice, some nurses are now undertaking additional training in tasks traditionally thought to be the responsibility of junior doctors. This includes training not only in intravenous therapy but also in many other areas including, counselling, chronic disease management, health education and promotion and audit. In some cases, with the support of the medical professionals involved, "nurse practitioners" have also taken over the diagnosis, investigation and treatment of minor injuries and illnesses. They work alongside junior doctors, but practice independently of them.

Nurse practitioners are also appointed and employed by GPs. Based in the community, they are mainly concerned with primary care and preventive medicine. Patients have direct access to the nurse practitioner, who refers patients to the GP as appropriate.

Both hospital and community based nurse practitioners aim to offer an holistic approach to patient care, but may differ in the type of training they receive. It is the responsibility of the doctors in charge to ensure that the nurse practitioner employed in this way is capable of fulfilling the tasks required and thus training must be the joint responsibility of the medical and nursing professions (see also the General Medical Council statement on the principle of delegation of duties in 11:3.2 below).

The Royal College of Nursing established a special interest group for nurse practitioners in 1992 which is producing guidelines on their role in 1993. Nurse practitioners, like all nurses must comply with the UK Central Council for Nursing, Midwifery and Health Visiting (UKCC) "Code of Professional Conduct" and "Scope of Practice" documents.

*11:2.2.3 Midwives*

Modern maternity care entails the services of a large variety of specialists, including, for example, obstetricians, paediatricians, anaesthetists, haematologists, radiologists, surgeons, midwives and general practitioners. All of these services need co-ordinating and this has usually been achieved by the consultant obstetrician acting as the focus for the various different interests.

289

Although the way in which ante-natal and post-natal care is provided depends on local arrangements, it is usual for GPs, community midwives and health visitors to share the patient's care whilst in the community and for consultants to supervise hospital visits and admissions. For many years, most births have taken place in hospital maternity units or in a GP cottage hospital. In early 1992, a House of Commons Committee on Maternity Services looked at this usual pattern of care and recommended some changes which have implications for the various professionals involved in maternity care.

It proposed that midwives should have the right to refer women directly to obstetricians or other appropriate specialists but drew attention to the need for GPs to be notified promptly of such referrals. The Committee drew attention to the conflict between different philosophies of care and saw evidence of a "damaging demarcation dispute between the professional groups over how labour should be organised". It saw no reason why midwives trained in the detection of congenital abnormalities should not be assigned routine examinations of apparently healthy newborns.

The effect of the many recommendations in the Committee's report is to acknowledge the status of midwives and their right to develop and audit their own professional standards. It also proposed a very different pattern of care, including the establishment of midwife- managed maternity units within and outside hospitals, and further proposed that midwives take full responsibility for the women under their care.

Although these recommendations are still under discussion, doctors are raising questions about the management of cases where doctors and midwives disagree about the safest management, or the desirability of a home birth in preference to hospital admission. GPs, for example, sometimes advise against home deliveries when this is the parents' preferred choice because of potential risks for the child and mother. The midwife, however, may be willing to supervise a home confinement in such circumstances. If a patient ignores the GP's advice, the doctor is not obliged to attend the patient during the home confinement. The doctor must, however, be available in emergency. It is important that the family do not feel abandoned by the doctor, who in most cases will resume health care after this episode. It must be made clear that the doctor's dissent to participating in a home delivery is solely on the grounds of patient interests and will not colour the future health care of the family.

## 11:3 Liaison with practitioners of complementary therapies

### 11:3.1 Shared care

In the United Kingdom, it is estimated that there are between 60 and 160 different forms of complementary therapies. Surveys of patients attending practitioners in such therapies indicate that the majority[313] are also consulting medical practitioners. It has therefore been concluded that "non-orthodox treatment was sought for a limited range of problems and used most frequently as a supplement to orthodox medicine". This indicates that many doctors will need to be informed about or liaise with complementary practitioners.

### 11:3.2 *GPs employing complementary practitioners*

As patients increasingly take control of their own health care, they often become interested in exploring options outside the scope of conventional medical practice. There is a growing demand by patients for access to complementary medicine. Many doctors are interested in acquiring such knowledge or employing complementary therapists to provide it. Following GP contractual changes in 1990, general practitioners received Government encouragement to consider employing complementary therapists. In a Parliamentary statement in 1991, the Junior Minister for Health stated that such therapies could be delivered either by the doctor or by a therapist treating the patient under the doctor's clinical authority.

In the latter case, the GMC makes clear that:

"a doctor who delegates treatment or other procedures must be satisfied that the person to whom they are delegated is competent to carry them out. It is also important that the doctor should retain ultimate responsibility for the management of these patients because only the doctor has received the necessary training to undertake this responsibility. For these reasons, a doctor who improperly delegates to a person who is not a registered medical practitioner, functions requiring the knowledge and skill of a medical practitioner, is liable to disciplinary proceedings".[314]

Therefore a doctor who delegates patient care to a non-medically-qualified practitioner must take steps to ensure that the latter is competent to perform the required procedures. For therapists who are subject to a recognised registering and disciplinary body this poses little problem. The majority of therapies, however, are not subject to a recognised training procedure, disciplinary code and registering body. In such cases, the employing doctor must use his or her judgement about the skills of the individual practitioner and also ensure that adequate supervision is given.

### 11:3.3 *Referral to practitioners who are not medically qualified*

With any referral, the GP must assess whether the proposed therapy is likely to benefit the patient. When the doctor does not consider that the treatment the patient requests would be beneficial, this must be explained to the patient and the reasons discussed.

The GP must also consider whether the practitioner is competent to

291

give the treatment required. As a general rule, it is inadvisable for a doctor to refer a patient to any practitioner who is not subject to a registering and disciplinary body. In cases where the doctor knows the un-registered practitioner and is confident of that person's competence to carry out the particular treatment required, the doctor may decide to make a referral in the knowledge that the doctor is likely to bear some liability if any harm results.

### 11:3.4 *Referral to doctors and nurses who provide complementary therapies*

There is no problem in referring to a complementary practitioner who is also medically qualified and thus subject to the discipline of the General Medical Council. It is apparent that many doctors are interested in acquiring complementary skills. A 1986 survey in Avon indicated that 38 per cent of GPs responding to a questionnaire claimed to have received some training in complementary therapy and a further 15 per cent wished to obtain training. These findings have been repeated by later studies.

The Royal College of Nursing has also established a Complementary Therapies in Nursing Special Interest Group whose statement of beliefs is based on the idea that "all patients have the right to be offered and to receive complementary therapies either exclusively or as part of orthodox nursing practice". This implies that, in future, many nurses will be qualified in complementary therapies. Since nurses are professionally regulated by the UKCC, a doctor can send patients to them with confidence for such therapies, when the doctor believes the patient can benefit from that treatment.

### 11:3.5 *Sharing information*

Doctors should only release patients' personal health information to complementary therapists with the patient's consent and when they believe this to be in the patient's best interests.

## 11:4 Liaison with social workers

The BMA receives lots of enquiries about liaison with social workers, in particular to do with the management of suspected cases of abuse of children; the abuse or exploitation of elderly people; the abuse or exploitation of mentally disordered people in the community and in residential facilities; and the neglect of people unable to care for themselves. The Children Act 1989 and Community Care Act 1990 emphasise the need for liaison between professionals caring for such client groups. The leading agency in the care of such individuals will often be the Social Services Department. Doctors are often concerned about confidentiality provisions covering the disclosure of information to such agencies, particularly when it concerns very sensitive issues such as sexual abuse or the HIV status of people who cannot consent to disclosure. Some of the issues have already been explored in chapter 2 on confidentiality (section 2:4.2.3) and chapter 3 on children (section 3:5.1.2), where emphasis is placed on the sharing of such information as is necessary, relevant and in the individual's interest but without disregarding a competent individual's right to confidentiality.

### 11:4.1 *Protection of children and young people*

The importance of inter-agency co-operation for the protection of children and young people has been emphasised in recent years. Such co-operation requires openness between professionals and seeks the active involvement of parents and minors. The BMA receives many enquiries concerning telephone requests by social workers for information from the medical file of a child or young person. Doctors are concerned that in such circumstances, there is often no urgency which would preclude the seeking of consent to disclosure from either the individual or a parent. Also the doctor has no written record of the request, or the reasons for it, or even any proof of the identity of the enquirer. In cases where doctors are not convinced there is urgency or risk, they should insist that all requests for information be written and seek the views of the individual about whom the details are sought.

It is essential that a medical contribution is made at all stages of child protection procedures. The role of the doctor includes attempting to prevent abuse, raising awareness, diagnosing, assessing risk, recommending therapy and continuing to treat the family unit. Liaison with social workers is likely to be essential during most of these stages. Doctors are not empowered to intervene to protect a child whom they believe to be at risk and will need to co-operate with social workers who are the statutory agents. One of the most frequently debated areas concerns the sharing of medical information at child protection case conferences. In this context, the GMC's advice is:

> "where a doctor believes that a patient may be the victim of physical or sexual abuse ... the patient's medical interests are paramount and may require a doctor to disclose information to an appropriate person or authority."

As has been mentioned in previous chapters, doctors often worry that the confidentiality of the information they give in child protection cases conferences cannot be guaranteed. The Department of Health advises that all those in receipt of such information from health professionals must treat it as confidential but there is still profound concern about the attendance of various lay people and participants who are not bound by professional codes of ethics, as well as about subsequent access to social work records by still other people not bound by professional codes.

293

Doctors will be faced by situations where they are asked to share information concerning not only the child, but possibly other family members, with a wider forum which includes non-professionals. The doctor can ask that certain information be given only within a limited group or only in writing to the chairman of the conference. In some circumstances, parents can be excluded from part of the conference and the need to maintain the confidentiality of medical information could be a criterion. Each case must be judged on its merits.

In conjunction with the Department of Health, the BMA is producing guidance on doctors' participation in child protection case conferences. This will be available in late 1993.

## 11:5 Liaison with carers

Doctors must often liaise with people caring for people who are not able to look after themselves. Such patients may be mentally disordered, physically handicapped or elderly and infirm. As is discussed in chapter 2 (section 2:4.2.1), it is recognised that in some circumstances doctors will have to share information with the patient's family or other carers in order for the patient to be properly looked after. There is a danger, however, that the confidentiality owed to individuals who are in a situation of dependency may be under-respected in that information regarding the patient's condition and treatment is directed to the carer without full consideration being given to the patient's interests.

Doctors are sometimes asked to provide confidential medical information about patients to managers or employees of hostels or residential homes, or to test residents for HIV infection. In some cases, the individual cannot give consent or is under pressure to consent, for instance, when this is made a requirement for residence. Where the patient is incapable of giving consent to a procedure or authorising disclosure of information, the focus must be on the best interests of the patient. The BMA emphasises that the confidentiality of all patients must be respected. Only information necessary and relevant to the care of the individual should be disclosed. Where the patient is in a residential facility, medical information should be restricted to the responsible health professional or director. Identifying only some individuals as a potential source of risk to others may mean that adequate precautions to prevent cross-infection are not routinely implemented in every case. Attempts to identify certain individuals as a potential health risk to others should never be an excuse for relaxing routine precautions or for poor standards of hygiene in other cases.

## 11:6 Doctors' relations with pharmacists

Doctors and pharmacists both advise patients concerning their areas of professional expertise. For many years, however, the BMA advised that the independence of doctors and pharmacists was best demonstrated by their refraining from sharing premises or having close financial connection, such as a doctor investing in a pharmacy within the practice area. In the early 1990s, changes in the provision of primary health care led to many GPs offering a range of additional services on their premises, including dispensing facilities. Rural GPs had long been able to dispense for their own patients and this did not appear to give rise to unethical practices. The BMA withdrew its objection to GPs owning pharmacies, employing pharmacists or sharing premises with pharmacists, providing doctors informed their patients of their financial interest in the pharmacy and that there was no direction of patients to the pharmacy in question.

An increasing number of pharmacists are working in closer relationship with doctors, as GPs employ pharmacists to work on their surgery premises or in pharmacies owned by the doctor. With specific patient consent, many pharmacists have established links with particular surgeries so that, for the convenience of patients, repeat prescriptions can be passed automatically to the pharmacist. The BMA advises doctors that they should not initiate such schemes or direct patients to a particular pharmacy but they can co-operate with schemes agreed between patients and pharmacists. The patient must be aware of the amount of information being passed to the pharmacist, as many patients have objected to the BMA about a variety of projects which involved pharmacists collecting information regarding the prescriptions issued to their regular customers.

Accompanying this evidence of greater co-operation between doctors and pharmacists is a growing number of complaints and disputes, as some pharmacists fear being put out of business by doctors opening their own pharmacies. In some, it is to be hoped exceptional, cases reported to the BMA, business rivalry has led to bad feeling between doctors and pharmacists being expressed through the local media. The BMA regrets this development and considers that implied criticism or unsustainable questioning of the competence of other professionals is unethical and undermines public confidence.

## 11:7 Doctors' relations with the pharmaceutical industry

### 11:7.1 *Gifts and hospitality*

Members of the public have a right to be concerned if they feel that the professional advice they receive may have been influenced by financial or other benefits offered to doctors by commercial organisations. The medical profession has an obligation to assure the public that treatment offered is appropriate and is justified by its intrinsic merit, uninfluenced by commercial or financial interests. This is especially important in relation to pharmaceutical products.

Promotional activities aimed at individuals may raise serious ethical problems. The pharmaceutical industry recognises this and the Association of the British Pharmaceutical Industry has a strict Code of Practice which refers specifically to what is acceptable practice where gifts and hospitality are concerned. Doctors would be well advised to consider the degree to which they may compromise themselves when an offer looks likely to put at risk their ability to defend themselves against the accusation of being unreasonably influenced.

The GMC offers the following advice:[315]

*"Gifts and loans*
It may be improper for an individual doctor to accept from a pharmaceutical firm monetary gifts or loans or expensive items of equipment for his personal use. No exception can, however, be taken to grants of money or equipment by firms to institutions such as hospitals, health care centres and university departments, when they are donated specifically for purposes of research.

*Acceptance of hospitality*
It may be improper for individual doctors or groups of doctors to accept lavish hospitality or travel facilities under the terms of sponsorship of medical postgraduate meetings or conferences. However, no exception is likely to be taken to acceptance by an individual doctor of a grant which enables him to travel to an international conference or to acceptance, by a group of doctors who attend a sponsored postgraduate meeting or conference, of hospitality at an appropriate level, which the recipients might normally adopt when paying for themselves."

The DHSS has issued a Health Note (HN(62)21) about gifts and hospitality, drawing the attention of hospital staff to the Prevention of Corruption Acts 1906 and 1916. Independent contractors, for example, general practitioners, are not under any contractual duty to comply with the instructions of this note as they are not employees. However, they, like all other citizens, are subject to the provisions of the Prevention of Corruption Act 1906 and 1916 and they would therefore be wise to consider the underlying principles, as laid out in the Health Note.

As prescribers of pharmaceutical products, they also have an ethical responsibility to satisfy themselves that their prescribing is responsible. These basic principles concerning inducements apply equally to doctors who are working in private, general or psychiatric hospitals. As a profession, doctors must be seen to be uninfluenced by any non-scientific promotion directed towards them by the pharmaceutical industry.

## 11:7.2  *The influence of pharmaceutical promotions*

The degree to which individual doctors may be influenced by the promotion of pharmaceutical products varies considerably. Some doctors may accept relatively uncritically presentations made by the pharmaceutical industry; others critically analyse the presentations and published literature. Those who have conducted trials on drugs would be expected to have analysed the advantage and risk factors carefully, regardless of the presentation of the product by the industry.

There does not appear to have been extensive analysis of the degree to which doctors may be subliminally influenced by promotional methods used by the industry. It must be recognised that the substantial support of the pharmaceutical industry in promoting continuing medical education has been of benefit not only to the industry, but also to the profession and patients.

Whether doctors prescribe a new product or not, they must clearly rely on and maintain their scientific and clinical integrity when considering the information provided by the company. The GMC emphasises that "prescribing doctors should not only choose but also be seen to be choosing the drug or appliance which, in their independent professional judgement, and having due regard to economy, will best serve the medical interests of the patient".[316]

## 11:7.3  *Payments for meeting pharmaceutical representatives*

It is unacceptable for doctors to demand payment for meeting and listening to pharmaceutical representatives. It is also contrary to the Code of Practice for the Pharmaceutical Industry for a medical representative to pay a fee in return for an interview. Doctors have an obligation to keep abreast of pharmaceutical developments and may do this by attending a presentation by a company representative or by scrutiny of the literature.

## 11:7.4  *Research*

Payments are made by pharmaceutical companies to doctors who conduct research on their behalf. There is a demand for more guidance from both sides. Doctors want to know what they may ethically accept and the pharmaceutical industry needs to know what may reasonably be offered. Joint advice has been issued by the BMA and others on subjects such as "Clinical Trials in General Practice" and "Post Marketing Surveillance".[317]

The General Medical Council has stated:

"It may be improper for a doctor to accept per capita or other payments from a pharmaceutical firm in relation to a research project such as the clinical trial of a new drug, unless the payments have been specified in a protocol for the project which has been approved by the

297

relevant national or local ethical committee. It may be improper for a doctor to accept per capita or other payments under arrangements for recording clinical assessments of a licensed medicinal product, whereby he is asked to report reactions which he has observed in patients for whom he has prescribed the drug, unless the payments have been specified in a protocol for the project which has been approved by the relevant national or local ethical committee. It is improper for a doctor to accept payment in money or kind which could influence his professional assessment of the therapeutic value of a new drug."

## 11:8 Summary

1 All professionals have some responsibility for ensuring the competence and proper functioning of other team members.
2 Support measures for justified "whistle-blowers" should be established.
3 The BMA emphasises the need for proper communication between professionals for the good of the patient.
4 The doctor is responsible for medical treatment and overall management of the patient but must recognise that other team members have skills which they can exercise without reference to the doctor.
5 It is for the individual nurse or midwife to decide what procedures are within his or her competence.
6 Doctors must also ensure that the nurse is not required to undertake a task beyond the nurse's experience or ability. This is usually adequately established by asking the nurse's opinion. The nurse has a reciprocal duty to ensure that the doctor is competently carrying out treatment.
7 It is clear that nurses and doctors should respect each other's area of expertise.
8 Doctors should make sure that the people to whom they refer patients are professionally registered.
9 A doctor who delegates treatment or other procedures must be satisfied that the person to whom they are delegated is competent to carry them out.
10 Doctors can refer patients with confidence to therapists who are subject to a registering and disciplinary body.
11 Where a doctor believes that a minor or incapacitated person may be the victim of physical or sexual abuse, the patient's medical interests are paramount in questions of liaison with other professionals.

# 12 Rationing and Allocation of Health Care Resources

*This chapter looks at the issues which arise in relation to the rationing and allocation of health care resources. It notes areas where needs have traditionally been poorly met and patients deterred from making explicit demands. It briefly considers the role of government, the public, the medical profession and individual doctors. Various models are considered for how just decisions could be made. A few conclusions are put forward for further consideration in the continuing debate on these issues.*

## 12:1 Introduction

### 12:1.1 *Background to the debate*

There has been debate for some time now about whether the National Health Service was ever really expected to pay for itself. Some[318] assert that in the post-war period, the reforms ushered in with the setting up of the health service were widely envisaged as self-financing through compulsory contributions from those in work, topped up by assistance from public revenue. Aneurin Bevan joked about his aim of making all doctors unemployed and did apparently believe that one general effect of disease prevention would be a more effective and continuously employed workforce to fund the insurance necessary to pay for medical care.[319] Others perhaps foresaw how, in Powell's words, an "illimitable volume of demand would be released by the magic wand of public provision".

In practice, rationing of health care has always existed within the NHS, although rationing decisions have frequently not been taken openly. In recent years, a number of measures to reform the NHS and transfer aspects of care into the community have resulted in greater focusing on costs and priorities. The BMA believes that discussion about rationing needs to take place in the public arena and involve people who are sick as well as the healthy, health professionals and Government. Traditionally priority has often been given to medical need and welfare maximisation. Thus, the most seriously ill and those likely to live longest or those who had the most dependents were given preference at the cost of services to other groups, such as people with learning disabilities, mental illness, physical disability and the elderly. Recent reforms have drawn attention to hidden assumptions and sought to rectify some aspects of these unacceptable inequalities but with variable degrees of success, largely related to the funding committed to them.

In 1991 the NHS was reorganised along lines that divided its providing and purchasing roles. A corollary of the purchaser-provider system was to bring out into the open the varying criteria used for prioritising the provision of care in certain areas. Purchasing contracts required explicit judgements to be made, and revealed which services were not sought because purchasers gave them low priority. Thus the introduction of systems for needs assessment and contracting made prioritisation and rationing decisions more visible. It gave added urgency to the rationing debate.

### 12:1.2 *Quality, cost and audit*

A prerequisite for justifiable rationing is that existing resources are used as effectively as possible. Wastage of resources is unethical because it diminishes society's capacity to relieve suffering through the other uses that could be made of the wasted resources. Doctors working within the NHS need to be aware of cost-effectiveness as well as clinical effectiveness in the care provided for the patient. But quality is multi-dimensional, embracing both the quantitative, in terms of measurable improvements and the qualitative, as experienced by the patient and the community. Quality is not absolute but relative. A different perspective, new data or revised clinical guidelines change our perceptions of what constitutes good quality care.

Cost, like quality, is a complicated concept. In discussing rationing and resources, it is inevitable that we think primarily in terms of financial cost but health care economists[320] remind us that the cost of something is not necessarily, or only, a monetary consideration. "What is the cost?" means "What will have to be sacrificed to achieve this?" and the sacrifice may be more than simply cash. Those who argue that clinical decisions should not be influenced by cost may be saying that medical decisions for one patient should ignore the sacrifices imposed on others. It has been argued that doctors can perhaps justify such an attitude on bureaucratic or legalistic grounds, saying "they are not my responsibility" but that they cannot then call such views ethical. On the other hand, those who advocate the desirability of low-cost services are probably only thinking of the financial aspect and not the hidden costs. Low morale, stress, loss of compassion in health care providers, and reduced quality of relationship with patients may also be elements of the overall cost if we focus on finance alone.

A number of measures are emerging as tools intended to improve the quality and cost-effectiveness of care but they could also be used for rationing. Among these are disease-specific clinical guidelines, which are proliferating in Britain and the USA. Studies[321] have shown that direct medical participation in guidelines set in accord with local priorities is an important factor in their use and success, whereas nationally set standards have limited impact. It has been suggested that setting priorities and monitoring the implementation of guidelines should be a collaborative activity, involving family health services authorities (FHSAs), purchasing authorities, medical audit advisory groups, health professionals and patient groups. The argument is that good practice is better implemented from the roots upward rather than imposed from the top down. Duplication, however, could be avoided by collection and dissemination of successfully implemented guidelines by a central agency.

Quality control measures, medical audit, peer review and efforts to validate the efficacy of accepted practices and promote good practice are all relevant to the resources debate. They are not new but are receiving increased attention. Doctors have always looked to ways of promoting good practice and long ago many GPs set up systematic annual reviews of aspects of practice without labelling the activity "audit". To be of value, however, such measures require adequate funding and scientific methodology. Over the last decade the BMA's annual meetings have passed several resolutions supporting medical audit which is buttressed by adequate financial resources. It is recognised, however, that audit will only be effective in producing change when its methods are as rigorous as those of the best research. Such measures improve medical practice by giving a clear understanding of what is actually happening. They pave the way for judgements about the appropriateness of current practice and assessments of medical, managerial and financial efficiency.

### 12:1.3 *Changing focus*

Thus, in this chapter we look at some of the elements involved in the rationing and allocation of scarce resources but we cannot hope to provide an exhaustive analysis of this rapidly developing and sometimes contentious subject. Our focus is the renewed debate about resources with reference to the changes introduced into the NHS, but it must be noted that long before the introduction of the new system the development of various economic models in health care provided the impetus for much discussion within the profession about the moral and practical issues of resource allocation. The question of how best to allocate limited resources is only part of the picture, since how to develop resources is also seen as a legitimate medical concern. Such development involves more aggressive political canvassing than some have thought appropriate to the profession. This is a continuing debate in which the traditional ethical preoccupations of doctors are meshed with the demands of the market economy.

#### 12:1.3.1 *Prevention versus treatment*

The focus on prevention of disease involves educating the public to take responsibility for its health, and issues of preventive measures versus treatment lie at the heart of the resource allocation debate. It is clearly

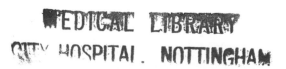

important that there be extensive consultation within the profession and society at large on how, as a nation, we adapt and develop the health care system for the next century. It may be helpful, however, to look at the various models for deciding health care priorities and to see how the same problems are tackled in other countries. To this end, we draw below upon some of the recommendations of the Dutch report issued by the Dunning Commission in 1992 (see sections 12:2.1 and 12:4.1(b) below).

### 12:1.4 *Allocating national resources to the health care sector*

All health care systems ration care by some method. Health care is rationed in two ways: firstly, through the proportion of national resources spent on the health care sector and secondly, through the distribution of those resources within the health care sector. This internal rationing and distribution is the main focus of our discussion below.

#### 12:1.4.1 *The bottomless pit*

It should be noted that the BMA has consistently argued for a substantial increase in overall funding, which it considers would resolve some of the current problems of rationing. It is recognised, however, that this would provide only a temporary solution and that simply allocating a greater share of national resources to health care will never satisfy the public's demand for health services. According to the so-called "bottomless pit" theory, expectations will always grow faster than the resources available to meet them. Within the BMA,[322] however, it has been argued that the "bottomless pit" analogy is misleading insofar as it might imply that there should be a bottom to the pit, ie that there could be a final goal of complete and perfect care towards which we should be moving. The BMA view is that this is false in that there is no final goal - but always the possibility of more change and a need for further evolution.

That said, some form of rationing within any health sector is likely to be inevitable. This view is supported by macrostatistical research, which shows that the gap between possible services and what can be afforded is ever widening. Advances in medical technology are constantly increasing the range of services potentially available, public expectations are rising in parallel and the ageing of the British population is resulting in ever-increasing demands on health care services. Many experts believe that the NHS and community care services can never meet all patient needs and that cost-containment measures must be found.

### 12:1.5 *BMA views on rationing*

As mentioned above, it has often been argued that permitting considerations of cost to influence clinical decisions is unethical. Such considerations have been seen as conflicting with doctors' duty of beneficence, which obliges them to do the best for the individual patients in front of them. A doctor, it is said, who changes the way he or she practises medicine because of cost rather than purely medical considerations "has embarked on the slippery slope of compromised ethics and waffled priorities".[323] Yet the ethics of ignoring the possibly adverse implications for other patients are questionable. The BMA's view has traditionally been to emphasise the clinician's professional duty to the individual patient and the ethical duty to use the most economic and efficacious treatment available. Some responsibility exists for those waiting outside the surgery door as well as those who cross the threshold. The Association has also long stressed the doctor's duty to co-operate with research into the rational use of resources.

In 1992, BMA members[324] recognised the inevitability of the rationing of health services as an unfortunate fact of life and resolved that:

a)   rationing should be done openly;

b)   agreement should be reached between the Department of Health and clinically active members of the profession concerning its scope and the priorities within the service;

c)   whilst doctors should be involved in deciding priorities they cannot be held responsible for the consequences of political decisions about rationing;

d)   rationing decisions should involve full consultation among health care professionals, the Government and the public;

e)   that the BMA should give publicity to the issues;

f)   that no patient should be denied medical diagnosis and treatment just because of advanced age.

While specifically excluding age as the sole criterion for rationing treatment, the BMA has not proposed alternative criteria: discriminatory measures which disadvantage any group of patients is to be avoided. Doctors would generally be unhappy with any rationing system which defined treatment options by implicitly labelling some sorts of patient as less worth treating than others: they would want a system which considered patients as individuals. Defining criteria for treatment, however, is not the function of professional associations or doctors alone, but must be a joint and open enterprise in which patients and the public participate.

## 12:2 Approaching the problem

In many parts of this book we have touched upon rationing problems which raise ethical dilemmas and have emphasised the need for informed public and professional debate about them. In chapters 4 and 8, for

303

example, we have drawn attention to scarce resources for infertility treatments and to how research requirements may be in competition with treatment. In chapter 6, it has been noted that while heroic technological measures should not be used to prolong dying, open discussion is needed about the use of scarce resources to maintain indefinitely, patients in a persistent vegetative state.

The concept of Quality Adjusted Life Years (QALYs) was developed by health economists[325] as a crude indicator of the success of different forms of treatment, to help solve dilemmas by calculating cost-benefit ratios. Many fear that QALYs provide only a superficial solution and manipulate statistics to give an appearance of scientific validity which ignores the complexities of moral decision-making in real life. Another major criticism of QALYs, which also applies to some other decision-making mechanisms, is that the individuals who calculate how resources should be used have no contact with the patients whose futures are affected by their decisions.

We know that many unmet needs exist. There are people who never receive services and people who must wait to receive services. The following areas have presented particular problems:

- the extent to which age is used as a criterion in deciding which patients receive certain life-saving procedures such as transplants, by-pass operations and kidney dialysis, is a matter of debate. (Almost no one over seventy receives kidney dialysis in the UK. In other European countries, the over seventies make up as many as 20 per cent of those on dialysis programmes);[326]

- we treat fewer people with renal failure than in many other countries and numbers vary from region to region within Britain;

- only 3 per cent of those who could be helped by specialist treatment for infertility actually receive such treatment;

- access to psychotherapeutic treatment is severely limited;

- rates for coronary-artery bypass surgery are lower than in many other developed countries;

- rehabilitation services are sparse;

- waiting times for minor plastic surgery procedures are indefinite;

- many carers are left to look after elderly, disabled or mentally ill relatives with minimal or no support.

These unmet needs are sometimes not translated into demands either because people do not receive information about services that could benefit them, or the demands that they do make are deflected.

### 12:2.1 *Dealing with patient demand*

A 1992 report from the King's Fund College[327] suggested four main ways in which demand for care has been countered within the NHS:

i)  **Deterrence**: patients may be discouraged from making their demands effectively at their first point of contact with the NHS, their general practitioner, through the behaviour of receptionists and deputising services in general practice. The Government also rations explicitly by setting charges for NHS dental care, optical care, prescriptions and for new types of diagnostic tests and treatments.

ii) **Deflection**: Doctors may refer patients to other agencies.

iii) **Dilution**: The need for NHS managers to satisfy demand may lead to services being spread so thinly that standards are inevitably reduced.

iv) **Delay:** Waiting lists operate for many out-patient clinics and operative procedures.

Given that rationing is inevitable, it is important that attention is given to such methods of dealing with patient demand. They cannot be dismissed out of hand. Many would see deflection and delay as legitimate measures for coping with demands which outstrip supply. The Dunning report,[328] for example, sees waiting lists as an acceptable way of rationing but considers that they should be regulated. Explicit criteria for admission to, and progression along, such lists are therefore essential.

## 12:3 Who decides?

### 12:3.1 *Decisions taken by the Government*

Government decides the overall proportion of national resources to be spent on the health care sector. The National Health Service Act 1977 obliges the Secretary of State to provide services to meet "reasonable requirements". He or she has discretion as to how financial resources are used but is not held directly accountable for failure to provide certain services. This was shown by a legal case brought in 1980[329] when four patients sued the Secretary of State for failure to provide an efficient and comprehensive health service. The patients argued that the Secretary of State's duty to provide services was not limited by considerations of Government finances, but the courts rejected the argument. A later case[330] confirmed that the courts would only intervene if there was an unreasonable failure to allocate resources.

Each year the Department of Health issues a statement of priorities, which is sometimes criticised for its imprecision.[331] Recurring priorities such as day surgery and waiting lists are mentioned but no clear hierarchy is established between the various priorities. Nor is there any indication of how performance is publicly monitored or how medical audit is to be integrated into the listed priorities.

Government also establishes what proportion of the health care budget should be spent on management and administration, as opposed to direct patient care. In the past, Britain's NHS and community care services have spent proportionately little on management and administration in comparison with systems in other countries. The 1991 NHS reforms increased the proportion of the NHS budget spent on management and administration, as they introduced a need for sophisticated costing and billing systems, as well as for information on the health care needs of populations, and the costs and outcomes of treatment.

### 12:3.2 *Decisions taken by health care purchasers*

Purchasers include NHS health authorities and general practitioners managing their own budgets. Purchasers are confronted by the necessity of estimating needs and assigning priorities. These include the following main areas of decision-making:

- Allocation of health care resources to broad groups. Assessment must be made as to whether all groups, such as the young, the old, people with young children and those whose illnesses are perceived as self-inflicted, should receive differing priority.

- The way in which health care resources should be allocated to specific services, particularly those which require investment in new facilities. This includes decision-making on whether treatment, prevention and community care services should receive equal or special priority. Government policy, as indicated in the White Paper "Health of the Nation", is to focus attention on prevention and thus shift resources from treatment to prevention and community care.

NHS managers generally have neither formal training in ethics nor a code of practice on ethical decision-making, although plans are afoot for a code of conduct to be drawn up for managers by the Institute of Health Services Management, which will cover decisions on rationing. Public education in this area, not only for managers, should be a matter of urgency.

### 12:3.3 *The medical profession*

As implied by the resolution passed at its 1992 annual meeting, the BMA believes that doctors and their professional associations have an ethical duty to advise governments on the appropriateness or otherwise of particular forms of rationing. This implies the existence of adequate mechanisms for providing medical input at the national and local level into decisions involving rationing. One way of combining medical and managerial opinion in decision-making about rationing and resource allocation in the NHS is to involve more health professionals, particularly doctors, in management. This obviously presents problems, some of which are touched upon in chapter 9 on dual obligations, since doctors are likely to face conflicts between their professional and managerial roles.

### 12:3.4 *Decisions taken by individual doctors*
*12:3.4.1 Decisions for individual patients*

Traditionally, doctors have played a large part in rationing decisions. Such decisions have taken the form of individual clinical decisions as part of the doctor-patient relationship, rather than collective decisions made on the basis of identifiable criteria and open to public scrutiny. Some medical sociological literature[332] has pointed out that doctors' usual criteria for treatment decisions is often based on factors other than strictly medical ones. While it is usual for doctors to take into account the overall interests of the patient rather than only the individual's clinical prospects, medical training does not qualify them to make value judgements about factors such as merit or social worth. On the other hand, questions such as whether the last bed in intensive care should be given to the drunken driver or the child he injures are probably debated more as theoretical examples than as real dilemmas. A host of considerations, such as relative neediness, potential for full recovery and likely quality of life enter into medical prioritising in each individual case. Whether other non-medical factors, such as the patient's value to society, should be part of the equation is a matter for public debate. This is discussed further in 12:4.1(e) below.

Some argue that although weight must be given to an individual doctor's assessment of a patient's quality of life, this is not in itself an adequate ethical standard for rationing, since it will almost certainly be influenced by the doctor's subjective moral beliefs and personal preferences. There are several strands to this argument. The BMA and the World Medical Association (see 12:4.1(i) below) do not see advanced age or reduced mental capacity as valid criteria for excluding patients from necessary treatments. As we have also shown in chapter 6, when choices are to be made about whether life-prolonging treatment is to be provided, patients' views are the ones that matter and the law does give some guidance about quality of life aspects to be considered when the patient in question is incapacitated. Although there will still be problems about tailoring resources to meet some patients' demands for apparently futile life-prolonging treatment, these should be handled, as discussed in chapters 5 and 6, in accordance with clinical judgement of appropriateness and equity. No framework for the just distribution of resources is ever likely to encompass the provision of futile treatments unless it is based exclusively on the criterion of ability of pay.

### 12:3.4.2 Duties to others

The BMA believes that a doctor's ethical duty goes beyond the individual patient to all other patients and to society as a whole. The General Medical Council endorses:

> "the principle that a doctor should always seek to give priority to the investigation and treatment of patients solely on the basis of clinical need. Acknowledging this, doctors have to work within resource constraints and, whatever the circumstances, they must make the best use of resources available for their patients, recognising the effects their decisions may have on the resources and choices available to others."

The first implication of this is that doctors should not favour their own patients at the expense of other doctors' patients. Many argue that the 1991 NHS reforms increase this tendency of doctors to try to get better treatment for their patients at the expense of those of other doctors. Evidence from the USA[333] shows that when certain groups of patients and categories of care were specified as eligible for subsidised treatment, doctors became adept at fitting their patients into the defined categories to get care for them at the expense of others. Doctors, therefore, should be alive to the consequences for other patients of their efforts to do their best for one patient.

The second implication is that in the context of finite resources for health care, doctors have an ethical duty to understand the cost-effectiveness of the treatment that they recommend and of the main alternatives. Further, when alternative forms of treatment produce the same outcome, the doctor should choose the least costly alternative. This presents several problems: i) how to define what counts as a relevant difference in outcome when we do not have reliable data on outcomes; ii) how to define the limit in treatment beyond which a marginal increase in benefits does not justify further increases in cost, and iii) how certain doctors must be of the exactness of the calculations they make when dealing with i) and ii). We have already touched upon how doctors deal with such problems in chapter 7 on prescribing, (see particularly section 7:4.1 on prescribing in the patient's interest and 7:5.2 on clinical freedom and resources).

### 12:3.5 The public

The public have had little involvement in decision-making over rationing. In the absence of any official guidelines on how to make decisions about procedures such as extra-contractual referrals, each health authority has established its own priorities and criteria but these are not made public. Most health authorities are aware that public opposition to explicit rationing is likely to be strong. When it has become known that health authorities are trying to curtail certain medical procedures, such as cosmetic surgery, varicose vein treatment, in vitro fertilisation, reversal of vasectomy and sterilisation, the backlash of public protest has sometimes forced them to think again. And when a public health director rashly asserted that money should not be spent on drugs for "hopeless cases" of terminally ill patients, he was quickly obliged to recant by the force of public outrage.[334] On the other hand, there is a view that public money should not be directed as a priority to diseases perceived as self-inflicted, such as conditions related to smoking, alcohol or drug abuse.

Too often public opinion is only apparent as a reaction to a crisis. The BMA strongly supports public consultation. Representatives of the healthy majority and those who suffer particular forms of illness should be included, allowing for the articulation of the needs of the poor, the elderly, the mentally impaired as well as ethnic and other minority groups. There are, however, practical difficulties involved in public consultation, given that response rates to questionnaires are often poor and it is difficult to encapsulate complex issues into simple questions. Nevertheless, these difficulties should not deter efforts to involve the public in decision-making in a systematic way.

## 12:4 Criteria for decision-making on rationing

### 12:4.1 Selection criteria and strategies

In the absence of UK national guidelines on making rationing choices, decision-making on rationing is often inconsistent between district and regional NHS authorities and may not be based upon an adequate assessment of the local population's health care needs. Various models have been put forward for dealing with the problems of rationing in a just manner. We rehearse the various options here, although in our view some of them are clearly unacceptable, either ethically or in practical terms, or both.

a)  **Ability to pay for comprehensive health care** is a method of rationing used in some developed and developing countries. Where those who can afford to pay, do so, and there is a public health system to provide basic care for those who cannot afford to pay for comprehensive treatment, the public health system is often inadequate. This arrangement can lead to over-treatment at one end of the scale - for those who can afford to pay - and almost complete failure to treat at the other. This is perceived by many people to be both immoral and wasteful in terms of both material and human resources.

b)  **Care restricted to core services** can be seen as a humane variation on the ability-to-pay model. A defined range of basic health care services is made available through insurance, or funded by taxes. Patients requiring care outside the scope of the defined range must pay for it privately. A related concept is **care limited to optimum medical success**. Under this system priority to state-funded treatment is in effect given to those for whom such treatment has the highest probability of medical success in relation to financial cost. Medical success is also a criterion which is often combined with other selection techniques, since it is generally seen as the fundamental priority.

The Dunning report, which focuses on **necessary health care**, supports a detailed model based on these concepts. According to the report's proposals, the state should provide access to a basic range of necessary treatments. To qualify as necessary, treatment "must be effective, efficient and cannot be left to individual responsibility". To ensure that treatments meet these requirements, a series of "sieves" are envisaged to eliminate unnecessary care. The sieves filter out all treatments not documented as clinically effective, not demonstrably cost-effective and those which can be left to individual responsibility. Treatments which remain at the end of the filtering process are described as necessary and therefore worthy of state-funding.

c) **Conservation** supports giving priority to those who require proportionately smaller amounts of resources. This is also an important facet of QALYs, which rely on utilitarian arguments of maximising benefits for the greatest number by sacrificing the few for the many.

A well known example of incorporating community decision-making into decisions about rationing is provided by the Oregon public consultation exercise in which a commission examined the cost-effectiveness of over 700 treatments and the values which the community assigned to them. It was envisaged that available resources could only fund 587 of the 700 or so services available. Treatments which fell below the proposed cut-off point included those for cancer sufferers with low survival prospects and extremely low birthweight babies. In Britain too, debate has focused on similar groups. A report by the Office of Health Economics in 1993, for example, highlighted the use of resources for preserving the lives of extremely pre-term infants.[335] The BMA argues that there is clearly the same obligation to preserve the life of an infant as of any other patient. As will be clear throughout this report, the Association is unhappy with any proposal which attempts to classify patients into groups as regards decision-making, (this is discussed further in 12:5 below). Some might see the cost of excluding such treatments as unjustifiable if cost is assessed in terms other than the purely financial, such as of loss of compassion. While there is interest in this country in the Oregon methods of computing cost-effectiveness, public opinion shows little enthusiasm for exclusion of certain treatments from the NHS.

d) **Treatment according to merit**. There are various ways of assessing merit for medical treatment. For example, those who had previously donated blood might be considered first when needing a transfusion and patients demonstrating an aggressive determination to survive might merit more treatment than those who succumb prematurely to the inevitability of death. The practical effect of this notion is that most people would receive treatment unless they were considered to have contributed to their disease. Potentially excluded from state-funded treatments would be patients whose poor health was related to smoking, abuse of alcohol or drugs, high-risk sporting activities, bad dietary choices or unsafe lifestyles.

Practical considerations immediately show up the flaws in adopting such a notion as a criterion for treatment. For instance, predisposition to certain diseases may owe more to genetics than to lifestyle. And as Harris[336] points out, there are numerous ways in which a person may contribute to his or her predicament, and the task of deciding how far people are responsible for their misfortune would be formidable. Fire-fighters, miners and life-savers would risk exclusion from treatment, as might the elderly suffering from hypothermia. Non-treatment of addiction or sexually transmitted disease would put more people at risk and the innocent dependents of the sick would also bear the cost of non-treatment.

e) **Treatment according to social value** is a variation of the merit criterion. This would involve allocation of treatment according to the probable total future contributions that prospective patients would be expected to make to society. It is sometimes defended on the grounds that state-paid medical care, like state education, is an investment which expects and deserves some repayment. A variation of the social value notion is the special importance sometimes accorded to the **parental role**. The adoption of this criterion would mean that patients whose death or disablement would incur drastic difficulties for dependents would receive priority. The use of social value criterion is unacceptable because it devalues the principle of the intrinsic worth of the individual. In practical terms, it raises the prospect of having to quantify diverse contributions within a single set of values, with the result reflecting the prejudices of the decision-makers.

f) **Random selection** is sometimes justified[337] as an egalitarian approach but poses practical difficulties. Strictly random selection among all those requiring treatment cannot begin until all potential candidates for treatment are identified. We cannot begin treating any until all are present and we know the full extent of the demand. Random selection cannot be the first criterion since it can be overridden by other criteria, such as need or urgency.

Some, however, support random selection as a way of finally choosing among a group of similar patients who have all been judged suitable on other criteria. In this context, it has several advantages. It eliminates the possibility of judgements being made on subjective grounds, is an easy method of selection which relieves the decision-maker of heavy moral responsibility and maintains the self-respect[338] of the patients denied treatment, since it was bad luck rather than insufficient personal worth that excluded them.

g) **First come, first served.** This is a type of random selection which has operated throughout the history of the NHS. Those who present at an accident and emergency department or arrive in intensive care when beds are available will be treated. The next person might experience delays or even forgo treatment if beds are full. Some people feel changes within the NHS have increased reliance on first come, first served since the treatment(s) patients receive might depend on whether they present at the beginning or the end of the financial year. Another variation may be the allocation of resources according to the power of the demands of the patient's advocate. Fundholding GPs, for example, could bring financial pressure to bear to ensure that their patients receive earlier treatment than those of other doctors.

h) **Medical neediness** is the most widely used criterion for selection: those in most urgent need are given priority, with the proviso that there is a reasonable chance of success. Needs must be distinguished from wants and this might sometimes pose difficulties. Some define health care needs as needs it is necessary to meet in order to achieve normal functioning[339], while others describe it as a capacity to benefit. With this criterion it is necessary to be able to distinguish between the urgency of each case and the relative merits of dissimilar needs.

When patients with identically urgent needs present for treatment, other criteria come into play. Some argue that such cases of identical need are merely theoretical. However, if, for the sake of argument, a busload of identically fit footballers of similar age and background were equally severely injured in a crash outside a hospital to which they could be all simultaneously conveyed, then neediness would have to be combined with other criteria such as treating all equally, or if resources were lacking, random selection.

On the other hand, when patients with dissimilar needs present, judgements about the relative merits of, for example, cancer treatment and IVF would have to be made. We might see access to infertility treatments or cosmetic surgery as wants rather than needs, unless the psychological effects of denying treatment grew to be life-threatening. Judgements in such cases might then be seen as open to subjectivity and inconsistency: the values placed on infertility treatments or cosmetic surgery by the decision-maker being the basis for the defining of "want" as opposed to "need".

i) Subjectivity is avoided by a criterion which demands that patients be **treated equally**. This could be interpreted in at least two ways. In one system, all patients would receive equal attention regardless of urgency of need. A more acceptable version involves treating fairly and consistently all patients with similar needs; not providing second class treatment for "Cinderella" groups. Thus, this is a criterion which works in combination with other criteria, such as medical neediness, since "there is no greater injustice than to treat unequal causes equally".[340]

The concept of equal treatment does not rule out clinical discretion but demands that decisions are based upon consistency and universalizability. In its 1992 declaration,[341] the World Medical Association ruled as unacceptable "the rationing of medical care to individuals with persistent organic or mental disability based only on reasons of an economic nature and on the assumption that certain inactive groups of the population do not contribute resources to the society to which they belong". The moral arguments for treating equally are based on concepts of justice. In our view, treating equally, in the sense of fairly and consistently, is not necessarily in conflict with a case-by-case approach to resolving moral dilemmas.

### 12:4.2 *The combined package*

None of these models stands alone or is sufficient of itself as an adequate system of rationing. Many people would see the best strategy as combining some of these different concepts in a consistent package. There are obviously many ways of doing this and perhaps three main ways of approaching the establishment of a combined package.

### 12:4.2.1 *What core treatments should be provided?*

One approach, which is adopted by the Dutch report issued by the Dunning Commission in 1992 (see section 12:2.1 and 12:4.1(b) above), advocates the provision of a package of validated core treatments. Treatments whose value had not been strictly proven would be sieved out. All patients would have equal access to necessary core treatments but any

313

other procedures they required, including a conventional treatment which had not been validated, would have to be self-financed. The dominant emphasis is on i) identifying effective treatment as a way of deciding who receives care, and ii) the type of care to be provided.

Problems with this approach arise in the selection of treatments to be excluded from the core package. Among other things, judgements would have to be made as to whether a psychological benefit counted as a validation of treatment and whether the public could tolerate the non-treatment of emotive cases involving, for example, pre-term babies.

### 12:4.2.2 *Which patients come first?*

Another approach tries to establish a list of priority patients. Kilner,[342] for example, combines optimum medical success, neediness, social value, conservation and random selection. In his example, it is patients rather than treatments who are sieved out when the following combination strategy is implemented:

• only patients who will benefit medically are eligible to enter the selection pool;

• those at risk of imminent death unless treated take first priority;

• those with special responsibilities (dependents) or special skills come next;

• these are followed by those whose treatment consumes least of the available resources;

• remaining resources are then randomly allocated among the rest of the patients.

Many find this an unacceptable strategy because of the way in which it links need and merit, excluding any obligation to treat equally, thus disadvantaging the elderly and people with physical disability or learning disability.

### 12:4.2.3 *What rights do patients have to treatment?*

Some people, particularly in the United States, have tackled the problem from the point of view of patient rights. Dougherty,[343] for example, sees the right to health care as containing four elements:

• a negative right of health non-interference;

• a right to access to a decent minimum of care, including basic primary care, emergency care and whatever other treatment society considers minimally necessary and affordable for all;

• a right to interventions designed to sustain and restore normal functioning where that is feasible;

314

- a right allowing those with greater means to purchase other forms of health care to satisfy their own needs and desires.

A difficulty with this approach might be that patients with little hope of recovering normal functioning would receive no more than minimum care, however, that is defined. The concept of neediness only appears for those with means to pay: greater need for those without such means does not necessarily evoke greater provision of care.

## 12:5 Future debate

Any strategy for the NHS is likely to draw upon several concepts to make up a combined package. Some have speculated that rationing protocols which have the effect of excluding categories of patient are unlikely to be supported, since this would run counter to traditional NHS values of universal access to health care. Such a move was opposed in 1991, for example, by the Secretary of State for Health, who stated that while it was acceptable for doctors to make choices between patients to treat, on the grounds of clinical judgement, health authorities were not entitled to make policy decisions excluding categories of patients.[344]

Nevertheless, once rationing is accepted as inevitable, hard decisions have to be made about prioritising. While many believe that it is clearly unethical to deny any patient treatment and so condemn that person to suffering or early death, others suspect that rationing, no matter how it is packaged, boils down to deciding "which patients will be left to die and which patients will be left in pain and discomfort".[345] While the calls for public debate echo ever louder, it is clear that any challenge to the NHS ideal of access to comprehensive health care will inevitably arouse forceful and emotive opposition. Many look to developments abroad to find techniques for rationing in an acceptable way but an ideal rationing formula remains as elusive as the Holy Grail. According to some, experiments like Oregon "hold out a warning rather than offering a model for import into Britain: a warning that there are no ready made techniques for determining choices among competing priorities in health care".[346] The debate is likely to be a prolonged exercise.

## 12:6 Conclusions

a) An agreed moral framework is needed. Evolution of such a framework must involve doctors and other health professionals, managers, economists, healthy people and the sick.

b) Decision-making strategies must be based on factual evidence. This involves validation measures such as rigorous research and medical audit.

315

c)    Strategies must be decided openly.

d)    Decision-makers both nationally and locally must be accountable for decisions taken.

e)    Cost evaluations should include awareness of costs other than merely financial ones.

# 13 Aims and Philosophy

*At the beginning of this book, we mentioned how and why it was written. This final section briefly explains the reasoning behind the advice and why it has often not been possible to give definite solutions applicable to every case. A summary is given of the kind of factors likely to be important in the reasoned consideration of hard cases.*

## 13:1 Introduction

### 13.1.1 *Aims*

The aim of this book is to identify common ethical queries and suggest solutions which are both ethically acceptable and workable in real life situations. The substance of the text has been largely dictated by the needs of doctors. Our focus has been on the questions they ask and their demand for sensible advice which reflects good practice and current legal requirements. Our remit, laid out in the introductory chapter, was to combine practical advice with extrapolation of some of the relevant philosophical arguments. We have therefore drawn attention briefly to some of the main theories associated with each issue. Our approach is eclectic. We do not confine ourselves to just one method of moral reasoning but nor have we sought to produce a philosophy textbook. The footnotes and bibliography indicate sources we have found helpful although these, like the experts who kindly contributed views, do not necessarily accord with the BMA's policies on ethical issues.

Much of our advice stems from the simple notion that central to the ethical practice of medicine is a willingness to listen carefully to patients, engage in dialogue with them, and promote their interests but in so doing avoid the likelihood of harm to anyone. Some facets of this notion can be conveyed by reference to value systems based on patients' rights or doctors' duties or utilitarian theories of maximising good. It also fits in with the powerful and often quoted concept of resolving ethical dilemmas by reference to four basic principles, which are defined as respect for autonomy and justice and the duties of doing good and avoiding harm.

### 13.1.2 *Finding answers to ethical dilemmas*

Moral values are traditionally seen as arising from a variety of sources, which we cannot hope to discuss fully. In brief, some thinkers believe in the existence of a natural law, which may or may not stem from God.

317

Some political philosophers, for example, have seen natural law as co-existent with theological commitments while others consider that natural law and natural rights are quite separate from theological beliefs. For those who believe in the existence of a natural moral order, there is still the difficulty of ascertaining what it is and how it can be applied. Some of those who believe in a natural moral order consider that this is discoverable by observation, since man has the moral capacity to sense what the laws of nature consist of. Some might see this as an intuitive moral sense.

On the other hand, philosophers since Socrates have attempted to solve dilemmas by the application of reason, rather than by automatically opting for what appears to be intuitively acceptable, or by recourse to emotion or what others consider expedient. They have sought a moral course of action by appeal to very basic moral rules which they believe all accept as valid, such as we should not harm others or tell lies. Much of recent western philosophy has been influenced by what Kant termed "practical reason", which is based on the notion that there are certain rules of behaviour, or maxims, which represent universally accepted standards. We have tried to reflect some of the accepted standards as far as doctors are concerned and point to the theories which support them.

In our view, awareness of the moral arguments will often be helpful but common sense and a caring approach are always indispensable. Within any system of reasoning, there will be cases of uncertainty. Perhaps one cannot be sure what will produce the greatest good because, for example, the implications of the various factors are impossible to compare or conflicting rights or duties are invoked. The four principles, while offering a helpful encapsulation of what are widely held to be the important elements of medical decision-making, often clash and cannot be ranked in order of priority. We have made reference to such conflicts, for example, in chapter 6 (section 6:2.2). In any case where moral imperatives conflict, doctors and patients will have to weigh up the issues. Doctors may have to justify a decision assigning priority to one line of argument.

We have not envisaged any simple mechanism for problem solving. We share the reservations, which many people have expressed, about the application of abstract or formulaic responses to the untidy dilemmas of real life. Few dilemmas are likely to be resolved wisely or satisfactorily by a blinkered adherence to abstract principles alone. Solutions to most cases will be dictated by a combination of factors, among which the following considerations may figure: the accepted standards of the profession and the expectations of society at large, the individual patient's values, the expected benefits for the patient or anyone else, the degree of medical certainty regarding the diagnosis and all or any of the potential options, the likelihood of real or symbolic harm (to the patient, other people including health professionals, potential people or society), the availability or otherwise of various resources. In every case, it will be essential to clarify the facts and the morally relevant factors. Those which are relevant must be accommodated within the particular circumstances of the situation.

## 13:2 Signposts in the decision-making process

### 13.2.1 *Professional standards*

Among the things doctors need to know in order to resolve ethical dilemmas is what society expects of them and how the profession in general views the particular issue in question. Both of these factors can be considered aspects of professional standards.

Knowledge always confers power but this is particularly evident in the case of the doctor, whose power may ultimately relate to the life and death of the patient. It has long been accepted that the doctor-patient relationship cannot be governed only by the usual rules of professional contract, precisely because of the inequality of bargaining power between doctor and patient. Historically, doctors have bound themselves by additional constraints by agreeing to conform to certain standards. The perception of what constitutes appropriate professional conduct changes with time and with cultural context but awareness of a particular moral obligation to those in need is commonly expected of doctors. This has been exemplified, for example, by the Knights Hospitallers of Jerusalem who referred to their patients as "our lords the sick". Similar precepts have been expressed in other cultures.

The Hippocratic Oath and the World Medical Association's International Code of Medical Ethics[347] are probably the most widely known statements of medical commitment to the service of humanity. The Caraka Samhita, a Hindu code dating from about the first century AD, instructs doctors to "endeavour for the relief of patients with all thy heart and soul; thou shalt not desert or injure thy patient for the sake of thy life or living".[348] Not dissimilar instructions were given by early Islamic physicians and the modern Declaration of Kuwait[349] instructs doctors to focus on the needy be they "near or far, virtuous or sinner, friend or enemy". Thus, compassion is a long accepted facet of medical practice, counter-balancing the power accorded to doctors in their relationship with vulnerable patients. Doctors are expected to put patients' interests before their own. In the past, doctors often damaged their own health by treating plague victims and other infectious patients. In modern times also, the BMA has emphasised that doctors cannot refuse to treat patients simply for fear of risk to themselves.[350]

Doctors must be accustomed to being told that they should cultivate certain personal attitudes as well as medical proficiency. Nearly two centuries ago, Percival[351] was advising doctors "to unite tenderness with steadiness, and condescension with authority, as to inspire the minds of their patients with gratitude, respect and confidence". Such views are unlikely to have appeal for modern patients, who nevertheless want doctors to show something more than technical prowess. Maximally effective health care depends partly on health professionals taking a human approach which actively involves patients rather than, as in some other countries, making them recipients of what may be seen as a preoccupation with impersonal, high-tech procedures.

Part of our task is to try to apply to modern situations, traditionally accepted facets of a doctor's duty. A central aim of the BMA's ethical guidance has consistently been to listen to doctors and reflect back to the profession these standards to which doctors believe they should aspire. The BMA's views of these are established by debate at the Association's Annual Representative Meetings (ARM). In the past, these assemblies of doctors have passed a very wide range of resolutions on moral issues, not only on clearly medically relevant topics such as abortion, euthanasia or embryo research but also, for example, opposing all types of discrimination and torture, and voicing strong concerns about prison conditions in Britain and abroad. This supports our view that medical ethics are not simply a list of the duties owed within the professional fraternity but rather the articulation of the collective conscience of its members.

Professional standards should seek to be consistent and objective, not subject to the vagaries of subjective opinion. Thus, most doctors agree that when they take on a professional role, they should try to act in an objective manner. Medical advice should not project individual moral values unless the patient is seeking the doctor's personal view. Professional ethics are distinct from personal moral standards. Doctors, who regard sexual intercourse outside marriage as immoral, should nevertheless be able to give balanced medical advice to unmarried people if contraception is among the services those doctors provide. A doctor need not agree with a patient's proposed course of action but should not deliberately impede a patient's legitimate goal, for example, by delaying a referral for abortion advice or by withholding information a patient needs to make an advance directive.

Even where many members of the profession share a similar attitude, there is a duty to subject the grounds for that view to the scrutiny of analytical reasoning. Possible distaste for certain procedures, such as gender selection of an embryo for social reasons, does not diminish the importance either of conducting serious and reasoned analysis of both the potential advantages and disadvantages of such procedures, or of the examination of why people desire them. Nor does the fact of legislation or other regulation of some areas of medical practice prevent us from questioning whether a consistent logic is being applied to all issues of intrinsic similarity.

The BMA's ethical advice must be subject to continual scrutiny and, where appropriate, reflect factors such as recent legislation, changing views on personal liberty and multicultural influences in society. This is not to say that we believe there has been a change in the fundamental ethical principles of medicine, but rather that we must seek consistency in the application of traditional principles to changing practice.

### 13.2.2 *The patient's values*

Many moral theories give emphasis to individual autonomy, liberty and rights. We have alluded frequently to patients' autonomy, by which we mean their capacity to choose freely and control as far as possible what happens to them. Respect for patient autonomy has become a core principle of modern medicine, although some ethicists argue that this principle has always inspired health work and that the whole point of providing treatment is to enable people to direct their own lives and flourish. They maintain that all theories of health equate work for health in some way with the creation of autonomy.

Throughout this book, emphasis has been given to the importance of communicating with patients and understanding their viewpoints. Personal freedom, however, is not unlimited and sometimes the outcome the individual would like to choose is not a practical possibility. The law, society's views, the rights of other people, resources and an individual's circumstances, all restrict autonomy. Illness, addiction or other forms of physical or moral dependency also impinge on the individual's ability to exercise free choice. Fortunately, it is not necessary to be omniscient and free of all constraints in order to be able to decide which of the options on offer is most acceptable to the individual who must choose.

In all cases, individuals should exercise to the limits whatever decision-making capacity they have, if this will not harm others. Some harm is held to be so great, such as killing or gratuitous mutilation, that people cannot legally consent to it being done to them, no matter how carefully they have reflected upon it. Nor can they choose an option that seriously offends the commonly held values of society. Patients may make a valid choice apparently to harm themselves by refusing potentially life-saving treatment, since this reflects a generally held right of the individual to be free of interference. They cannot, however, oblige others to comply with a demand for euthanasia, because the implications of being able to do so might damage the security of vulnerable people and so impinge upon their rights.

Respect for people obliges us to give due weight to their deliberated choices made in accordance with their own values. Such choices may be expressed in anticipation of incapacitating illness through an advance directive, as is discussed in chapter 6 (section 6:3.3). Protecting patients' dignity and integrity, maintaining an honest and open approach, and only making promises which can be kept are aspects of this respect.

In many parts of the book, we have discussed how individual desires come into conflict with other important considerations. In the context of consent, for example, (chapter 1, section 1:1.4) the potential for conflict

321

between the autonomy of the patient and that of the doctor was noted. Cases of so-called maternal-fetal conflict (chapter 4, section 4:7.2), requests for euthanasia (chapter 6, section 6:2.2.1) and the equitable distribution of scarce NHS resources (chapter 12, section 12.4) are all areas where the importance we give to one person's wishes may be modified.

### 13.2.3 *The possibility of harm*

The possibility of harm to anyone, including the patient is an important factor to be weighed. Quite often the doctor's duty to avoid harming a patient comes into conflict with what the patient wants. We have discussed this in particular in relation to patients who insist on drugs that are demonstrably bad for them in the long run (chapter 7, section 7:5.1.4). In considering young people who refuse treatment, we have considered how avoiding harm might involve doctors in wronging patients in another sense by denying those patients' wishes (chapter 3, section 3:2.4). Imposing one's own moral values on others is wrong. Obviously, wherever it is possible, doctors must avoid harm and do this by following a course of action likely to bring most medical benefit to the patient and also avoid wronging patients by not overriding their views. Sometimes it is not possible to do both and common sense will often indicate which is the lesser evil if no acceptable compromise can be found.

The infliction or risk of harm, including the risks of medical practice, can only be justified by the pursuit of other important moral values. These must consist principally of benefits to the individual patient sufficient to outweigh the harm. Much of the debate about tissue donation by children or people who are unable to consent depends upon assessing the validity of claims that the benefit for the individual in preserving the life of somebody close to him or her outweighs the physical effects. In discussions about non-therapeutic research, the emphasis is on the individual's consent, since potential risks without anticipated benefit for that individual can usually only be compensated by the person's agreement in the knowledge that others are likely to benefit.

Most doctors consider it wrong to lie to a patient but acknowledge that there are circumstances when they would hold back information on the grounds that it would harm the patient to know it. The law acknowledges the importance of clinical discretion in such cases, although it maintains they should be exceptional. Some philosophers, however, argue that to fail to tell the full truth is a manifestation of dishonesty no less wrong than telling an outright lie. The view that we have expressed in chapter 5, on the dying and chapter 4, on genetic screening, is that truth-telling in a sensitive manner is essential in most cases but that to insist on telling patients the full truth when they make it clear they are not ready to know it, conflicts with both reason and intuition. It denies respect for the patient's autonomy to choose not to know. This is an area where common sense and the ability to strike a rapport with patients are likely to be most valuable in making a wise pragmatic decision.

The possibility of harm is not only a question of physical or psychological damage to an individual but may also involve an indignity or symbolic harm which stretches beyond the particular case: for example, the way you treat one member of a particular group may have implications for all other members of that group. Throughout society we see the rights of the elderly or of incapacitated people compromised or precariously balanced against other considerations. The doctor's traditional role is to respond to the needs of the vulnerable. Some patients cannot be seen as less valuable or less worthy of doctors' best endeavours. Doctors' efforts must be tailored to meet the requirements and best interests of all patients. Like any other damage, therefore, symbolic harm must be avoided unless to do so would permit a greater wrong. This is discussed in chapter 3 where it is envisaged, for example, that a doctor might justifiably override the wishes of a mature minor in order to preserve that person's life. In other cases the risk of symbolic harm to some apparently may be outweighed by some very desirable benefits for others. An example may be seen in the discussion in chapter 1 (section 1:7.1.4), of the ventilation of moribund patients for organ donation. We recognise the risk of appearing to undervalue, and thus symbolically harm the status of dying patients, but believe that the important and tangible benefits to others may justify the action. We welcome further discussion within the profession and among the public on such issues.

As a final consideration of the injunction to avoid harm, we note that the principle of double effect, often espoused by duty-based moralists, supports the view that actions which bring about a harmful result but which are undertaken with the aim of benefiting the patient are not reprehensible. Thus, in chapter 6 (section 6:2.2.2) for example, we discuss the ethics of providing relief of pain and distress at the end of life in order to improve the quality of the time the patient has left even though a foreseeable effect will be to shorten that life.

### 13:2.4 *Implications for other people*

Doing the best for one patient may have implications for others. Some of these implications are not necessarily harmful and indeed may be beneficial if the person who is the subject of the procedure is willing to share information about it with others who want to know and for whom it may also be important. Examples are given in chapter 1 (section 1:9) where we discuss the importance of consent and confidentiality in relation to sterilisation, genetic screening, HIV and paternity testing.

Sometimes, however, protecting the confidentiality of one patient could be disastrous for others and the doctor may be obliged by other moral considerations to override the usual rights of one patient. This overlaps with the previous section on assessment of harm. In chapter 2 (section 2:4.2.3) for example, we consider the dilemmas which may arise with the abuse of vulnerable people whose silence may have immense implications for other people.

The BMA's objection to euthanasia partly hinges on its implications for society at large. For the person seeking a right to be killed, euthanasia arguably brings no harm, but its practice may affect the fabric of society.

### 13:2.5 *The circumstances of the case*

As mentioned above, our aim has not been to set up a blueprint for resolving ethical dilemmas but rather to explore some of the factors which are likely candidates for consideration. Even if one hoped to provide a standard formula for obtaining the correct ethical response, such an enterprise would be confounded by the variability of individual cases, which must be a vital factor in resolving them. As we have discussed throughout the book, few values can be considered absolute and in assessing the relevance of various factors in individual cases, common sense and clinical judgement are indispensable. In chapter 4 (section 4:7.2), we have drawn attention to one model for analysing conflicting claims to rights. Among other things, this involves not only weighing the relevant harms and benefits but the degree of harm in the individual case and the strength of the arguments for risking it.

In general, we have considered it regrettable where conflict of values or viewpoint have led to confrontation, and cases involving aspects of patient's rights going before the courts. What we suggest is that in some of these there may be scope for negotiation and for the balancing of conflicting imperatives to lead to constructive and creative decision-making.

## 13:3 Conclusion

In our consideration of ethical dilemmas we have sought to look at a number of factors. Our arguments are based primarily on accepted professional standards but whose application to particular situations may sometimes seem unclear because of changing technology and ever-evolving expectations. In our view, the difficulty is not in identifying ethical standards, which many have done previously against a background of well known principles, codes and declarations, but in relating these standards to everyday dilemmas. The difficult task is often how to decide upon a practical course of action in a situation of uncertainty where moral imperatives are in conflict with one another. These must be addressed individually, accepting that individual circumstances and patient preferences have an important bearing in most cases. We have sought to point to factors which it is hoped will permit doctors and patients jointly to resolve their dilemmas and reminded doctors that they may be called to account for the priority they give to some principles over others.

We have attempted to be consistent in recognising the underlying ethical arguments of each case, while at the same time recognising the limits of theory when faced with difficult practical situations which require action. We have emphasised individual autonomy but recognise that there are constraints upon it. The period of preparation of this book has been punctuated by a series of complex legal cases regarding treatment of young people, people whose competence fluctuates and pregnant women (see chapters 3 and 4). We have discussed the implications of such cases and the fact that they appear to contradict the values of respect for the individual which society claims.

Anomalous attitudes exist and it would be unwise to pretend they do not. Thus, while there is an undoubted value in the exercise of submitting medical intuitions about what is "ethical" to the rigorous test of logic, it must be recognised that in human affairs little is ruled by such consistent logic and few would want it to be. One of the suggestions arising in this book, particularly in chapter 5 where we discussed care of the dying, is that informed intuition has a place in some circumstances and there is no shame in steering a reasoned middle course where such an action appears an appropriate and sensitive response to the situation.

Finally, we note that the progress of biomedical sciences and medical technology and their application to medical practice has brought new ethical dilemmas. Discussions of "medical ethics", "bioethics" and "health policy ethics" have proliferated, not only among those directly involved in scientific research or the provision of health care but also in university departments of philosophy, theology, law and social policy. Experts in these fields have contributed greatly to the debate and dispelled the impression that medical ethics is something which only interests those working directly to provide health care.

The subject, and the study of medical ethics is blossoming as never before and medical ethicists find a steadily growing demand for their skills, but where does this leave doctors? All too often, there appear to be gaps between the important theories to which ethicists urge doctors to aspire and the messy complexities of real patients who somehow fail to fit neatly with those theories. These gaps and potential inconsistencies are matters which the BMA has made efforts to recognise and debate. In some cases we have not been able to provide conclusive answers but we have sought to guide the busy doctor towards possible solutions which would be endorsed within the profession. Meanwhile the debate must continue. Many issues will not be resolved by doctors alone and, although our advice is primarily directed to them, the Association welcomes wider informed public discussion of medical ethical problems as the most helpful way forward.

325

# Appendix One

## The Hippocratic Oath

The methods and details of medical practice change with the passage of time and the advance of knowledge. However, many fundamental principles of professional behaviour have remained unaltered through the recorded history of medicine. The Hippocratic Oath was probably written in the 5th century BC and was intended to be affirmed by each doctor on entry to the medical profession. In translation it reads as follows:

I swear by Apollo the physician, and Aesculapius and Health, and All-heal, and all the gods and goddesses, that, according to my ability and judgement, I will keep this Oath and this stipulation - to reckon him who taught me this Art equally dear to me as my parents, to share my substance with him, and relieve his necessities if required; to look upon his offspring in the same footing as my own brothers, and to teach them this Art, if they shall wish to learn it, without fee or stipulation; and that by percept, lecture and every other mode of instruction, I will impart a knowledge of the Art to my own sons, and those of my teachers, and to disciples bound by a stipulation and oath according to the law of medicine, but to none other. I will follow that system of regimen which, according to my ability and judgement, I consider for the benefit of my patients, and abstain from whatever is deleterious and mischievous. I will give no deadly medicine to anyone if asked, nor suggest any such counsel; and in like manner I will not give to a woman a pessary to produce abortion. With purity and with holiness I will pass my life and practise my Art. I will not cut persons labouring under the stone, but will leave this to be done by men who are practitioners of this work. Into whatever houses I enter, I will go into them for the benefit of the sick, and will abstain from every voluntary act of mischief and corruption; and, further, from the seduction of females, or males, of freemen or slaves. Whatever, in connection with my professional practice, not in connection with it, I see or hear, in the life of men, which ought not to be spoken of abroad, I will not divulge, as reckoning that all such should be kept secret. While I continue to keep this Oath unviolated, may it be granted to me to enjoy life and the practice of the Art, respected by all men, in all times. But should I trespass and violate this Oath, may the reverse be my lot.

# Appendix Two

## International Code of Medical Ethics

One of the first acts of the World Medical Association, when formed in 1947, was to produce a modern restatement of the Hippocratic Oath, known as the Declaration of Geneva, and to base upon it an International Code of Medical Ethics which applies in time of both peace and war. The Declaration of Geneva, as amended by the 22nd World Medical Assembly, Sydney, Australia, in August 1968 and the 35th World Medical Assembly, Venice, Italy, in October 1983, reads:

At the time of being admitted as a member of the Medical Profession:

I solemnly pledge myself to consecrate my life to the service of humanity;

I will give to my teachers the respect and gratitude which is their due;

I will practise my profession with conscience and dignity;

The health of my patient will be my first consideration;

I will respect the secrets which are confided in me, even after the patient has died;

I will maintain by all the means in my power, the honour and the noble traditions of the medical profession;

My colleagues will be my brothers;

I will not permit considerations of religion, nationality, race, party politics or social standing to intervene between my duty and my patients;

I will maintain the utmost respect for human life from its beginning even under threat and I will not use my medical knowledge contrary to the laws of humanity;

I make these promises solemnly, freely and upon my honour.

The English text of the International Code of Medical Ethics is as follows:

*Duties of physicians in general*

A PHYSICIAN SHALL always maintain the highest standards of professional conduct.

327

A PHYSICIAN SHALL not permit motives of profit to influence the free and independent exercise of professional judgement on behalf of patients.

A PHYSICIAN SHALL, in all types of medical practice, be dedicated to providing competent medical service in full technical and moral independence, with compassion and respect for human dignity.

A PHYSICIAN SHALL deal honestly with patients and colleagues, and strive to expose those physicians deficient in character or competence, or who engage in fraud or deception.

The following practices are deemed to be unethical conduct:

a) Self advertising by physicians, unless permitted by the laws of the country and the Code of Ethics of the national medical association.

b) Paying or receiving any fee or any other consideration solely to procure the referral of a patient or for prescribing or referring a patient to any source.

A PHYSICIAN SHALL respect the rights of patients, of colleagues, and of other health professionals, and shall safeguard patient confidences.

A PHYSICIAN SHALL act only in the patient's interest when providing medical care which might have the effect of weakening the physical and mental condition of the patient.

A PHYSICIAN SHALL use great caution in divulging discoveries or new techniques or treatment through non-professional channels.

A PHYSICIAN SHALL certify only that which he has personally verified.

*Duties of physicians to the sick*

A PHYSICIAN SHALL always bear in mind the obligation of preserving human life.

A PHYSICIAN SHALL owe his patients complete loyalty and all the resources of his science. Whenever an examination or treatment is beyond the physician's capacity he should summon another physician who has the necessary ability.

A PHYSICIAN SHALL preserve absolute confidentiality on all he knows about his patient even after the patient has died.

A PHYSICIAN SHALL give emergency care as a humanitarian duty unless he is assured that others are willing and able to give such care.

*Duties of physicians to each other*

A PHYSICIAN SHALL behave towards his colleagues as he would have them behave towards him.

328

A PHYSICIAN SHALL NOT entice patients from his colleagues.

A PHYSICIAN SHALL observe the principles of "The Declaration of Geneva" approved by the World Medical Association.

Subsequently, the World Medical Association has considered and published material on a number of ethical matters.

# Appendix Three

## Declaration of Helsinki

### Human experimentation

In 1964, the World Medical Association drew up a code of ethics on human experimentation. This code, known as the Declaration of Helsinki, as amended by the 29th World Medical Assembly, Helsinki, Finland, in 1975, and by the 35th World Medical Assembly, Venice, Italy, in 1983, reads:

> It is the mission of the medical doctor to safeguard the health of the people. His or her knowledge and conscience are dedicated to the fulfilment of this mission.

> The Declaration of Geneva of the World Medical Association binds the physician with the words, "The health of my patient will be my first consideration", and the International Code of Medical Ethics declares that "A physician shall act only in the patient's interest when providing medical care which might have the effect of weakening the physical and mental condition of the patient".

> The purpose of biomedical research involving human subjects must be to improve diagnostic, therapeutic and prophylactic procedures and the understanding of the aetiology and pathogenesis of disease.

> In current medical practice most diagnostic, therapeutic or prophylactic procedures involve hazards. This applies especially to biomedical research.

> Medical progress is based on research which ultimately must rest in part on experimentation involving human subjects.

> In the field of biomedical research a fundamental distinction must be recognised between medical research in which the aim is essentially diagnostic or therapeutic for a patient, and medical research, the essential object of which is purely scientific and without implying direct diagnostic or therapeutic value to the person subjected to the research.

> Special caution must be exercised in the conduct of research which may affect the environment, and the welfare of animals used for research must be respected.

330

Because it is essential that the results of laboratory experiments be applied to human beings to further scientific knowledge and to help suffering humanity, the World Medical Association has prepared the following recommendations as a guide to every physician in biomedical research involving human subjects. They should be kept under review in the future. It must be stressed that the standards as drafted are only a guide to physicians all over the world. Physicians are not relieved from criminal, civil and ethical responsibilities under the laws of their own countries.

## I    *Basic principles*

1   Biomedical research involving human subjects must conform to generally accepted scientific principles and should be based on adequately performed laboratory and animal experimentation and on a thorough knowledge of the scientific literature.

2   The design and performance of each experimental procedure involving human subjects should be clearly formulated in an experimental protocol which should be transmitted to a specially appointed independent committee for consideration, comment and guidance.

3   Biomedical research involving human subjects should be conducted only by scientifically qualified persons and under the supervision of a clinically competent medical person. The responsibility for the human subject must always rest with the medically qualified person and never rest on the subject of the research, even though the subject has given his or her consent.

4   Biomedical research involving human subjects cannot legitimately be carried out unless the importance of the objective is in proportion to the inherent risk to the subject.

5   Every biomedical research project involving human subjects should be preceded by careful assessment of predictable risks in comparison with foreseeable benefits to the subject or to others. Concern for the interests of the subject must always prevail over the interest of science and society.

6   The right of the research subject to safeguard his or her integrity must always be respected. Every precaution should be taken to respect the privacy of the subject and to minimize the impact of the study on the subject's physical and mental integrity and on the personality of the subject.

7   Physicians should abstain from engaging in research projects involving human subjects unless they are satisfied that the hazards involved are

believed to be predictable. Physicians should cease any investigation if the hazards are found to outweigh the potential benefits.

8    In publication of the results of his or her research, the physician is obliged to preserve the accuracy of the results. Reports of experimentation not in accordance with the principles laid down in this Declaration should not be accepted for publication.

9    In any research on human beings, each potential subject must be adequately informed of the aims, methods, anticipated benefits and potential hazards of the study and the discomfort it may entail. He or she should be informed that he or she is at liberty to abstain from participation in the study and that he or she is free to withdraw his or her consent to participation at any time. The physician should then obtain the subject's freely-given informed consent, preferably in writing.

10   When obtaining informed consent for the research project the physician should be particularly cautious if the subject is in a dependent relationship to him or her or may consent under duress. In that case the informed consent should be obtained by a physician who is not engaged in the investigation and who is completely independent of this official relationship.

11   In case of legal incompetence, informed consent should be obtained from the legal guardian in accordance with national legislation. Where physical or mental incapacity makes it impossible to obtain informed consent, or when the subject is a minor, permission from the responsible relative replaces that of the subject in accordance with national legislation. Whenever the minor child is in fact able to give a consent, the minor's consent must be obtained in addition to the consent of the minor's legal guardian.

12   The research protocol should always contain a statement of the ethical considerations involved and should indicate that the principles enunciated in the present Declaration are complied with.

## II  *Medical research combined with professional care*
(Clinical research)

1    In the treatment of the sick person, the physician must be free to use a new diagnostic and therapeutic measure, if in his or her judgement it offers hope of saving life, re-establishing health or alleviating suffering.

2    The potential benefits, hazards and discomfort of a new method should be weighed against the advantages of the best current diagnostic and therapeutic methods.

3  In any medical study, every patient - including those of a control group, if any - should be assured of the best proven diagnostic and therapeutic method.

4  The refusal of the patient to participate in a study must never interfere with the physician-patient relationship.

5  If the physician considers it essential not to obtain informed consent, the specific reasons for this proposal should be stated in the experimental protocol for transmission to the independent committee (I.2).

6  The physician can combine medical research with professional care, the objective being the acquisition of new medical knowledge, only to the extent that medical research is justified by its potential diagnostic or therapeutic value for the patient.

**III**  *Non-therapeutic biomedical research involving human subjects*
(Non-clinical biomedical research)

1  In the purely scientific application of medical research carried out on a human being, it is the duty of the physician to remain the protector of the life and health of that person on whom biomedical research is being carried out.

2  The subjects should be volunteers - either healthy persons or patients for whom the experimental design is not related to the patient's illness.

3  The investigator or the investigating team should discontinue the research if in his/her or their judgement it may, if continued, be harmful to the individual.

4  In research on man, the interest of science and society should never take precedence over considerations related to the wellbeing of the subject.

# Appendix Four

## Declaration of Tokyo

*Torture and other cruel, inhuman or degrading treatment or punishment*

In 1975 the World Medical Association adopted the following guidelines for medical doctors concerning Torture and Other Cruel, Inhuman or Degrading Treatment or Punishment in relation to Detention and Imprisonment (Declaration of Tokyo):

### Preamble

It is the privilege of the medical doctor to practise medicine in the service of humanity, to preserve and restore bodily and mental health without distinction as to persons, to comfort and to ease the suffering of his or her patients. The utmost respect for human life is to be maintained even under threat, and no use made of any medical knowledge contrary to the laws of humanity.

For the purpose of this Declaration, torture is defined as the deliberate, systematic or wanton infliction of physical or mental suffering by one or more persons acting alone or on the orders of any authority, to force another person to yield information, to make a confession, or for any other reason.

### Declaration

1   The doctor shall not countenance, condone or participate in the practice of torture or other forms of cruel, inhuman or degrading procedures is suspected, accused or guilty, and whatever the victim's belief or motives, and in all situations, including armed conflict and civil strife.

2   The doctor shall not provide any premises, instruments, substances or knowledge to facilitate the practice of torture or other forms of cruel, inhuman or degrading treatment or to diminish the ability of the victim to resist such treatment.

3   The doctor shall not be present during any procedure during which torture or other forms of cruel, inhuman or degrading treatment is used or threatened.

4    A doctor must have complete clinical independence in deciding upon the care of a person for whom he or she is medically responsible. The doctor's fundamental role is to alleviate the distress of his or her fellow men, and no motive, whether personal, collective or political, shall prevail against this higher purpose.

5    Where a prisoner refuses nourishment and is considered by the doctor as capable of forming an unimpaired and rational judgement concerning the consequences of such a voluntary refusal of nourishment, he or she shall not be fed artificially. The decision as to the capacity of the prisoner to form such a judgement should be confirmed by at least one other independent doctor. The consequences or the refusal of nourishment shall be explained by the doctor to the prisoner.

6    The World Medical Association will support, and should encourage the international community, the national medical association and fellow doctors, to support the doctor and his or her family in the face of threats or reprisals resulting from a refusal to condone the use of torture or other forms of cruel, inhuman or degrading treatment.

# Appendix Five

## Useful addresses

**British Medical Association**, BMA House, Tavistock Square, London WC1H 9JP.

**General Medical Council**, 44 Hallam Street, London W1N 6AE.

**Medical Defence Union**, 3 Devonshire Place, London W1N 2EA.

**Medical Protection Society**, 50 Hallam Street, London W1N 6DE.

**National Library of Medicine**, 8600 Rockville Pike, Bethesda, Maryland, MD 20894 - USA.

**National Counselling Service for Sick Doctors**, 3rd Floor, 26 Park Crescent, London W1N 3PB.

**World Medical Association**, PO Box 63, 28 Ave des Alpes, 01212 Ferney-Voltaire Cedex, France.

# References

## Chapter 1

1. The law on consent is fully detailed in chapter 1 of *Rights and Responsibilities of Doctors*, BMA, 1992.

2. Re R (a minor) [1991] 4 All ER 177; Re J (a minor)(medical treatment) [1992] 4 All ER 614; Re T [1992] 4 All ER 649. All 3 cases are also detailed in *Medical Law Reports*, 1992, 3.

3. Slater v Baker and Stapleton, 95 Eng Rep 860 (KB 1767).

4. The phrase was coined by Katz J, in 'Duty and caring in the age of informed consent and medical science', *Humane Medicine*, vol 8, no. 3, July 1992, 187-194.

5. Lord Donaldson, MR, in Re J (a minor)(medical treatment) [1992] 4 All ER 614.

6. See case of Bolam v Friern Hospital Management Committee [1957] 2 All ER 118. The implications of the case are discussed in the BMA publication *Rights and Responsibilities of Doctors*, 1992, p.19.

7. Sidaway v Board of Governors of the Bethlem Royal Hospital and the Maudsley [1985] AC 871, 1 All ER 643. The full legal position regarding all aspects of consent is given in the BMA publication *Rights and Responsibilities of Doctors*, 1992.

8. The variations in the Mental Health legislation in force in Scotland, Northern Ireland and England and Wales are explored in chapter 8 of *Rights and Responsibilities of Doctors*, BMA, 1992.

9. A view of the law on this matter was stated by Lord Donaldson in the case of an adult Jehovah's Witness, Re T [1992] 4 All ER 649.

10. Gillick v Norfolk & Wisbech AHA [1985] 3 WLR 830, 3 All ER 402.

11. The Access to Health Records Act 1990 gave children and young people under 16 full access to their health records if the record-holder judged them capable of understanding the nature of their application.

12. Re R (a minor) [1991] 4 All ER 177; Re J (a minor)(medical treatment) [1992] 4 All ER 614.

13. See case of Re W (a minor)(medical treatment) [1992], 4 All ER 627.

14. Reported by Counsel and Care (originally the Elderly Invalids Fund), a charitable organisation providing advice to older people and carers in its 1992 report *What If They Hurt Themselves*.

15. *The Independent*, 25 June 1991.

16. This principle was stated by Lord Goff of Chievely in the House of Lords' hearing of F v West Berkshire HA and another [1989] WLR 1086 at B.

17. per Lord Donaldson in Re T [1992] 4 All ER 649.

18. The modern use of tutors dative is discussed in Scottish Law Commission discussion paper 94 on *Mentally Disabled Adults, Legal Arrangements for Managing their Welfare and Finances*, September 1991, Edinburgh.

19. See Re T [1992] 4 All ER 649.

20. Moore v Regents of the University of California [1990] 793 P 2d 479 (Cal).

21. The Nuffield Bioethics Committee has undertaken a study on the current and prospective medical and scientific uses made of sub-cellular structures, cells and their products, tissue and organs. Its report is anticipated in 1993.

22. The BMA's views on these subjects are fully debated in its publication *Medicine Betrayed*, Zed Press, 1992.

23. This policy was established at the 1988 Annual Representative Meeting of the BMA.

24. per Lord Templeman in Sidaway v Board of Governors of the Bethlem Royal Hospital and Maudsley Hospital [1985] AC 871 at 904, 1 All ER 643.

25. Lord Donaldson in Re T [1992] 4 All ER 649.

26. The BMA welcomed the initiative of the British Paediatric Association in setting up a working party on neonatal resuscitation in 1992.

27. The Human Organ Transplants Act 1989 restricts transplants between people who are not genetically related. The Act does not cover bone marrow donation. The law is fully discussed in *Rights and Responsibilities of Doctors*, BMA, 1992, p.5.

28. See, for example, the comments by Lord Goff in the House of Lords' hearing of Re F (mental patient: sterilisation) [1990] 2 AC 1.

29. This is quite a different matter, however, to the generation of a pregnancy with the aim of later aborting the fetus to provide material for transplantation.

30. *Report of the Working Party of the Conference of Medical Royal Colleges and their Faculties in the United Kingdom on Organ Transplantation in Neonates,* 1988.

31. This, for example, is the view taken by Mason and McCall Smith in *Law and Medical Ethics,* third edition, Butterworths, 1991.

32. See, for example, 'Anencephalic babies as heart donors', *BMJ*, vol 303, September 7, 1991, p.538.

33. The law is set out in full in chapter 1 of *Rights and Responsibilities of Doctors*, BMA, 1992.

34. *Review of the Guidance of the Research Use of Fetuses and Fetal Material*, Cmnd 762, London, HMSO, 1989.

35. McCullagh P, 'Some ethical aspects of current fetal usage in transplantation', in *Ethics and Law in Health Care and Research*, (ed) Byrne P, Wiley, 1990.

36. The Mental Health Act 1983 (including reference to variation in Scotland and Northern Ireland) is discussed in chapter 8 of *Rights and Responsibilities of Doctors*, BMA, 1992.

# Chapter 2

37. Lord Wilberforce in the case of British Steel Corporation v Granada Television [1981] 1 All ER 417 at 455.

38. WMA code is appended.

39. The Access to Health Records Act 1990 permits limited disclosure after the patient's death. The legislation is discussed in chapter 4 of *Rights and Responsibilities of Doctors*, BMA, 1992, and a BMA guidance on the Act is available from the BMA's Ethics Division.

40. The notifiable diseases and legal provisions concerning disclosure in the public interest are laid out in full in chapter 3 of *Rights and Responsibilities of Doctors*, BMA, 1992.

41. The Data Protection Act 1984 and the eight principles it contains are set out in chapter 4 of *Rights and Responsibilities of Doctors*, BMA, 1992. The General Medical Services Committee of the BMA has also issued guidance on the practical implications of the Act for GPs.

42. The General Medical Services Committee of the BMA has produced guidance on this and other aspects of the use of computers in general practice.

43. The legal position is laid out as far as it can be clarified in chapter 4 of *Rights and Responsibilities of Doctors*, BMA, 1992.

44. These statements were formally adopted as BMA policy at the Association's Annual Representative Meeting, 1990.

45. The full provisions of the Access to Medical Reports Act 1988 and the Access to Health Records Act 1990 are given in the BMA's guidance note available from the BMA's Ethics Division and further discussed in chapter 4 of *Rights and Responsibilities of Doctors*, BMA, 1992.

46. The term "parents" should be understood as including those, such as a guardian, who are legally recognised as exercising a parental role.

47. Available from the BMA's Ethics Division.

48. Kings College Hospital Unit Survey, quoted by Peter Thurnham, House of Commons, *Official Report*, 20 June 1990.

49. The recommended retention times for various types of record are given in chapter 4 of *Rights and Responsibilities of Doctors*, BMA, 1992.

50. *Working Party Report on the Health Care of Remand Prisoners*, BMA, 1990.

51. See, for example, the Control of Substances Hazardous to Health Regulations 1988.

52. Court proceedings and pre-trial disclosure of documents are fully discussed in chapter 3.2 of *Rights and Responsibilities of Doctors*, BMA, 1992.

53. *Working Together Under the Children Act* 1989, HMSO, 1991, p.42

54. *The Law Commission Consultation Paper No.119*, HMSO, 1991, p.183.

55. *Professional Conduct and Discipline: Fitness to Practise*, GMC, January 1993, para 83.

56. The law on these matters is set out in *Rights and Responsibilities of Doctors*, BMA, 1992, chapters 3, 5, 6, 9 and 12.

57. This provision applies only in England and Wales. Again the legal position is fully explained in chapter 3 of *Rights and Responsibilities of Doctors*, BMA, 1992.

58. Attorney General v Mulholland and Foster [1963] 1 All ER 767.

59. 'Doctors, drivers and confidentiality', 1974, 1 *BMJ* 399.

60. W v Egdell [1990] 1 A ER 648. The facts of the case are summarised in *Rights and Responsibilities of Doctors*, BMA, 1992, p.45.

61. X Health Authority v Y [1988] 2 All ER 648. The statement was made by Rose J at 653.

62. This is discussed in Brazier M, *Medicine Patients and the Law*, Penguin, 1992, p.108.

63. *Professional Conduct and Discipline: Fitness to Practise*, GMC, January 1993, para 89.

64. *Eighth Report of the Data Protection Registrar*, HMSO: London, June 1992, p.9.

# Chapter 3

65. See, for example, Alderson P, 'In the genes or in the stars? Children's competence to consent', *Journal of Medical Ethics*, 1992, 18, 119-124.

66. The Act is discussed in chapter 7, *Rights and Responsibilities of Doctors*, BMA 1992.

67. See Mental Health Act 1983, s131(2).

68. The Family Law Reform Act 1969 is discussed in chapter 7 of *Rights and Responsibilities of Doctors*, BMA, 1992.

69. See, for example, Skegg P D G, 'Consent to medical procedures on minors', 1973, 36 *Medical Law Reports* 370.

70. Gillick v Wisbech & W Norfolk AHA [1984], 1 All ER 365; revised [1985] 1 All ER 533, CA; revised [1985] 3 All ER 402, HL. The Gillick case is discussed in detail in chapter 1 of Kennedy I and Grubb A, *Medical Law: Text and Materials*, 1989, Butterworths; and a very helpful summary is given by Brazier M, in chapter 15 of *Medicine, Patients and the Law*, Penguin, 1992. A very brief summary of the legal implications is given in chapter 7, *Rights and Responsibilities of Doctors*, BMA 1992.

71. Mill J S, 'On Liberty', in Warnock M (ed) *Utilitarianism*, Fontana, London, 1972.

72. Law Commission consultation paper 119, *Mentally incapacitated adults and decision-making: an overview*, HMSO, London, 1991.

73. This is discussed further by Alderson P, 'In the genes or in the stars? Children's competence to consent', *Journal of Medical Ethics*, 1992, 18, 119-124.

74. See, for example, Solberg A, 'Negotiating childhood' in James and Prout, (eds), *Constructing and Reconstructing Childhood*, Basingstoke: Falmer Press, 1990.

75. These recommendations were stated by Lord Fraser in the Lords' hearing of the Gillick case, [1985] 3 All ER at 413.

76. In 1990, the conception rate in the 13-15 age bracket was 10.1 per 1000. (OPCS statistics provided by Brook Advisory Centres).

77. The RCGP has drawn particular attention to this option for consumer choice in its December 1991 policy statement on *Family Planning and Sexual Health*.

78. Lord Templeman in the Sidaway case [1985] AC 871 at 904.

79. Chatterton v Gerson [1981] QB 432.

80. Re T [1992] 4 All ER 649.

81. In 1983, the BMA's Annual Representative Meeting resolved to seek legislation against female circumcision and to prohibit the practice unless carried out as part of the necessary treatment of an existing disease in the child.

82. Virginia Bottomley drew attention to the Department's guidance in answer to a Parliamentary question, *Hansard*, 586, 13 November 1991. The DoH publication, *Working Together under the Children Act*, 1991, reminds authorities of the effect of the Prohibition of Female Circumcision Act 1985.

83. Re J (a minor)(wardship)(medical treatment) [1990] 2 WLR 140.

84. Re B (a minor)(wardship: medical treatment)[1981][1990] 3 All ER 927.

85. The case of R is discussed further in chapter 7, section 7:7.2.3 of *Rights and Responsibilities of Doctors*, BMA, 1992.

86. Re W (a minor)(medical treatment) [1992] 4 All ER 627.

87. We note that anorexia nervosa can be regarded as a psychiatric illness rendering the patient incapable of making a true decision. Such cases are sometimes treated under the provisions of the Mental Health Act. In this particular case, however, the patient was deemed competent.

88. To distinguish between diagnostic and therapeutic interviews with a child, and interviews for forensic purposes, see *Memorandum of Good Practice for Video-Recorded Interviews*, HMSO, 1992.

89. The discussion in this section applies to the situation in England and Wales only.

90. Formal guidance has been published, in *Working Together Under the Children Act* 1989, HMSO, 1991, see also *Child Sexual Abuse, a Guide to the Law*, published by the Children's Legal Centre, 1992 and Mitchels B and Prince A, *The Children Act and Medical Practice*, Family Law, 1992.

91. The Human Organ Transplants Act 1989 restricts transplants between people who are not genetically related. It is discussed in chapter 1 of the BMA publication *Rights and Responsibilities of Doctors*, 1992. In the case of children, organ donation is usually only proposed when there is a close genetic relationship.

341

92. See, for example, chapter 14 of Mason J K and McCall Smith R A, *Medical Law and Ethics*, 3rd edition, Butterworths, 1991.

93. Skegg P D G, 'Consent to medical procedures on minors' 1973, 36 *Medical Law Review* 370, 370-375.

94. Schoeman F, 'Parental discretion and children's rights: background and implications for medical decision-making', *Journal of Medicine and Philosophy*, 1985, 10, 45-62.

95. See for example Buchanan A E and Brock D W, *Deciding for Others: the Ethics of Surrogate Decision-Making*, Cambridge University Press, 1989.

96. See Re W (a minor)(medical treatment) All ER 627.

97. Veatch R, *Case Studies in Medical Ethics*, Cambridge, Mass: Harvard University Press, 1977: 222-223.

98. See Startzl T E, 'Will live organ donations no longer be justified?', *Hastings Center Report*, 5, 1986, quoted also in *Health Policy, Ethics and Human Values*, papers from the XXIst CIOMS Conference in 1987, (eds) Bankowski and Bryant.

99. This is discussed by Brazier M, *Medicine, Patients and the Law*, 1992, Penguin, p.398.

100. MRC publication, *The Ethical Conduct of Research on Children*, December 1991.

101. *Medical Research with Children*, (ed) Nicholson R H, Oxford University Press, 1986.

102. See, for example, Harth S C and Thong Y H, 'Sociodemographic and motivational characteristics of parents who volunteer their children for clinical research: a controlled study', *BMJ*, vol 300, 26 May 1990, 1372-1375.

## Chapter 4

103. Lady Saltoun in the first Lords' debate on the Warnock report, *Official Report*, 31.10.84; col.563.

104. *Report of the Committee of Inquiry into Human Fertilisation and Embryology*, Cmnd 9314, HMSO, 1984.

105. *Report of the Committee on the Ethics of Gene Therapy*, Cmnd 1788, HMSO, 1992.

106. This is the conclusion reached in the report *Infertility, Guidelines for Practice*, Royal College of Obstetricians and Gynaecologists, 1992.

107. Jones, E F et al, 'Teenage pregnancy in developed countries: determinants and policy implications', *Family Planning Perspectives*, 1985, vol 17, no.2, p.53-63.

108. For under-16s total conceptions fell from 9,108 in 1979 to 8,382 in 1989 but for 17 and 18-year-olds pregnancy figures remained much the same and abortion rates rose. Office of Population Censuses and Surveys (OPCS), *Birth Statistics 1990*, HMSO, 1992.

109. *Annual report of the Chief Medical Officer on the State of Public Health*, 1991, HMSO, 1992.

110. *The Health of the Nation*, HMSO, 1992.

111. A joint statement by the BMA, RCGP, FPA and Brook Advisory Centres on confidentiality and teenage contraception is available from the BMA's Ethics Division.

112. The Gillick case and principles regarding the provision of contraception to minors are both discussed in detail in chapter 3.

113. Kennedy, I, *Treat me right*, Oxford University Press, 1988, p.112.

114. *Human Reproduction*, British Council of Churches, 1962.

115. Policy to this effect was approved by the 1978 BMA Annual Representative Meeting.

116. BMA policy to this effect was made at the 1985 Annual Representative Meeting.

117. Thompson J J, 'A defence of abortion', in Singer P (ed), *Applied Ethics*, Oxford Readings in Philosophy, Oxford University Press, 1986.

118. Kuhse H and Singer P draw upon various studies showing that up to 302 societies have been said to practise infanticide at least occasionally, for reasons of self-preservation or to achieve those societies' long-range objectives. Kuhse H and Singer P, *Should the Baby Live?*, Oxford University Press, 1985.

119. Glover J, *Causing Death and Saving Lives*, Penguin, Harmondsworth, 1977, p.145.

120. Hursthouse R, *Beginning Lives*, 1987, Blackwell, Oxford.

121. Botros S in 'Abortion, embryo research and fetal transplantation: their moral interrelationships', in Byrne P (ed) *Medicine, Medical Ethics and the Value of Life*, Wiley, 1989.

122. Statistical surveys appear to show growing support for this view in groups traditionally opposed to abortion (see section 4:3.1.5).

123. Except in Northern Ireland. For a brief discussion of the law, *Rights and Responsibilities of Doctors*, BMA, 1992, p.67.

124. This shift has been noted, for example, by the Government Statistical Service in *Population Trends 64*, Summer 1991, Office of Population Censuses and Surveys.

125. This is discussed by Morgan D and Lee R in *Blackstone's Guide to the Human Fertilisation and Embryology Act*, Blackstone, London, 1991, p.19.

126. See for example, Henshaw R C and Templeton A A, 'Mifepristone: separating fact from fiction', *Drugs*, 1992, 44 (4) 531-536.

127. Report of the RCOG Working Party on Unplanned Pregnancy, September 1991.

128. *Official Report*, vol 201; No 37, Part II, 20 December 1991, col 355.

129. Janaway v Salford HA [1988], 3 All ER 1079 HL. This case is also discussed in *Rights and Responsibilities of Doctors*, BMA, 1992, p.70.

343

130. This policy was established at the 1992 BMA Annual Representative Meeting.

131. Re D (a minor) [1976] Fam 185, [1976] 1 All ER 326.

132. Re B (a minor)(sterilisation) [1988] AC 199, [1987] 2 All ER 206, HL.

133. Kennedy I and Lee S, 'This rush to judgement', 1987, *The Times*, 1 April 1987.

134. Lee R G and Morgan D 'Sterilisation and mental handicap: sapping the strength of the state?', *Journal of Law and Society*, 1988, 15, 229.

135. The debate is briefly summarised by Mason and McCall Smith in *Law and Medical Ethics*, 3rd edition, chap 4, Butterworths, 1991.

136. See, for example, *The Times*, 1 March 1987.

137. Re F (mental patient: sterilisation) [1990] 2 AC 1, [1989] 2 All ER 545.

138. Lord Brandon at AC 56.

139. The Official Solicitor's practice note is reproduced in *Rights and Responsibilities of Doctors*, BMA, 1992, p.109-112.

140. See for example, Snowden R, 'The family and artificial reproduction', in Bromham D, Dalton M and Jackson J (eds), *Philosophical Ethics in Reproductive Medicine*, 1990, Manchester University Press.

141. A 1990 study of female infertility suggested this figure over-estimates the reality of the problem. Templeton, Fraser & Thompson, 'The epidemiology of infertility in Aberdeen', *BMJ*, 301, 148.

142. Except in cases where society makes a judgement based on the learning disability of an individual (see section 4:4) where the argument for sterilisation or termination of pregnancy is usually grounded on the inability of the prospective mother to cope with pregnancy and childbirth.

143. *Report of the Committee of Inquiry into Human Fertilisation and Embryology*, Cmnd 9314, HMSO, 1984.

144. Jouannet P et al, 'Demandes d'AID faites par les couples dont l'homme a des anticorps seriques anti-VIH' ('Requests for donor insemination by couples in which the man is HIV-positive'), *Contraception, Fertilité, Sexualité*, 1990, vol 18, no7-8, p.603-604.

145. An exception is the interesting study by Douglas G published in 1992 by Cardiff Law School. The findings of this study will also be published in Freeman M D A ed. *Current Legal Problems*, Oxford University Press, 1993. It must be noted, however, that this has attracted some critical comment, in particular on its methodology and sample size.

146. R v Ethical Cttee of St Mary's Hospital, ex p Harriott, [1988] 1 FLR 512 , in which an ex-prostitute was refused fertility treatment.

147. The HFEA may reassess this view, however, in the near future.

148. BMA archive, London.

149. The courts have not always taken the same view. See Re S [1992] 4 All ER which concerned a case of enforced caesarean section.

150. Arnal F and Cohen J, 'Characteristiques des grossesses en fonction du nombre d'embryons transferes' ('Characteristics of pregnancies in relation to the number of embryos transferred'), in the French FIVNAT study, Testait J & Mouzon J D, (eds) Paris, 1989.

151. This was the conclusion of the Department of Health report, *Three, Four or More*, HMSO, 1990. The report found that in 6 per cent of cases of triplets and 16 per cent of four or more fetuses, the correct number of babies in the pregnancy was only discovered at birth.

152. Department of Health report as above.

153. Some of the issues concerning allocation of resources to preterm and low birthweight babies are raised in Griffin J, *Born Too Soon*, Office of Health Economics, January 1993.

154. This is discussed by Price F, 'Tailoring multi-parity: the dilemmas surrounding death by selective reduction of pregnancy', in Morgan D and Lee R (eds), *Death Rites*, 1993. Routledge, London.

155. Salat-Baroux et al argue, however, that most cases of fetal malformation cannot be related to the reduction procedure although there is some slight risk. 'Is there an indication for embryo reduction?' in *Human Reproduction*, 1992, 7, p.67-72.

156. Price F, as above.

157. Waterstone J, Parsons J, Bolton V, 'Elective transfer of two embryos', *Lancet*, 1991, 337, p.975-6.

158. See Page E, 'Taking surrogacy seriously' in Bromham D, Dalton M and Jackson J (eds), *Philosophical Ethics in Reproductive Medicine*, Manchester University Press, 1990.

159. *Surrogacy: Ethical Considerations*, BMA, 1990.

160. Glover J and others, *Fertility and the Family: The Glover Report to the European Commission on Reproductive Technologies*, Fourth Estate, London, 1989.

161. See for example Kolder V, Gallagher J and Parsons M, in 'Court-ordered obstetrical interventions', *New England Journal of Medicine*, 1987, 316, 19, 1192.

162. For example, in Re F (in utero) [1988] 2 All ER 193, the Court of Appeal concluded that it had no jurisdiction to intervene on behalf of an unborn child.

163. This is argued by Morgan D, 'Whatever happened to consent', *New Law Journal*, 23 October 1992, 1448.

164. Re S (Adult: refusal of treatment) [1992] 3 WLR 806.

165. See for example, Hewson B, 'When no means yes', *Law Society Gazette*, 45, 2, December 1992, and Grubb A, 'Treatment without consent: Adult' [1993], 1. *Medical Law Review*, 1992.

166. See Kennedy I, 'A woman and her unborn child', in *Treat me right*, Oxford University Press, 1988.

167. Sir Cecil Clothier in *Human Embryo Research: Yes or No?*, Ciba Foundation, Tavistock, London, 1986.

168. Harris J, 'Should we experiment on embryos?', Lee R and Morgan D (eds), *Birthrights*, Routledge, London, 1990.

169. See, for example, the 1985 Annual Report of the BMA Council and *BMJ*, 290, 255.

170. House of Lords, *Official Report*, 20 March 1990, vol 247.

171. Harris J, *Wonderwoman and Superman*, p.46, Oxford University Press, 1992.

172. Harris J, 'Is gene therapy a form of eugenics?', paper presented at the Inaugural Congress of the International Association of Bioethics, Amsterdam, October 1992, to be published in *Bioethics* in 1993.

# Chapter 5

173. The literature is briefly discussed by James N, 'From vision to system: the maturing of the hospice movement', in (eds) Lee R & Morgan D, *Death Rites: Law and Ethics at the End of Life*, Routledge, London 1993, in press.

174. See, for example, Thompson I, *Dilemmas of Dying: a Study in the Ethics of Terminal Care*, Edinburgh University Press, 1979.

175. R v Cox (unreported), Ognall J, Winchester Crown Court, 18 September 1992.

176. At the beginning of 1992, there were 2,890 hospice beds in the UK. The figure for England and Wales was 2,410. A few more hospices have opened during the year.

177. This issue is discussed by Thompson I, *Dilemmas of Dying: a Study in the Ethics of Terminal Care*, Edinburgh University Press, 1979.

178. *Percival's Medical Ethics*, (ed) Leake C D, Williams & Wilkins, Baltimore, 1927.

179. In 1992, the BMA's Annual Representative Meeting passed a resolution reaffirming its view that it is unethical and unacceptable for a doctor to withhold treatment from a patient on the grounds that the patient's condition may pose a risk to the doctor's health.

180. Kubler-Ross E, *On Death and Dying*, Tavistock publications, 1970; *Death as the Final Stage of Growth*, New Jersey, Prentice-Hall, 1975.

# Chapter 6

181. Mr Justice Devlin in the case of R v W Adams [1957] CLR 365.

182. Devlin as above.

183. See, for example, Lifton R J, *The Nazi Doctors*, 1986, Macmillan.

184. Medische Beslissingen Rond Het Levenseinde. I. Rapport van de Commissie Onderzoek Medische Praktijk inzake Euthanasie. II. Ondersoek voor de Commissie Medische Praktijk inzake Euthanasie (Medical Decisions about the End of Life. I. Report of the Committee to Study the Medical Practice Concerning Euthanasia. II. The Study of the Committee of Medical Practice Concerning Euthanasia) The Hague, 1991.

185. 'Arts Geeft Jongeren Dodelijke Pil Mee' ('Doctor supplies boys with deadly pills'), *Brabants Dagblad*, 10.10.87.

186. 'Grote Publieke Steun Voor Dokter Voute' ('Broad public support for Dr Voute') *Brabants Dagblad*, 31.10.87.

187. Van der Maas P, van Delden J, Pijnenborg L, Looman C, 'Euthanasia and other medical decisions concerning the end of life', *Lancet*, 1991, 338, 669-74.

188. 35 per cent of these deaths conform to current English law and practice because, for example, they involve a decision to cease futile treatment or not resuscitate a patient with a poor prognosis. Only in 3 per cent is there active killings as we would define it.

189. Potts S G, 'Euthanasia and other medical decisions about the end of life', *Lancet*, 1991, 338, 952-3.

190. All data concerning these 23,006 cases are published in the Remmelink report.

191. Segers J H, 'Elderly persons on the subject of euthanasia', *Issues in Law and Medicine*, 1988, 3: 429-437.

192. Fenigsen R, 'Mercy, murder and morality : perspectives on euthanasia. A case against Dutch euthanasia', *Hastings Center Report* 1989, 19 (1)(suppl) 22-30.

193. A Japanese study, for example, using WHO guidelines confirmed complete pain relief for 87 per cent of cases. Takeda F, 'Preliminary report from Japan on results of field testing of WHO draft interim guidelines for relief of cancer pain', *The Pain Clinic Journal*, No 2, 1986.

194. Dorrepaal K et al 'Pain experience and pain management among hospitalized cancer patients', *Cancer*, vol 63, 1989, 593-598.

195. Bonica J J, 'Importance of the problem', in *Advances in Pain Research and Therapy*, vol 2, New York, Raven; Marks R M & Sachar E J, 'Undertreatment of medical inpatients with narcotic analgesics', *Annals of Internal Medicine*, 1973, 78; 173-181.

196. Twycross R G, 'Analagesics', in *Clinics in Oncology*, 1984, vol 3, London, and the same author in *Symptom Control in Far Advanced Cancer Pain Relief*, Pitman, London, 1983.

197. As yet unpublished evidence given to the BMA by St Christopher's Hospice suggests that about 0.7 per cent annually of hospice patients with particularrly difficult pre-terminal pain cannot be relieved by conventional means.

198. This is discussed, for example, in Jecker N, 'Giving death a hand: when the dying and the doctor stand in a special relationship', *Journal of the American Geriatrics Society*, 1991, 39: 831-835.

199. Kuhse H, and Singer P, 'Doctors' practices and attitudes regarding voluntary euthanasia', *Medical Journal of Australia*, 1988, 148: 623, and anecdotal evidence given to the 1988 BMA Working Party on Euthanasia.

200. The law is set out in chapter 6 of *Rights and Responsibilities of Doctors*, BMA, 1992.

201. Although this is a matter under consideration by the English Law Commission.

202. GMC press release 17.11.92

203. Barlow P and Teasdale G, 'Prediction of outcome and management of severe head injury: attitudes of neurosurgeons', *Neurosurgery*, 1986, 19: 989-91

204. Kennedy I, *The Unmasking of Medicine*, Allen and Unwin, London, 1981, p.87.

205. It may be noted, however, that in a 1992 case involving the danger to the lives of a pregnant woman and her unborn child, a judge appeared to override the woman's competent refusal of life-saving treatment. See chapter 4 (section 4:7.1 and 4:7.2).

206. See remarks of Lord Donaldson in Re T [1992] 4 All ER 649.

207. A BMA guidance note on advance directives is also available on request from the BMA's Ethics Division.

208. Re T [1992]4 All ER 649; and Airedale NHS Trust v Bland [1993]1 All ER 859.

209. Airedale NHS Trust v Bland [1993]1 All ER 859.

210. The full proposal is available on request from the BMA's Ethics Division.

211. Lord Goff in the Lord's judgment of the Bland case, as above.

212. Re J (a minor) (wardship: medical treatment) [1990] 3 All ER 930.

213. These points are based on the Appleton Consensus on 'Guidelines for Decisions to Forgo Medical Treatment', published in the supplement of the *Journal of Medical Ethics*, September 1992, vol 18.

214. The BMA issued a discussion document on PVS in 1992 which reflected its initial analysis of the issues. Guidance for decision-making in cases of PVS was issued in 1993. Both of these documents are available from the BMA's Ethics Division.

215. Lord Goff in the 1993 Lords' judgement of the Bland case, Airedale NHS Trust v Bland [1993]1 All ER 859.

216. Details available from the BMA's Ethics Division.

217. Re W (a minor)(medical treatment) [1992] 4 All ER 627.

218. Available from the BMA's Ethics Division.

219. Letter from the Chief Medical Officer (PL/CMO (91) 22).

220. *Handbook of Declarations*, WMA, 1992, France.

221. Canadian Law Commission, *Working Paper 28*, Ottawa, 1982, p.54.

222. Wanzer S et al, 'The physician's responsibility towards hopelessly ill patients', *New England Journal of Medicine*, 1989, 320, 13, 844-849.

223. Hare R, then White's Professor of Moral Philosophy, Oxford, *Personality and Science: an Interdisciplinary Discussion*, 1971, Ciba Foundation, p.92.

# Chapter 7

224. In legal terms, the standard of care required by a doctor is the standard of the reasonably skilled and experienced doctor. In the case of Bolam v Friern Hospital Management Committee (1957) the judge said "The test is the standard of the ordinary skilled man exercising and professing to have that special skill. A man need not possess the highest expert skill; it is well established in law that it is sufficient if he exercises the ordinary skill of the ordinary competent man exercising that particular art".

225. The BMA has approved a statement by the Association of the British Pharmaceutical Industry (ABPI) on effective information for patients, published in *Medicines: Good Practice Guidelines*, 1990. This gives comprehensive guidance, primarily addressed to the matter of written information provided to patients by doctors or manufacturers.

226. Available on request from the BMA's Ethics Division.

227. *British National Formulary*, No 24, September 1992.

228. NHS Management Executive, *Responsibilities for Prescribing between Hospitals and GPs*, EL(91)127.

229. The British controls on the import and export of drugs are discussed in *Rights and Responsibilities of Doctors*, BMA, 1992, p.134. The import regulations in the country for which the drugs are destined must be obtained from the relevant embassy. Drugs which are mailed are subject to postage regulations.

230. BMA, *Complementary Medicine: New Approaches to Good Practice*, Oxford University Press, 1993.

231. The regulations are summarised in *Rights and Responsibilities of Doctors*, BMA, 1992, chapter 9. *The British National Formulary* gives detailed practical information about controlled drugs and the notification of addicts as well as advice for the prescribing of diamorphine (heroin), dipipanone and cocaine for addicts. Further help for doctors looking after patients with drug problems, whether in the general practice, hospital or other specialist setting can be found in *Drug Misuse and Dependence - Guidelines on Clinical Management*, issued by the Department of Health in 1991.

# Chapter 8

232. *Percival's Medical Ethics*, Leake C D (ed), Williams & Wilkins, Baltimore, 1927.

233. See, for example, Silverman W A, 'The myth of informed consent: in daily practice and in clinical trials', *Journal of Medical Ethics*, 1989, 15, 6-11.

234. *Report of the Committee of Inquiry into Human Fertilisation and Embryology*, HMSO, Cmnd 9314, chaired by Baroness Warnock, 1984.

235. Neuberger J, *Ethics and Health care: The Role of Research Ethics Committees in the United Kingdom*, King's Fund Institute, 1992.

236. See Appendix 3.

237. This is briefly discussed by Grubb A, 'The law relating to consent', in the *Manual for Research Ethics Committees*, King's College, London, 1992.

238. Personal communication to the BMA by Professor Michael Baum, Honorary Director of the Cancer Research Campaign Clinical Trials Centre, 1992.

239. Lorber J, 'Ethical problems in the management of myelomeningocele and hydrocephalus', *Journal of the Royal College of Physicians*, Vol 10, No 1, Oct 1975.

240. *Percival's Medical Ethics*, Leake C D (ed), Williams & Wilkins, Baltimore, 1927.

241. Bolam v Friern Hospital Management Committee [1957] 2 All ER 118, [1957] 1 WLR 582.

242. Wells F, 'Bioethics and industry', *International Journal of Bioethics*, Paris, January 1993.

243. Beecher, 'Ethics and clinical research', *New England Journal of Medicine*, 1966, 274, 1354.

244. Pappworth M H, *Human Guinea Pigs*, Routledge and Kegan Paul, London, 1967.

245. Neuberger J, *Ethics and Health Care: the Role of Research Ethics Committees in the United Kingdom*, King's Fund Institute, 1992.

246. This is discussed in the report, *Fraud and Malpractice in the Context of Clinical Research*, ABPI, 1992.

247. *WMA Declaration of Helsinki* is appended (Appendix 3).

248. The Nuremberg Code is given in the *Dictionary of Medical Ethics*, Duncan A S, Dunstan G R, Welbourn R B (eds), Darton, Longman and Todd, London, 1981.

249. *The Lancet*, editorial, 'Informed consent: how informed?', 1991, vol 338, September 14, p.665-666.

250. Neuberger J, *Ethics and Health care: The Role of Research Ethics Committees in the United Kingdom*, King's Fund Institute, 1992.

251. See, for example, Tobias J, 'Informed consent and the introduction of new cancer treatments' Williams C J (ed), *Introducing New Treatments for Cancer: Practical, Ethical and Legal Problems*, Wiley, Chichester, 1992.

252. Faulder C, *Whose Body is it? the Troubling Issue of Informed Consent*, p.26, Virago, 1985.

253. See, for example, Stenning S, 'The uncertainty principle: selection of patients for cancer clinical trials' Williams C J, (ed), *Introducing New Treatments for Cancer*, 1992, Wiley, Chichester.

254. See Botros S, 'Equipoise, consent and the ethics of randomised clinical trials' in Byrne P (ed), *Ethics and Law in Health Care and Research*, Wiley, Chichester, 1990.

255. Botros S, as above.

256. Baum M, 'The ethics of clinical research' in Byrne P, (ed), *Ethics and Law in Heath Care and Research*, Wiley, Chichester, 1990.

257. Burkhardt R and Kienle G, 'Basic problems in controlled trials' *Journal of Medical Ethics*, 1983, 9, 80.

258. Kennedy I, *Treat Me Right*, p.218, Oxford University Press, 1988.

259. Information about the regulations concerning supply of medicinal products for use in clinical trials is given in chapter 9 of *Rights and Responsibilities of Doctors*, BMA, 1992.

260. Angell M, 'Patients' preferences in randomised clinical trials', *New England Journal of Medicine*, 1984, 310, 1385.

261. *Guidelines for the Ethical Conduct of Medical Research Involving Children*, published by the Ethics Advisory Committee of the British Paediatric Association, London, August 1992.

262. British Paediatric Association as above.

263. *The Ethical Conduct of Research on the Mentally Incapacitated*, MRC, London, December 1991.

264. *Mentally Incapacitated Adults and Decision-Making: Medical Treatment and Research*. Consultation paper 129, Law Commission, April 1993.

265. *Guidelines for Ethics of Research Committees on Psychiatric Research involving Human Subjects*, Royal College of Psychiatrists, London, 1990.

266. The legislation is discussed more fully in chapter 5 of *Rights and Responsibilities of Doctors*, BMA, 1992.

267. Published by HMSO, Cmnd 762, 1989.

268. *Report of the BMA Working Party on No Fault Compensation*, January 1991.

269. *Professional Conduct and Discpline: Fitness to Practise*, GMC, January 1993, para 89.

270. Very similar points, for example, are made in the Department of Health guidance, *Local Research Ethics Committees*, 1991. This particular formulation is discussed by Wells, F in 'Bioethics and industry', *International Journal of Bioethics*, Paris, January 1993.

271. Available on request from the BMA's Ethics Division.

272. See, for example, the Department of Health guidance on *Local Research Ethics Committees*, HSG(91)5, 1991; and *Guidelines on the Practice of Ethics Committees in Medical Research Involving Human Subjects*, Royal College of Physicians, 1991.

273. The need for training and support for LRECs was the subject of a resolution passed at the BMA's 1991 Annual Representative Meeting.

274. Report of the Committee on the Ethics of Gene Therapy, Cmnd 1788, HMSO, 1992.

275. *International Guidelines for Ethical Review of Epidemiological Studies*, Council for International Organisations of Medical Sciences, Geneva, 1991.

276. *Guidelines for the Ethical Conduct of Medical Research Involving Children*, Ethics Advisory Committee of the British Paediatric Association, August 1992.

# Chapter 9

277. BMA guidance on the Act is available from the BMA's Ethics Division.

278. This gives factual information about aspects of insurance practice and incorporates ethical guidelines. The full guidance note can be obtained from the BMA's Private Practice and Professional Fees Committee.

279. *Our Genetic Future - the Science and Ethics of Genetic Technology*, Oxford University Press, 1992.

280. A full discussion of genetic screening in the workplace is given in the BMA's publication *Our Genetic Future - the Science and Ethics of Genetic Technology*, Oxford University Press, 1992, p.201-204.

281. Available from the BMA's Occupational Health Committee.

282. The 1948 Act and the National Assistance (Amendment) Act 1951 are fully explained in *Rights and Responsibilities of Doctors*, BMA, 1992.

283. *The Law and Vulnerable Elderly People*, Age Concern, 1986.

284. Neilson v Laugharne [1981] 1 ALL ER 829.

285. See Heir v Cmm of Police [1982] 1 All ER 335; Conerney v Jacklin [1985] Crim LR 234; Makanjuola v Cmm of Police [1989] NLJR 468.

286. Under the Police and Criminal Evidence Act 1984, the legal age of consent for a person in custody is 17 but for therapeutic treatment, age is irrelevant (see chapter 3).

287. The full guidance note regarding the provisions of the Act and BMA policy on the subject is available from the BMA's Ethics Division.

288. Personal communication from Principal Medical Officer, Northern Ireland Department of Health and Social Services, September 1992.

289. Duhamel O, 'Esquisse d'une typologie des greves de la faim' ('Sketch of a typology of hunger strikes') in *La Greve de la Faim* (The Hunger Strike), Paris: Economica, 1984.

290. *BMA, The Torture Report*, 1986; *BMA, Medicine Betrayed*, Zed Press, 1992.

291. The working party on the health care of remand prisoners reported in 1990 and the working party on medical participation in human rights abuses published its report, *Medicine Betrayed*, 1992, Zed Press.

292. E Dooley, 'Prison suicide in England and Wales 1972-87', *British Journal of Psychiatry*, 1990, 156, 40-45.

293. This Declaration is appended (Appendix 4).

294. These are available on request from the Foundation or from the BMA Ethics Division.

## Chapter 10

295. The law on this matter is laid out in *Rights and Responsibilities of Doctors*, BMA, 1992, p.25ff. See also the case of Wilsher v Essex Area Health Authority [1987] 2 WLR 425.

296. *BMA, Medicine Betrayed*, Zed Press, 1992, p.190.

297. *Professional Conduct and Discipline: Fitness to Practise*, GMC, January 1993, para 63.

298. The full regulations concerning sale of goodwill are outlined in *Rights and Responsibilities of Doctors*, BMA, 1992, p.144-146.

299. The General Medical Services Committee of the BMA has drawn up a basic framework for a medical partnership agreement, available from GMSC.

300. General Medical Services Committee, *The New Health Promotion Package*, BMA, February 1993.

301. *GP fund holding practices: the provision of secondary care*; HSG(93)14, NHS Management Executive.

302. *Professional Conduct and Discipline: Fitness to Practise*, GMC, January 1993, paras 116-7.

303. The BMA has published a guidance note on advertising which is available from the BMA's Ethics Division.

304. *Professional Conduct and Discipline: Fitness to Practise*, GMC, January 1993, paras 93-94.

305. See appendix 5 for address.

306. They are also set out in *Health Committee (Procedure) Rules 1987*, HMSO, statutory instrument, No 2174, 1987.

307. Department of Health circular HC(82)13.

# Chapter 11

308. *Percival's Medical Ethics*, (ed) Leake C D, Williams & Wilkins, Baltimore, 1927, p.112.

309. This is discussed further in Douglas G, *Law Fertility and Reproduction*, Sweet & Maxwell, 1991.

310. Midwives were regulated by the Midwives Act of 1902 but could still practise, even if they were unqualified, up to the 1930s.

311. Figures published by the Royal College of Nursing in 1992 in its factsheet, *Nursing Workforce*, indicated that there were over 600,000 qualified nurses and midwives registered with the nursing regulatory body, the UKCC.

312. *Professional Conduct and Discipline: Fitness to Practise*, GMC, January 1993 edition: there is similar wording in previous editions.

313. Thomas et al, 'Use of non-orthodox and conventional health care in Great Britain', *BMJ*, 1991, 302; 207-10, found that 64 per cent of 2437 patients seeking non-conventional treatments had received previous care from a GP or hospital.

314. *Professional Conduct and Discipline: Fitness to Practise*, GMC, January 1993, paras 42 and 43.

315. *Professional Conduct and Discipline: Fitness to Practise*, GMC, January 1993, paras 121 and 122.

316. *Professional Conduct and Discipline: Fitness to Practise*, GMC, January 1993, para 119.

317. Available from the General Medical Services Committee of the BMA.

# Chapter 12

318. Enoch Powell published an article to this effect in *The Independent*, 1.12.92.

319. Personal communication to the Working Party from Mr Michael Foot.

320. See, for example, Williams A, 'Cost-effectiveness analysis: is it ethical?', *Journal of Medical Ethics*, 1992, 18, 7-11.

321. See, for example, Haines A, Feder G, 'Guidance on guidelines', *BMJ*, 1992, 305, 785-786.

322. Presidential address by Professor J Howell to the 1989 ARM of the BMA in Swansea.

323. Loewy E L (correspondence), 'Cost should not be a factor in medical care', *New England Journal of Medicine*, 1980, 302, 697.

324. This was debated at the 1992 BMA Annual Representative Meeting where the resolutions on rationing listed in Chapter 12:1.5 were approved.

325. See Maynard A, 'Logic in medicine: an economic perspective', *BMJ*, 1987, 295, 1537-41.

326. Le Fanu J, 'Who to treat and who to allow to die', *Evening Standard*, 11 November 1991.

327. Heginbotham C, Ham C, Cochraine M and Richards J, *Purchasing Dilemmas*, Kings Fund College and Southampton and Hampshire HA, 1992.

328. *Choice in Health Care*, a report by the Government Committee on Choices in Health Care, the Netherlands, 1992.

329. R v Secretary of State for Social Services, ex p Hincks (18 March 1980 unreported) CA, discussed by Finch J, in *Health Services Law*, Sweet and Maxwell, London, 1981.

330. Re Walker's Application, *Times Law Report*, 26 November, 1987.

331. See for example, Maynard A, 'Priorities in Nether Netherland', *The Health Service Journal*, 27.8.92.

332. Kilner J F, *Who lives, who dies?*, Yale University Press, 1990.

333. Hunter D, 'Explicit rationing decisions - the pitfalls', paper presented at National Association of Health Authorities and Trusts Conference, The Oregon Experiment, October 1991, RIBA, London.

334. Moore W, 'Public health chief's drugs call sparks off row over rationing', *Health Service Journal*, 1992, 102 (5289) 6.

335. Griffin J, *Born Too Soon*, Office of Health Economics, 1993. This report estimated that in 1990 the cost of neo-natal care for infants weighing less than 1500g was between 42 and 70 million pounds out of a total NHS expenditure of £32,422 million but that many surviving infants continued to require additional resources throughout their lives.

336. Harris J, 'The Survival Lottery' in *Applied Ethics*, (ed) Singer P, Oxford University Press, 1986.

337. These arguments are put forward by Winslow G R, *Triage and Justice*, Berkeley: University of California Press, 1982.

338. See Childress J F, 'Who shall live when not all can live', in Wertz R, *Readings on Social and Ethical Issues in Biomedicine*, New Jersey, Prentice Hall, 1973.

339. Daniels N, *Just Health Care*, Cambridge University Press, 1985.

340. Aristotle, *The Politics*, book 3, chapters 9 and 12, Penguin Classics, 1962.

341. WMA *Statement on Allocation of Resources and Priorities in Medical Care*, discussed in Marbella, 1992.

342. Kilner J F, *Who lives, Who Dies?*, Yale University Press, 1990.

343. Dougherty C J, *American Health Care: Realities, Rights and Reforms*, New York, Oxford University Press, 1988.

344. Ewart I, 'A family matter', *Health Service Journal*, 1991, 101 (5251); 18-20.

345. Maynard A at a symposium held at the University of Manchester during the 33rd Annual Scientific Meeting of the Society for Social Medicine, September 1989. The proceedings of the symposium, 'The ethics of resource allocation', are published in *Journal of Epidemiology and Community Health*, 1990, 44: 187-190.

346. Baker R, 'Warning signals from Oregon', *BMJ*, 304, 1992, 1457-1458.

# Chapter 13

347. The Hippocratic Oath (and its modern re-statement as the Declaration of Geneva) and the WMA Code are appended.

348. Srikanta Murthy K R, 'Professional ethics in ancient Indian medicine', *Indian Journal of the History of Medicine*, 1973, 18; 46.

349. Adopted in Kuwait by the International Conference on Islamic Medicine, January 1981 (1401 in the Islamic calendar).

350. In 1992 the BMA's Annual Representative Meeting adopted the resolution that "it is unethical and unacceptable for a doctor to withhold treatment from a patient on the grounds that the patient's condition may pose a risk to the health of the doctor".

351. Leake C D (ed), *Percival's Medical Ethics*, Williams and Wilkins, Baltimore, 1927.

# Bibliography

## Publications by organisations

Many bodies have published a wide series of documents which provide helpful views. In this brief bibliography, we have only selected a very limited list of those which are particularly relevant to the issues in this book.

Association of British Pharmaceutical Industry (ABPI), *Medicines: Good Practice Guidelines*, 1990

Age Concern & Centre of Medical Law and Ethics, *The Living Will*, Edward Arnold, 1988

BMA, *Rights and Responsibilities of Doctors*, revised 1992

BMA, *Our Genetic Future: The Science and Ethics of Genetic Technology*, Oxford University Press, 1992

BMA, *Medicine Betrayed: the Participation of Doctors in Human Rights Abuses*, Zed Press, 1992

BMA, *Surrogacy: Ethical Considerations*, 1990

British Paediatric Association (BPA) *Guidelines for the Ethical Conduct of Medical Research Involving Children*, 1992

Department of Health HSG(91)5 *Local Research Ethics Committees*, 1991

GMC, *Professional Conduct and Discipline: Fitness to Practise*, January, 1993

Home Office & DoH, *Working together under the Children Act 1989*, HMSO 1991

King's College, *Local Research Ethics Committees*, 1992

King's Fund Institute, Neuberger J, *Ethics and Health Care: the Role of Research Ethics Committees in the UK*, 1992

Law Commission, *Mentally Incapacitated Adults and Decision-Making: an Overview*, HMSO, 1991

World Medical Association, including *Handbook of Declarations*, 1992

## Publications by individuals

Beauchamp T L and Childress J F, *Principles of Biomedical Ethics*, Oxford University Press, New York, 1983

Brazier M, *Medicine, Patients and the Law*, Penguin, London, 1992

Campbell A V, *Moral Dilemmas in Medicine*, Churchill Livingstone, Edinburgh, 1975

Chadwick R (ed), *Ethics, Reproduction and Genetic Control*, Routledge, London 1990

Duncan A S, Dustan G R, Welbourne R B, (eds), *Dictionary of Medical Ethics*, Darton, Langman & Todd, London, 1981

Dyer C (ed), *Doctors, Patients and the Law*, Blackwell, Oxford, 1992

Faulder C, *Whose Body Is It? The Troubling Issue of Informed Consent*, Virago, London, 1985

Finnis J, *Natural Law and Natural Rights*, Oxford University Press, London, 1980

Frankena W K, *Ethics*, Prentice Hall, New Jersey, 1963

Freeman M D A (ed), *Medicine Ethics and Law*, Stevens, London, 1988

357

Gillon R, *Philosophical Medical Ethics*, Wylie, Chichester, 1986

Glover J, *Causing Death and Saving Lives*, Penguin, Harmondsworth, 1977

Harris J, *The Value of Life*, Routledge and Kegan Paul, London, 1985

Harris J, *Wonderwoman and Superman*, Oxford University Press, 1992

Hursthouse R, *Beginning Lives*, Blackwell, 1987

Kennedy I, *The Unmasking of Medicine*, Allen and Unwin, London, 1981

Kennedy I & Grubb A, *Medical Law: Text and Materials*, Butterworths, London, 1989

Kennedy I, *Treat Me Right*, Oxford University Press, 1988

Kuhse H & Singer P, *Should the Baby Live?*, Oxford University Press, 1985

Lockwood M (ed), *Moral Dilemmas in Modern Medicine*, Oxford University Press, Oxford, 1986

Mackie J, *Ethics*, Pelican, Harmondsworth, 1977

Mason J K & McCall Smith R A, *Law and Medical Ethics*, third edition, Butterworths, London 1991

Morgan D & Lee R (eds), *Birthrights: Law and Ethics at the Beginning of Life*, Routledge, London, 1990

Morgan D & Lee R (eds), *Death Rites: Law and Ethics at the End of Life*, Routledge, 1993 in press

Morgan D & Lee R G, *Blackstone's Guide to the Human Fertilisation and Embryology Act 1990*, Blackstone, London, 1991

Nagel T, *Mortal Questions*, Cambridge University Press, Cambridge, 1979

Nicholson R H (ed), *Medical Research with Children: Ethics, Law and Practice*, Oxford University Press, 1986

Paton H J, *The Moral Law*, Routledge, 1948

Phillips M and Dawson J, *Doctors' Dilemmas*, Harvester Press, London, 1984

Rachels J, *Moral Problems*, Harper & Row, New York, 1975

Seedhouse D, *Ethics: the Heart of Health Care*, Wiley, Chichester, 1988

Shelp E E (ed), *Virtue and Medicine*, Reidel Publishing Co, Dordrecht (NL), 1985

Singer P, *Practical Ethics*, Cambridge University Press, Cambridge, 1979

Singer P (ed), *Applied Ethics*, Oxford University Press, 1986

Skegg P D G, *Law, Ethics and Medicine*, Clarendon Press, Oxford, 1984

Steinbock B, *Killing and Letting Die*, Prentice-Hall, Englewood Cliffs, 1980

Thompson I (ed) *Dilemmas of Dying*, Edinburgh University Press, 1979

Tooley M, *Abortion and Infanticide*, Oxford University Press, London, 1983

Veatch R M, *A Theory of Medical Ethics*, Basic Books, New York, 1981

# Index